COURAGE:

The Choice That Makes the Difference

COURAGE:

The Choice That Makes the Difference

Your Key to a Thousand Doors

Dwight GoldWinde

—with Trish Coffey—

To order additional copies of this book, contact:
Xlibris Corporation
1-888-795-4274
www.Xlibris.com
Orders@Xlibris.com
22788

Acknowledgments

Dwight GoldWinde is author, philosopher, and life coach to the movers and shakers of this planet. This book represents the insights Dwight has gleaned from 17 years of assisting earth's citizens manifest their goals, step into their challenges, and create the lifestyles they are passionate about. For more about Dwight see the back cover, the Foreword (page 17), the Introduction (18), Who I am (29), Is Dwight just lucky? (38), and the Journal section of this book (587).

Trish Coffey, co-author of this book, partnered with Dwight in the development of the Introduction and the Journal section.

Trish, at age eight, found herself alone with her five-year-old brother in the heart of West Africa. Her adventures in Cameroon included being a hostage at gunpoint during Cameroon's terrorist war for independence from France. By adulthood she had been influenced by nine cultures on four continents.

As a young mother, Trish needed all her resilience, resourcefulness, and stubbornness to bring her ten-day-old son through one-in-a-million odds of living. In December 2003 that brain-damaged baby had become Todd Coffey, recipient of the John von Neumann Fellowship, walking across the stage to receive his Ph.D. in applied mathematics.

Trish's joy as a life coach comes from partnering with clients to remove the blinders that have kept them playing small, so that they can celebrate their strengths, new-found freedom, and zest for life, as they express who they are and harvest the benefits.

When Dwight invited Trish to co-author this book, she was eager for the opportunity to internalize these life concepts to choose the courage to publish her own memoir.

Trish is quick to tell people that the process of working with Dwight GoldWinde on this project was one of the most fulfilling and life-transforming gifts to her life. (courage@trishcoffey.com)

Athena Xin designed and implemented the book cover. As a leading graphic designer working for a major publishing company, Athena has designed covers for a number of best-selling books, including *The Sweater Letter*, *King Winston and the Knights of the Square Table*, and *Immokalee's Fields of Hope*, winning high praise from her clients. She was born and lives in Shanghai, China (athenaxin@yahoo.com)

See additional acknowledgments on page 664

What is courage?

Courage is the will and the willingness
to embrace and fully feel your fear
as you take actions and risks
in service to your highest commitments
and deepest desires.

Courage is created; it is chosen.
And it is chosen *in the moment.*
It is *always* available to you.
It is *always* an open door,
you can *always* walk through it *or* not.
Courage *cannot* be stored or built up.
It's inaccurate to say that you "have courage"
or you "don't have courage."
It's accurate to say that you "choose courage"
or "choose to feel safe in the moment
rather than choose courage."

Many of us appear to choose courage when,
in fact, the courage we choose
is only "standing on one of three legs."

Almost all of us are masters
at suppressing, denying, camouflaging,
contracting against, and/or pushing away
(or trying to argue away) our fear.
We do this for the deadening, anesthetic effect
we expect it to have on our fear.

Full courage includes
full acknowledgment, experience,
and illumination of our fear,
while we are taking the appropriate actions.
It also includes an acknowledgment and honoring
of ourselves for choosing the courage—
regardless of the outcome.

Courage exists *independent* of the outcome.
Choosing courage (or not choosing courage)
is neither good nor bad, neither right nor wrong.
It is simply a choice,
with associated benefits and costs.

A life *primarily* oriented
toward the choice of courage
will give you one kind of life—
a life you will love.
A life *primarily* oriented
toward the choice of feeling safe and secure
will give you another kind of life—
a life of survival and withdrawal.
It's *okay* to want to feel safe and secure.
We all want that.
But, when feeling safe and secure becomes
your *primary* orientation
(usually by default),
then you are living a life of avoidance,
rather than a life of inspiration.

—J. Dwight GoldWinde, October 24, 1991—

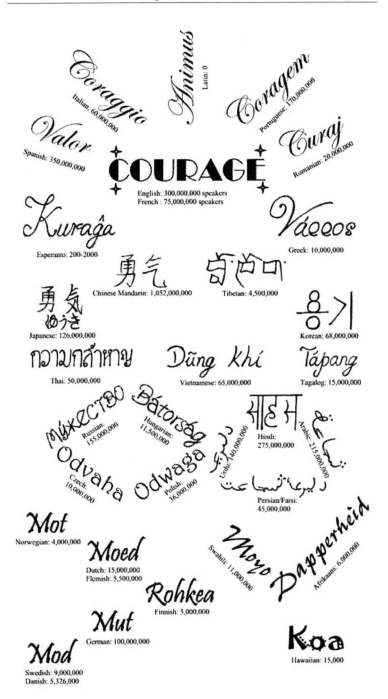

Latin: 0

Italian: 60,000,000 — *Coraggio*

Portuguese: 170,000,000 — *Coragem*

Spanish: 350,000,000 — *Valor*

Romanian: 20,000,000 — *Curaj*

COURAGE

English: 300,000,000 speakers
French : 75,000,000 speakers

Esperanto: 200-2000 — *Kuraĝa*

Greek: 10,000,000 — *Váeeos*

Chinese Mandarin: 1,052,000,000 — 勇气

Tibetan: 4,500,000

Japanese: 126,000,000 — 勇気 ゆうき

Korean: 68,000,000 — 용기

Thai: 50,000,000 — ความกล้าหาญ

Vietnamese: 65,000,000 — *Dũng khí*

Tagalog: 15,000,000 — *Tápang*

Russian: 155,000,000 — *Мужество*

Hungarian: 11,500,000 — *Bátorság*

Hindi: 275,000,000 — साहस

Arabic: 215,000,000

Urdu: 140,000,000

Czech: 10,000,000 — *Odvaha*

Polish: 36,000,000 — *Odwaga*

Persian/Farsi: 45,000,000

Norwegian: 4,000,000 — *Mot*

Dutch: 15,000,000 — *Moed*
Flemish: 5,500,000

Swahili: 11,000,000 — *Moyo*

Afrikaans: 6,000,000 — *Dapperheid*

Finnish: 5,000,000 — *Rohkea*

German: 100,000,000 — *Mut*

Hawaiian: 15,000 — *Koa*

Swedish: 9,000,000 — *Mod*
Danish: 5,326,000

To my mother,

Dorothy Ingman Minkler,

who has always been selfish
in her love, respect, and enjoyment
of her three children.

We thrived in the confidence that she received
selfish enjoyment from our presence in her life.

Mama, what an incredible gift that was
and always will be.

You might wonder why my last name, GoldWinde, is not the same as my parents'.

In 1993 when I got married, my wife and I made an announcement at our wedding that we would create a new last name to signify our partnership. Within the year we'd created a name that resonated in a significant way for both of us: GoldWinde. Whenever I see or speak my last name, I picture gold dust blowing around the world in the jet stream, touching people everywhere and anywhere with valuable and powerful insights.

A judge in the Phoenix, Arizona courthouse smiled at the two of us with amusement as she declared,

"Your new last name is GoldWinde."

When my wife and I divorced in 1997, my appreciation for my last name continued undiminished. It symbolizes my mission in life and that's never wavered. It's so right for me that it's candy for my spirit.

My first and second names (Jackson Dwight) remain the same, as I was named after my father.

&

Table of Contents

—*Abridged Version*—

This Table of Contents has two versions. First the abridged version gives a quick overview of the book. On page 673, near the back of this book, is the unabridged version that doubles, in some ways, as an index. An asterisk* is used to indicate that a web site link is provided for further non-essential reading.

On page 673, near the back of this book, is the unabridged version
of the Table of Contents that doubles as a non-alphabetized index.

᭱

_____

_____

_____

_____

_____

_____

_____

_____

_____

_____

_____

_____

_____

_____

_____

_____

_____

_____

_____

Glossary

I have introduced some new words in this book. I've kept the new words to a minimum and I've put the glossary up front so you can review it first before you jump into the later sections.

Most glossaries go at the end of the book. I felt it important that this glossary be placed here because several important words/distinctions in this book either take on a modified meaning (different from our everyday understanding) or they represent new words (or acronyms) altogether. I have indicated those words that I have coined with three asterisks [***].

Action Agreement *** This is an agreement made within the framework of the Consider It Done technique (see definition below).

Action Essay/Poetic Essay Much of the content of this book consists of short-to-medium length essays, formatted as poetry is often formatted. Sometimes I will refer to these as Action Essays. This emphasizes that they are all action/results oriented. These essays are not "just for learning" or "just for a different way to see things." They are about seeing a new opening for action and taking it. Other times I will refer to the essays as Poetic Essays. This just emphasizes their poetic format and encourages reading out loud, as you might read poetry, in order to effect the maximum impact on your life.

Consider It Done™ (CID) *** What difference might it make in your life if you could keep any agreement that you made with yourself? The Consider It Done technique will guarantee this for you. See page 272 for a full explanation.

Courage See the distinction of courage on the first page of this book.

Couragee *** A choice of courage that involves confronting a small amount of fear.

Coverage *** The antonym of courage. Coverage is the choice to feel safe (not necessarily be safe) in the moment at the expense of not going for what you really want and/or are committed to.

There is nothing wrong with choosing coverage. You will accrue certain costs and benefits from choosing coverage. You will accrue different costs and benefits from choosing courage. Most often coverage provides the benefit of feeling safe in the moment at the expense of longer-range safety and results.

Cross-Cultural Freedom Effect *** An experience of interpersonal freedom and safety that often occurs when two people of different cultures speak together. I call this the Cross-Cultural Freedom Effect. See page 365 for a full explanation.

Daily Adventure™ *** Normally we wait for fear to come to us, hoping it doesn't. With the Daily Adventure, we turn the tables on fear. We start looking for it so that we can play with it and exercise our courage muscles. See page 332 for a full explanation.

Deep Awakening Renewal™ **(DAR)** *** The most powerful process to dissolve and release suppressed fear and pain. See page 148 for a full explanation.

Divide and Conquer™ *** How can you ever keep your desk clean? Even if you're able to spend several hours and make a dent in the pile, it seems like only a temporary victory, right? With Divide and Conquer you can handle this problem once and for all. See page 264 for a full explanation.

Done Deal™ *** With the Done Deal technique, taking only one minute per day, you can take the brakes off, creating power behind any result or goal that you set. See page 267 for a full explanation.

Embrace, Honor, Action, Honor (EHAH) *** The acronym EHAH serves as a useful reminder of the steps for choosing full courage. See page 53 for a detailed explanation.

EnChanting™ *** A process of nonsensical, extemporaneous soundings which express non-conceptually the current mood or feeling. It is a de-repression process designed to dissolve calcified fears and uncover the natural joy and buoyancy of human beings. For a full description, see page 141.

Factbelief/Fatebelief *** See essay on page 431 for a full explanation of this important distinction.

Fear + Oxygen = Energy and Excitement (FOE) *** The acronym FOE reminds us that what we normally call fear is not pure fear; it is resisted fear. And that what we normally think of as our enemy may in fact be a powerful ally. When we take some deep breaths, accepting and embracing resisted fear, then we are able to feel (and use) its energy and excitement. See page 54 for a full explanation.

Fear, Embracing the Embracing fear means proactively taking the mental and physical actions so that the energy of fear is not resisted and is instead encouraged and allowed to flow through you. When you embrace fear, the energy that formerly stopped you becomes available to serve you. There are four specific processes to assist you in obtaining this result. See page 131.

Fear, Non-Specific See essay on page 107.

Fear, Paper-Tiger See essay on page 106.

Fear, Red-Herring See essay on page 106.

Fear, Validated See essay on page 105.

Fears, Hidden See essay on page 107.

Five Cs *** Choose courage, creativity, curiosity, and context. See the essay on page 81.

Goft *** The antonym of the word gift. A gift is something that occurs in our life that we want, that we are happy about, that inspires us, that gives us pleasure, that relieves our pain or fear, etc. A goft is something that occurs in our life that we don't want, that we are unhappy about, that discourages us, that takes away some pleasure, that adds to our pain or fear, etc. We might typically say, "It was a real gift to me that I got hired for the job." We might say, "What a goft that I got fired!"

How Others See Me (HOSM) *** A process whereby you can learn how others see, think, and feel about you. See page 291 for a full explanation.

Life Inspirations *** Once you discover your Life Inspirations you will be able to choose your directions and your actions with more certainty and clarity. See page 241 for a full explanation.

Neuro-Linguistic Programming (NLP) Developed by John Grinder and Richard Bandler, NLP has been called "The Science of Subjective Experience." For a fuller explanation, see the Recommendations on page 671.

Opportunity for Courage (OFC) *** Any situation that is recognized as a choice between courage and coverage. OFCs can be categorized many different ways. One way to categorize them is as (1) forced, (2) optional, and (3) created. See "The Three Types of OFCs" on page 77.

Quitaverance *** We all know the power of perseverance. But are you fully familiar with the power of Quitaverance? Perseverance and Quitaverance work hand in hand as great partners. See page 398 for a full explanation.

Reluctant and Frightened to Share (RAFTS) *** If I say to you, "I have a RAFTS," it means that I am about to choose courage to share a thought or feeling with you that I might normally keep to myself because of the resisted fear associated with sharing that thought or feeling. It also means that my intention in sharing with you is to assist in our better understanding each other, as well as having a better connection together. See the essay on page 336.

Refusal I use this word to denote any type of action that says "no" and thereby declines a request (either explicitly or implicitly) or maintains a boundary. Appropriate refusals can be important choices of courage.

Resistance Non-acceptance of the way things are. Resistance does not necessarily mean that we don't take action to change things we want to change. Actually, if we did not take action to change the things we want to change, most probably we would be resisting our fear of taking those actions. Ultimately, all resistance is a resistance to pain and/or fear. Again, however, we can take actions to reduce or eliminate pain or fear without necessarily resisting it. The most powerful place to stand in order to change something is to fully accept it first.

s/he, h/im, h/is, h/imself *** In this book I will use the following as generic pronouns:

write	pronounce	in place of
s/he	**she-he**	**"she or he"**

e.g., "When a person enters the building, s/he should turn left."

h/im	**her-him**	**"her or him"**

e.g., "Whoever meets you at the airport, please give this to h/im."

h/is	**her-his**	**"her or his"**

e.g., "Has the person who lost h/is money discovered that it's missing yet?"

h/imself	**her-himself**	**"herself or himself"**

e.g., "Each of us can easily blame h/imself."

Courage Now™ *** This is the name of the e-mail newsletter service I authored and distributed, the success of which stimulated the writing and publishing of this book.

Toxic Words *** Words that can often create unintended and/ or hidden costs for those who speak them as well as those they are directed toward. An awareness of their possible toxicity can provide a level of protection against these costs. See the section on Toxic Words starting on page 545.

Victimhood *** The state or process of making yourself wrong (self-blame and guilt), making others wrong (blame, resentment, and righteousness), and/or making the universe or God wrong (resignation and cynicism).

Whine List™ *** A process you do with a friend who will be your special listener for a whining session. You whine to your friend with nothing held back and with no sugarcoating. This process helps to clear out repressed pain and fear. See page 153 for a full explanation.

ᔆ

How To Read This Book

A powerful way to read this book

In reading a new book, some of us are jaded from the start, essentially saying, "Why should this book be any different? I probably already know this. It can't possibly make a big difference for me."

In reading a new book, others are "gullibility waiting to happen," essentially saying, "This man has all the answers! I'll believe anything he says."

Instead of either of the above approaches, I invite you to bring five basic attitudes to your reading of this book: curiosity, inventiveness, selectivity, critical thinking, and testing it out.

Curiosity

What might I discover just around the next sentence?

What insight might I get from this next essay that could change my life?

What new and powerful way of looking at things might I discover here?

What surprises or miracles might occur in my life out of reading this?

Inventiveness

What is the central idea here? How might I apply it in different areas of my life?

Is there a way to use this idea different from that suggested?

What other potentially valuable insights does this idea suggest to me?

Selectivity

What elements of this idea can I accept and use immediately to add to my life?

What elements of this idea seem unworkable in my life and must I reject, at least for now?

Critical Thinking

Is this thinking sound?

What evidence do I have to support this line of thinking?

What evidence do I have to contradict this line of thinking?

What circumstances exist that might be exceptions to the point being made here?

In what ways is this idea either an over-generalization or under-generalization?

What fears do I have; what about my own way of looking at things might be preventing me from discovering something of value here?

Testing it out

How might I test this idea easily and quickly and notice what results I get?

Am I clear enough about the idea so that I can give it a valid test?

If I get some desirable results from my first tests, how might I put some structures in place to expand upon and continue with the "testing" process?

What shall I read first?

You can choose from at least three different "orders" in which to read this book (listed below). Whichever way you choose to read (or reread) it, though, I strongly recommend that certain portions be read first to provide an adequate foundation for the rest of the book.

These are the sections that I consider to be either essential or at least very important as a foundation for the rest of this book:

How to Read this Book (this section)

Courage Definition, (found on the first page)—Read and study, as a minimum, this definition/distinction of courage; the essays in the section, "Courage: The Views from Many Windows," starting on page 34, also provide important sub-distinctions of courage.

Introduction (page 18)

Glossary (page 7)—Not only does the glossary put a new face on several common terms, it also introduces some terms that have been coined for this book.

Ways to Embrace Your Fear and Make it Your Friend (page 131)—This section provides four specific and complementary techniques to implement the first of the three cornerstones of courage.

Honoring Yourself for Choosing Courage (page 158)—This section provides examples and methods of how to honor yourself for choosing courage, the second cornerstone of courage.

Journal (page 587)—I recommend you read most of the essays in this book before moving on to this section. You will then have the best context in which to understand the viewpoints and actions expressed throughout the journal.

You can read this book in at least three different "orders," depending upon your purpose and/or your state of mind.

From front to back—Reading this book in sequential order has a lot of advantages: (1) You will ensure that the foundational material and distinctions are digested first, thereby making the later material more clearly relevant and understandable. (2) You will not miss any important parts of the book, making it easy to keep track of what you've read and haven't read.

On an as-needed or an as-interested basis: Once you've read the foundational material, then you can select a specific poetic essay or other section of the book either by (1) flipping through the pages and seeing what strikes your interest or (2) scanning the Table of Contents on page 673.

The "random method"—Just flip a coin to choose a topic, or turn to a page randomly and start reading. Wherever you turn, you will very likely find something relevant to your life right now.

Take notes

At the end of some essays and sections there are one or more lines for note taking. Jot down your own ideas to stimulate the deepest and most profound understanding of your own life and behaviors. Challenge yourself to discover access points for courage in each and every moment and issue of your life. Also, mark this book up. Put notes in the margins. Underline. Insert exclamation points and question marks. Use this book.

Recite the poetic essays

The essays have been formatted to facilitate ease of reading and understanding, providing for the possibility of a more immediate impact on the quality and direction of your life. You will probably find that reading the essays out loud, with some drama and flair, will add to both your comprehension and the ability of the essays to make an immediate difference in your life and behaviors.

Agree to disagree

You will probably discover that you disagree with some ideas in this book. That's great. Please don't get stopped by this. Use the ideas in this book more as stimulations for your empowerment and growth rather than to validate or invalidate what you already believe or think you know.

Also, especially in the journal portion of this book, you will get some candid insights into my day-to-day life. Be careful not to dismiss the power and value of the principles in this book because of the particular ways that I may apply (or misapply) them to my own life.

More than you bargained for

At various points throughout this book you will find a sub-link to my web site (www.GoldWinde.com). These links will take you to over 200 pages of additional materials that would not fit into this 700-page "tome." These links are strategically placed so that the material linked relates most directly to the material you've just finished reading. Don't worry. The printed form of this book is whole and complete by itself. This additional material is provided only for those whose appetite and curiosity leads them further. SPECIAL NOTE: when keying the web address links, key them EXACTLY, paying special attention to UPPER and lower case.

If you'd like to simplify your web access (and minimize your Internet connect time), go to www.GoldWinde.com/Cbook/More. Download each of the links there and use the "Save As" command (e.g., with MS Internet Explorer) under the "File" menu so that all these additional materials are later available to you without an Internet connection.

Duplicate Quotations

Sprinkled throughout this book are quotations (as below) from other authors. You will notice that a few of these quotations appear in more than one place. This is intentional.

༞

_____
_____
_____
_____
_____
_____
_____
_____
_____
_____
_____
_____
_____
_____
_____
_____
_____

Reading without reflecting is like eating without digesting.
—*Edmund Burke (1729-1797,*
British statesman, parliamentary orator, political thinker)

Take what you can use and let the rest go by.
—*Ken Kesey (1935-2001, American novelist)*

When I met Dwight GoldWinde, my marriage was busy unraveling and I had been working unhappily in my family business for over 20 years. Dwight worked with Jim and me in that time period and it is because of him that our marriage is so incredibly alive and passionate. Dwight asks the hard questions to be sure, but he does so with an elegance that leaves you powerfully awakened! We've just celebrated our twentieth anniversary and our life is rich and playful! Dwight's presence in our lives was the reassurance that we needed to face what had become of "us" and choose the courage to recreate "us"!

Dwight has the wisdom of a sage, and the powerful magic guiding you to create the life that you hunger for, the one that you think is far beyond your reach. Dwight took all that I shared with him and gave me strong roots and the wisdom to grow large! Because of many conversations with him I was able to choose the courage needed to take our son out of a traditional system of education that no longer fit him! I have also chosen the gift of the courage that I need so that I can walk away from the family business that I had made my whole life. Without Dwight's powerful coaching, and subsequently the incredible love and support of my husband, such a life decision would not have been possible and the probable outcome would be that I would still be trapped in the cage of my frustration, hating my work and struggling against my own stories of what a "good daughter, wife or mother" would do.

Dwight always says, "that courage is the only choice that we've got" and he exercises that daily in his own life. I always hear his voice when I am making decisions for myself. He's got this lovely southern drawl, edged with just the right tinge of steel that makes you feel safe. He knows how to help you create a life that you'll love; he's created that for himself! Enjoy this book and take it completely into your heart! If you choose the courage to look at whatever his words stir, you will be richly rewarded with opportunities that seconds ago seemed like impossibilities!

—Beth Schreibman Gehring, Former President of Schreibman Jewelers East, August 2, 2003—

Introduction

The bad news is that fear will be with you forever.
The good news is that fear can be your friend forever.

Me, a killer?

At age four, I cowered in bed while my mother pleaded for rest and my father, in one of his manic episodes, insisted she listen to him talk. I didn't understand what was happening, and in that moment fear became my ever-present companion. When I was in first grade, my father moved our family six times—the next town always looked better to him than the one we were living in. I became a scrapper, and at one party I bloodied the noses of three other kids.

When I was eight, I had another life-changing experience, this time during school recess. In the middle of a game of "King of the Dirt Pile," one of the boys I was playing with fell down and lay motionless. My classmates pointed at me (the new kid) and screamed,

"You killed him!"

They prodded him, but he just lay there, inert. I ran. My teacher found me scrunched into a ball on the school steps, arms around my head, my knees wet with tears. The vision of my classmate's motionless body, and all those accusing faces and fingers, flashed repeatedly. I felt defenseless. "I'm only eight years old and I've already killed someone," I thought. "No! I don't want to be a killer!" In the melee that characterized that game I didn't even know whether I had pushed him or if someone else had.

"You shouldn't have left," my teacher declared.

I breathed in ragged gasps. For the rest of the day no one was able to console me. This incident proved pivotal; force and violence were no longer options for me to achieve the status I craved as king of the dirt pile. Days later a teacher announced that my classmate was okay; I wasn't a killer after all, but the trajectory of my life had shifted.

I couldn't invent a better mother

The kids of that small South Carolina town applauded those who were strong and violent, and teased those who earned good grades by taunting, "Teacher's pet!" The kid with the scrappy courage of a house cat, the burning curiosity and aspirations of a scientist—namely me—discovered a resolve to never fight unless a life was threatened. I had to find my own way. Fortunately I had the gift of a creative, resourceful mother who supported me. Mama allowed my siblings and me to follow our childhood whims, blessing us with benign neglect. She let us construct dams in road ruts during gully washers (as long as we didn't ask for clean clothes more than three times in any one storm); she let me organize the annual neighborhood "Great Leaf" parties; and she allowed me to order a baby alligator from Florida and a horned toad from Arizona.

We lived in an impoverished South Carolina town and my clothes were scruffier than average. We had no indoor toilet or running water until I was eleven. But Mama nurtured a richness in our spirits and expanded our horizons with fine novels that she read to us for an hour or more at a time. We were encouraged to take things apart and understand them. And my parents assisted us with science projects.

My dad made a different difference

Dad was a great starter and founded the school rocket club, taught fencing, built a solar oven, and constructed a motor, all from scratch, but he lacked what it took to perfect or run things, or even hold a job. And we argued constantly. He provided the intellectual grit with which I polished my thinking and debating skills. This is one of several gifts for which I'm grateful to him. My father died in 1991.

At school, intelligence was suspect and sex was considered a lecherous, dirty subject, but my mom and sister had my utmost regard and I developed a respectful, gentle attitude toward girls. The brilliant minds that created tape recorders, airplanes, and hi-tech gadgets were my heroes.

Why has no one invented a technology of human behavior?

During my teen years I became fascinated with the fact that humans had harnessed the incredible power of synthesis (i.e., combining individual elements to make a coherent whole) through the discovery and isolation of the basic components of matter and energy. I noticed, however, that this process of isolation and synthesis had yet to be powerfully developed and applied within the realm of human behavior. In fact, it seemed that human beings were still acting like savages even as they held grenades and the atomic bomb. I asked myself, "What power might we reap in the realm of human behavior and human choice if we could identify and isolate those essential 'behaviors' that give rise to wanted and unwanted results in our lives? What powerful synthesis might then be available to us? What virgin continent might then be open for our exploration and use?"

Discover the essential "atoms" of human choice

Today, as an adult, I'm aware that we have only begun to tap the surface of what there is to discover. However, I am certain that the distinction I identify and explore in this book—the choice of courage—represents a fundamental element of human life that opens the door to almost any possibility.

The choice of courage is available to us all, no matter what our past or current circumstances, in each and every moment of our lives. Courage is elemental in nature. *It's not something we have. It's something we choose.* It can be supported and encouraged. But, at its core, *courage is a fundamental, first-cause act of creation, through the power of choice.* Many, many things lie outside our direct control or choice. Yet, within our direct control and choice, the possibilities for courageous action are everywhere.

In high school, I was on the swimming team. One day I wondered what it would be like to jump off the high diving board. "I'll just climb up there and see what it looks like," I thought. From the top, looking down onto the glassy water below, I felt fear raising every hair on my body as it rippled through me; instinctively, I tensed against it. A torrent of spontaneous thoughts rushed through my mind: "I don't need to do this. What's the purpose anyway?" I knew I was at a choice point. I could choose to jump, or I could choose to climb back down the ladder. I could list many influences "pushing me" toward either of these options. But beyond all those influences, I knew that I was the "first cause." I knew that it was *my choice* to jump or not to jump.

Choose courage and get everything you want

In this book I show how empowerment, self-esteem, self-confidence, resourcefulness, accomplishment, loving relationships, romance, breakthroughs, vitality, excitement, passion, creativity, gratitude, decisiveness, dignity, healthy vulnerability, spontaneity, integrity, compassion, a great career, great relationships with friends and colleagues, good health, enough money, enough time, and living a life you fully love are direct and often immediate consequences of choosing courage.

I used to be very shy around the women I was attracted to. I yearned for the self-confidence that some other men seemed to possess in approaching attractive women. Today I have that self-confidence. How did I develop it? By making individual choices of courage again and again (going step by step) to approach women I feared to approach.

Avoid choosing courage and get everything you don't want

I also show how feeling betrayed, just trying, depression, cynicism, guilt, resentment, hatred, oppressive governments, laziness, low self-esteem, lack of self-confidence, feeling overwhelmed, not feeling resourceful, stress, indecisiveness, procrastination, worry, shame, bitterness, blaming others, over-controlling, lying, self-suppression, boredom, complaining, crankiness, resignation, impatience, defensiveness, protectiveness, racism, religious intolerance, ingratitude, perfectionism, obsessiveness, petulance, stubbornness, inflexibility, self-consciousness, righteousness, animosity, criticalness, arrogance, rebelliousness, rudeness, jealousy, whining, insensitivity, unsatisfactory relationships, poor health, not enough money, not enough time, and having a life you'd rather not have are direct and often immediate consequences of the choices to feel safe in the moment *(not choosing courage)*, instead of a willingness to feel the fears and take the actions that will enhance your life and your passions *(choosing courage)*.

I had a client who had a problem with perfectionism. She agonized, over-prepared, and spent hours over the specific words in a paragraph or essay. Once she embraced her fears that someone would criticize her for a mistake and chose the courage to "under-prepare," her perfectionism became less and less an issue in her life, and finally disappeared.

While *not choosing courage* is the most frequent key cause of these unwanted conditions, I acknowledge the possibility of other contributing factors. But, if courage is chosen first, then the other factors, if they still exist, are more easily isolated and addressed.

Step by step into courage, one essay and action at a time

One hundred sixty-six essays in this book explore the distinction of courage. The opportunity to choose courage affects every corner and aspect of your life. While each essay is complete in itself, several will repeat themes covered in other essays, but from a slightly different standpoint. This is important because your results and the quality of your life rest upon a network of beliefs, ideas, and viewpoints, which have been arrived at through your automatic thoughts, and/or through conversations with others. It is my intention that this book will transform your life as you read through it, so that you can begin to approach your commitments and desires through the choice of courage.

This book is designed

to give you access to fun and playfulness in all parts of your life,

to stimulate your thoughts,

to inspire great office and party discussions,

to propel you into the life you want.

At the end of almost every essay, I offer suggestions for specific actions. Take these on, and this book will be a powerful partner in your life.

Every behavior has benefits

I started my career as a life coach over seventeen years ago. Through this work I have discovered that almost all unnecessary human suffering has, at its roots, the resistance to fear and the avoidance of the choice of courage. In working with over a thousand clients, I've found the following question more powerful than any other in addressing unwanted results and behaviors:

"What might be a benefit of having that result, that behavior, that feeling, that belief, that thought?"—where the result, behavior, feeling, belief, or thought is an unwanted one. Here are some specific examples:

> "What is a benefit of not doing everything you can to get that job?"
> "What is a benefit of interrupting your wife?"
> "What is a benefit of feeling guilty?"
> "What is a benefit of believing you're not good enough?"
> "What is a benefit of feeling resigned?"
> "What is a benefit of having the thought, 'What will others think of me?'"

At first, my clients often have a difficult time with this type of question. But, after a little probing, they begin to discover some amazing benefits. After asking questions like these thousands of times, I saw a pattern: almost every benefit comes down to the avoidance of the experience of fear (the resistance to fear).

This book is dangerous to your beliefs

What is the common denominator, or focus, of *all* the belief systems that shape our lives from cradle to grave? Our parents, teachers, culture, peers, religion, philosophy, and government have thrust upon us the importance of, and strategies to achieve, (feelings of) security and safety. No matter their differences, the common denominator among these beliefs and life rules is that they make us *feel* safer. But we confuse *feeling* safe with *being* safe. And what is the end result? We're actually in more danger, *especially the danger of not having the life we truly want*. These beliefs (both explicit and implicit) attempt to reassure us that "if you will just follow these simple rules, you will be safe and successful." However, more often than not, these same beliefs dampen and damage our spirit, our self-esteem, our self-confidence, our vitality, our self-expression, our innocence—and seldom help us attain the results we would really like to have in our lives.

My approach to life marks a major departure from the focus on security being of primary importance. Adoption of my approach will *not* make you feel safe, at least in the short run. I intend that you experience your fear more; I want to wake you up. I'll encourage you to stimulate your fear, to embrace your fear, to actually make friends with your fear, and have your fear serve you in support of your deepest desires and most exciting passions. My approach to life is a full acknowledgment that life is risky, and the most foolhardy course we consistently select is to resist and deny the risk that life is.

Are you living a life of inspiration or a life of avoidance?

At issue is what we consider to be the foundation of our life. Is security of primary importance, or are our life inspirations primary? Is security a value in the service of our desires and passions, or does security take on a life of its own and become an end unto itself?

In almost all other life systems security takes precedence. However, if you adopt *courage* as primary in your approach to life, then your life inspirations will motivate you to create the life you truly want.

I'm afraid to reveal some of the things in this book

Many of my views are controversial. I don't expect (or even want) you to always agree with me. It is a human tendency to dismiss the ideas of someone who holds views with which we disagree. We lose if we indulge this tendency. Perhaps your first choice of courage will be to keep reading, to stay curious even after you've found something significant in this book that disturbs you. Some of the most useful ideas I've acquired were from people whose views were quite divergent from my own.

You'll find that I'm more forthcoming about my private life

(especially in the journal section of this book) than most authors typically are. Although there are risks involved with this openness, I do it in the hope that the drama and detail of my personal life will provide some compelling examples of how the choices of courage have given me the life that I want (and therefore, by extension, could give you the life you want). Please know that I chose *considerable* courage to share so openly with you.

I did it my way (the definition of courage)

Over the years, I've enjoyed many discussions with clients, friends, and colleagues about courage. Sometimes we uncovered "disagreement" about the definition of courage. In using any pre-existing word, we borrow from already existing ideas (which vary from person to person) of what that word means. I do not dispute any other particular definition for the word "courage." However, to *really* understand and get the most value from this book, you will have to take on *my* definition of courage. Although it contains elements of the generally accepted definition, it diverges in important ways. When you read the word "courage" in this book, bring yourself back to *my* definition (see the first page of this book).

Courage is not moral. Courage is not immoral.

Although the definition of courage used in this book is unique, it has broad similarities to the idea of courage as we know it in the English language. One of the issues in using the already existing word courage (as contrasted with coining a new word) is that it conveys connotations from its general usage. One of these unfortunate connotations is the idea that courage is *morally good,* courage is *right,* courage is a *virtue* (as opposed to a sin). In this book I show again and again how it disempowers us to view courage as a moral issue. I show, instead, the benefits and costs of choosing courage or not choosing courage. There is nothing inherently right about the choice of courage. Like everything else, it has benefits and costs. However, as we become clearer and clearer about these benefits and costs, we choose courage more and more. These choices increase the benefits and decrease the costs, both in our lives and in the lives of others.

This book is dangerous to your current way of life

It is not dangerous to your life; it is dangerous to the pseudo-safety that has kept you from living the life you once dreamed about, but have relinquished hope of ever experiencing in the real world.

Courage is most often associated with physical acts involving a risk of life. Those acts of courage (assuming they fit my definition of courage) are, by far, the least important opportunities for courage in our lives. The courage that counts is the choice to embrace fear and take action when the "adversary" is society, our customers, our colleagues, our classmates, our teachers, our bosses, our siblings, our parents, our children, our lover, the man or woman in the street, our own identity, or our own automatic ideas of the way we "should be" and "should feel" and "should act." The opportunity to choose courage is *right here, right now!*

Precision or clarity: Must I choose?

"What is the opposite of clarity?" a teacher once asked me.

"Vagueness, . . . ahhh . . . blurriness," I bumbled.

"Precision," he declared.

"Precision?! I don't understand!" I blurted.

At the time, I was trying to make a statement about what my "Consider It Done" technique would accomplish (see the essay on page 272). The statement went something like this, "For about 95 percent of the population, when implemented rigorously by both the action partner and accountability partner, the Consider It Done technique will guarantee that at least 98 percent of the promises made to oneself will be kept." He suggested that I say instead, "Consider It Done guarantees that you will keep any promise you make to yourself." The latter statement is powerful and clear. Yet it lacks some precision. Throughout this book I have tried to provide a balance between clarity and precision, because both must be served.

Everyone is frightened

Since 1987 I've had the privilege of working with approximately five thousand people, whether for a single gift coaching session or through my regular four-month, one-on-one coaching program. These people have often shared themselves more deeply with me than they would with any other person in their life. I've worked with single moms on government support, psychologists and counselors, doctors and lawyers, famous authors, a vice president of Intel, a woman responsible for yearly revenues of $6,000,000,000 and five thousand employees, actors and actresses, international team-building consultants, kids as young as seven and adults as old as eighty-two. The one fundamental issue that all of these clients brought to the table was the issue of resisted fear, although they most often did not recognize it as such at the beginning. Everyone is frightened and everyone is resisting it. And we all try to hide it. Often the number one person we try to hide it from is ourselves.

Vive le courage!

As an eight-year-old, my working paradigm burst and I was thrust on thought trails less traveled. My chosen path of courage has added zest, adventure, and recognition to my life, given me freedom from money worries, and liberty to live in any country that has a telephone, with only a twenty-five hour work week. My lifestyle is characterized by leisure, connection, writing, romance, and work that is play for me. I've guided thousands to the achievement of dreams they never expected to accomplish. Many pay a thousand dollars per month (U.S.) for the truths in this book. I invite you to integrate the ideas in this book into your life and thrive on the gifts of courageous decisions.

I want to be at your bedside!

The choice of courage is broad in application and powerful in creating both the immediate and future life that you want. This book is not one that can be mastered. I wrote it, yet I am still aware of how much I need to "get into my bones" both the essence and form of what I say. Keep this book by your bedside. Read it, skim it, mark it up, jump from here to there in it. Use it so that it begins to use you.

I want you to have what you want!

**"Courage may be dangerous,
but it's the safest choice we've got"™**

৯০

_____
_____
_____
_____
_____
_____
_____
_____
_____
_____
_____
_____
_____
_____
_____
_____
_____
_____
_____
_____
_____
_____
_____
_____
_____
_____
_____
_____
_____
_____
_____

Who I am . . . Dwight GoldWinde

The following eleven "poems" express who I am. The first five are the most fundamental. I wrote these originally with the idea that no one but me would ever read them. This gave me the freedom to write only my truth without considering how it might impact or be evaluated by others. Only later did I choose the courage to share these poems with others. I invite you to choose the courage to take the first steps to write who you are. Let the words flow with only the intention that they inspire you, as they resonate profoundly with your deepest being and desires. Then read your poems daily out loud to yourself or another.

For some assistance in identifying your fundamental life inspirations, read the essay "Discover Your Life Inspirations" on page 241.

—Play—

I am play.
I am the dance and tease of the wind.
I bring the lightness and frivolity of the gods
to brighten and charm the heaviest of hearts.
I am playful about seriousness and serious about play.
Play is the essence and bubbling spirit
of every moment and nuance of my life.
Laughing through the tango,
horsing around in my play world,
mocking the drama of it all
is who I am
and am.

—Adventure—

I am adventure.
Each moment of thought, conversation, and movement,
I explore the unexplored,
I step again into the new and the unknown.
The dance of adventure and intrigue courses through my blood,
as I embrace and revel in the play-by-play repartee
between order and chaos.

—Connection—

I am connection.
I am the soul of humanity.
I know that you are there.
I feel your desire for safety
and your passion for life.
I touch your essence with my eyes.
Whether our paths cross
for a moment or a lifetime,
I feel your heart in mine.
I am awed by
my respect and admiration,
my affection and adoration,
my empathy and compassion
for you and for us.

—*Innocence*—

I am innocence.
The newness, the freshness of life assaults my being;
my senses come alive in the ever-roiling surge
of timeless events and happenings.
Each moment brings virgin beginnings to my life,
to my eyes, to the sensuousness of it all.
I live in expectation of the unexpected.
My eyes are awash in the glory and surprise
of life after life.

—*Romance*—

I am romance.
I am the enchanter. I am the enchanted.
To drown in her eyes, to steal a touch of her flesh,
to create a safety where all can be dared, this is my destiny,
this is my ever-awakening desire for exquisite connection.
To bring her, to bring us again and again to that point of
timeless union,
dancing, moving, back and forth,
always in the rhythm of chasing and surrender
in that ageless ritual that brings meaningless meaning,
now and forever more.
In thought, feeling, spirit, action, and affection—
intimately adoring, warmly embracing,
worshiping and revering, tenderly caressing,
while she bewitches and entrances me
with the thrill of her wild abandon,
allowing herself to be ravished to the edges
of full-body melt-down and mind-erasing pleasure,
this is who I am.

—Presence—

I am presence.
Every nuance of the world abides
in my eyes, ears, nose, and touch.
The essence of every being embraces my soul.
This moment invades me with all its shapes,
textures, colors, tones, reverberations, sensations, and flavors.
My present runneth over,
leaving space for neither the past nor the future.
I live in the timeless eternity of now,
my senses and soul filled to the brim.
This is who I am.

—Gratitude—

I am gratitude.
The present washes me in her love.
Whatever this moment brings,
I exalt in this gift of awareness
and my miracle of existence.
All those who have come before me have blessed me
with unfathomable support and opportunity.
Both the miracle of man and of God
suffuse each glorious moment.
How can I be me!?—In this world!?
In this time in history!?—With my country!?
With my parents!?—With my friends!?
Now living in Shanghai!?—With all that is given to me!?
With my mind, body, feelings, and spirit!?
How could have I chosen anything with more magnificence
and with more possibility!?

—Divine Bliss—

I am divine bliss.
The river of ecstasy runs through me.
Both the peace and glory of the ages reside within me.
In speechless awe, I am both the creator and the created.
My world is awash with the splashes of miracles.

—Discovery—

I am discovery.
What was unseen, I will see.
What was unheard, I will hear.
What was unacknowledged, I will acknowledge.
I live with sight, sound, scent, touch, and mind,
brimmed with curiosity and fascination
for just around the corner.
This is who I am.

—Invention and Design—

I am invention. I am design.
What was previously packaged, I will un-package.
What was previously un-combined, I will combine.
See if you can keep up with me.

—Awakening—

I am the awakening.
Whether for only a moment or a lifetime,
I will startle you from your sleep,
stimulating you to discover that indeed you were asleep.
Wake up and join me.
We have just begun.

Courage: The View from Many Windows

What Value will You Get from this Section on Courage?

The essays in this section examine in detail, and from many angles, what courage is and what courage is not. Once you have digested the basic ideas from these essays, you will find yourself easily distinguishing both when you choose courage and when you don't choose courage.

You will discover how courage is **always a choice.** It is never something that you "have" or "don't have." (This is both good news and bad news.)

You will grasp that courage is **independent of the results.** (If the results were guaranteed, it wouldn't be called "courage.")

You'll also understand that courage may be dangerous, but it's the **safest choice you've got.**

Furthermore, you'll become clear how **courage is the one "virtue"** that underlies all other true virtues.

Very importantly, you'll see that courage is not simply taking an action that you're afraid of taking; it *also includes* aligning with the energies of your fear and honoring yourself for choosing courage.

Perhaps surprisingly, when you choose courage (including aligning with the energy of your fear and honoring yourself for that choice), you will learn that **choosing courage is amazingly easy.**

As with everything else in life, the **step-by-step** approach makes a critical difference; when you apply it to choosing courage, you can build monuments out of molehills.

You'll learn about the power of the 5Cs: **Choosing Courage, Creativity, Curiosity, and Context.**

Opportunities for courage **(OFCs) will start to appear in numbers, places, and circumstances that will astound you.**

You'll also see how **it is never fear that stops you;** it is only your resistance to fear that stops you.

Specifically, you will understand the **five types of fear.**

You'll develop special insight into **Paper-Tiger Fears** and **Hidden Fears.**

Interestingly, you'll even begin to understand the benefits we derive by **not choosing courage.**

Finally, and of paramount importance, you'll appreciate how **fear need not be your enemy;** it can be your strongest ally.

Refer back to the definition of "courage" on the first page of this book as needed. Every idea that I share with you in this book depends upon your complete understanding of this definition.

ॐ

_____
_____
_____
_____
_____
_____
_____
_____
_____
_____
_____
_____
_____
_____
_____
_____
_____
_____
_____
_____
_____
_____
_____

Are you still tolerating your fear?

Or are you grateful for your fear?

How can I emphasize this enough!
    If you want to *really* experience life differently,
    you must have fun with fear,
    you must see and feel fear as something
        that adds juice, aliveness, and verve to your life,
    you must *give up* the notion that a life without fear
        might hold any attraction for you at all.

When I asked a client about her recent choices of courage,
    she told me that, if the risk did not seem too big,
    she would go for it.
    I then asked her if she were
        tolerating the fear that she was confronting
        or if she were grateful for that fear.
        She said she was tolerating it.

This is why choosing "courage" is still difficult for her.
    She is still resisting her fear.
    She is not looking at her fear
        as a source of energy and excitement.
    She is holding onto the notion
        that *somehow* she can have the life she wants
        by avoiding and minimizing the fear in her life.

Don't bulldoze through your fear.
    Don't see it as some "price"
        you have to pay to get what you want.
    Treat your fear as a gem.
        Breathe into it.
        Tap its energy.
        Unleash its excitement.
        Honor yourself for your capacity to do this.
        Above call, create gratitude for your fear.

This is a new habit.
    This is a new attitude.
    Step by step. Keep at it.

But as you make friends with your fear,
    your fear will make friends with you
    and *together* you will *fly!*

And the difficulty that was your life before
    will seem as to have never been.

Welcome to *life!*

☙

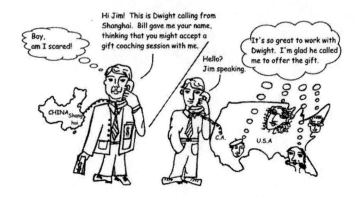

Is Dwight just lucky?

"But you're lucky, Dwight."

I often hear this refrain from my friends and clients,
    as they compare their lives negatively to mine or
    as they argue for their own limitations and the circumstances
    they say prevent them from living the life they truly want.

In large measure, especially since my 30s,
    I have had the life that I have wanted.

In the past few years
    my life has turned into an absolute cornucopia,
    nurtured by the clarity I have developed
    regarding the power and importance
    of choosing courage.

Certainly, I have used my intelligence
    in choosing courage (courage is *not* foolhardiness),
    but, I say, *courage* has played the deciding role
    in creating the life that I want.

Maybe I should tell my friends about the time that
    I chose courage to quit college
        (risking my parents' disapproval)
    because I could not see its relevance to the rest of my life
        (and college was boring).

Maybe I should tell them about the time that,
    at the age of 22, I chose courage
    to borrow $200 from my parents
    and take the bus to New York City,
        not knowing a single person there,
        but intending to build my life there.

Maybe I should tell them about the time that,
    at the age of 24, after two years of working for IBM,
    I chose courage to quit IBM
    and start working for myself
        as a freelance computer programmer,
        not having a single client before I quit my corporate job.

Maybe I should tell them about the time that
    I chose courage to take dancing lessons,
        even when I felt awkward and self-conscious.

Maybe I should tell them about the times that
    I chose courage to participate
    in human potential workshops
        that forced me to look deeply into myself.

Maybe I should tell them about the time that
    I chose courage to move (within two weeks of thinking of it)
    from New York City (after living there for 14 years)
    to Tempe, Arizona,
        driving a UHaul van 2,600 miles by myself over five days.

Maybe I should tell them about the time that
    I chose courage to walk into
    a computer department without an appointment,
    and say to the manager,
    "You should give me some work,"
        resulting in a six-month contract
        with the first company I approached in Arizona.

Maybe I should tell them about the time that
    I chose courage to ask
    my (then future) wife to marry me.

Maybe I should tell them about the time that
    I chose courage to change careers,
        after 20 years as a computer software consultant,
    to my new career as a life coach
        (which I've now enjoyed for 17 years).

Maybe I should tell them about the many thousands of times that
    I chose courage to call strangers on the telephone
        to offer them a gift coaching session,
            thereby making my business viable and deeply satisfying.

Maybe I should tell them about the time that
    I chose courage
        (perhaps the biggest choice of courage in my life)
    to initiate a divorce with my (now former) wife.

Maybe I should tell them about the time that
    I chose courage to ask for help when I really needed it.

Maybe I should tell them about the time that
    I chose courage to feel my pain and fear completely
    (crying more in a month than I had cried in all my life before)
    when my deepest love chose to end our romance.

Maybe I should tell them about the time that
    I chose courage to plan and implement
    a 40-day odyssey through Japan,
        living with 18 different home-stay families
        in 18 different cities from Yokohama to Nagasaki.

Maybe I should tell them about the time that
    I chose courage to move from Arizona
        (after living there for 18 years)
    to Hermosa Beach, California.

Maybe I should tell them about the time that
    I chose courage
    to move from California to Tokyo, Japan,
        relocating myself and my business
        into a totally new country and culture.

Maybe I should tell them about the time that
    I chose courage to ask Dawn,
    a Chinese student at Tokyo University, for directions.
        She ended up becoming one of my best friends ever,
        and is responsible for my living in Shanghai now.

Maybe I should tell them about the time that
    I chose courage to move
    from Tokyo, Japan to Shanghai, China.

Maybe I should tell them about all of the times that
    I chose courage to honor my own deepest desires,
        even when others disapproved or considered me selfish.

When a friend says I'm "lucky,"
    maybe I should tell h/im about the time that
    I chose the courage that resulted
    in my knowing h/im!

Maybe I should tell h/im that the reason
    that many things are so easy for me now
    is because I was willing to choose courage
    when they were still difficult for me.

How, indeed, can s/he really understand that
    it was not luck that has given me the incredible life that I have,
    but the courage that I continue to choose?

How, indeed, can s/he really understand that
    s/he has the power of choosing courage
    in h/is life just as I do in mine?

Do you fully realize the power
    that choosing courage can have on *your* life?

Do you know that it is never too late
    to begin choosing courage *now*.

❧

_____

_____

_____

_____

_____

_____

_____

Courage is always a choice

Our common expressions
    "He had courage,"
    and "he didn't have courage"
    are totally erroneous.

Courage is *not* something we *have.*
    It is something we *choose.*
    It is a choice made in the moment.
    We can choose courage.
    Or we can *not* choose courage.
    Choosing courage
        is just as much of a choice as not choosing courage.
But what does the word "choice" really mean?

Can we say that we chose courage
    because others gave us support to do so?
No.
Certainly others may have influenced us
    to choose courage;
but we also could have *not* chosen courage.

Can we say that we didn't choose courage
    because it was too frightening to choose courage?
No.
Certainly the level of fear may have influenced us
    to not choose courage;
but we still could have chosen courage.

The choice of courage is a *first cause;*
    no other causes precede it.
    To say it is a choice
        and to say our choice was caused by something else
        means it was not really a choice
        because something else caused it.

How can we know that we have a choice about something?
By simple introspection and experimentation.
    It is easy to demonstrate to yourself
        that you can cause yourself to choose courage
        or not choose courage
        in any given circumstance that presents
        an opportunity for choosing courage.

A simple example (illustrated on the cover of this book):
You are standing in line at the bank.
You think it would be nice to strike up
    a conversation with the person next to you.
Then, you notice the fear.
    "What if s/he doesn't want to be bothered?"
    "How will I feel if s/he ignores me?"
    "What if s/he's not interesting anyway?"
Now you are aware of the opportunity for choosing courage.
In this moment, you are presented with the understanding
    that you can move the universe with your choice.
You can *choose* to feel safe in the moment
    by not trying to strike up a conversation
or you can choose to feel the fear
    and go for what you really want.
Nothing, short of *you*, causes you to do either.
You are the first cause in the matter.

In this regard, you and I are like God.

Welcome to the good news and the bad news of life.

It's all your choice.

Honor yourself for choosing the courage to choose courage.

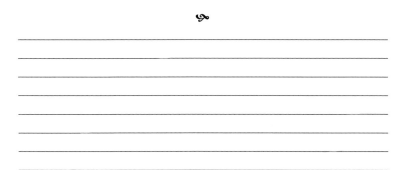

Most people fail in the art of living not because they are inherently bad or so without will that they cannot lead a better life; they fail because they do not wake up and see when they stand at the fork in the road and have to decide.

—*Erich Fromm (1900-1980,*
German-born social scientist and philosopher)

Life cannot wait until the sciences may have explained the universe scientifically. We cannot put off living until we are ready. The most salient characteristic of life is its coerciveness: it is always urgent, 'here and now' without any possible postponement. Life is fired at us point blank.

—*Jose Ortega y Gasset (1883-1955,*
Spanish philosopher and essayist)

The refusal to choose is a form of choice; disbelief is a form of belief.

—*Frank Barron (1890-1964)*

You don't have courage

"He had no courage."
"She had the courage to leave him."
"I had the courage to ask for a raise."
"He didn't have the guts to speak up."

All these statements are *false*.

When we speak about courage in this manner,
    we hide from the fact
        that courage is *not* something we have or don't have.
It is false and inaccurate to say
    that someone has or doesn't have courage,
    that someone has or doesn't have guts.

We *choose* courage.
    Courage is a choice in the *moment*.
    It is a creation of the human spirit.

It is that moment at the end of the diving board
    when we choose to jump.
It is that moment during the meeting with our boss
    when we choose to ask for raise.
It is that moment after something has been requested of us
    when we choose to say "no."
It is that moment during a conversation with an attractive person
    when we choose to ask h/im for a date.
It is that moment after considering a new project
    when we choose to go for it.

Courage is not something that can be stored or built up.
But as you step into the same fearful action again and again,
    the fear that you feel in taking that action will diminish,
    and therefore the amount of courage
    required to take the action will also diminish.

But because courage is a *choice in the moment,*
    how much courage you chose yesterday
    has no connection with how much courage
    you will choose today.

But the opposite is also true (this is the good news):
    how much courage you *did not* choose yesterday
    has no connection with how much courage
    you *will* choose today.

It is *all* a choice, *your choice,*
    for every moment in your life.

I invite you to create clarity
    in your speaking and listening by always putting the words
    "choose" or "did not choose" before the word "courage."

Notice the new opening this provides to you
    in living the life you really want.

⎈

_____

_____

_____

_____

_____

_____

_____

_____

It would not be courage if the results were guaranteed

The issue of results in choosing courage
    looks different depending on our point of view—
    whether we are looking forward
        (before the action and results have occurred),
    or whether we are looking backward
        (after the action is taken and the results become obvious).

Before we choose courage, we must consider the probability
        of obtaining the desired outcome from our actions.
    If it were *guaranteed* that the projected action
        could *never* provide any of the desired outcomes,
        then our proposed opportunity for choosing courage
        might be a choice of foolishness or blindness.
    In considering the option of choosing courage,
        part of the consideration must include a weighing of
        the certain-to-probable-to-possible-to-unlikely
        costs and benefits of a particular choice.
        Without such consideration,
        the choice of courage is *not* a choice of courage.

Whereas, *after* we have chosen courage,
    the fact that we chose courage
    does not change as a result of the outcome.
    Courage exists *independent* of the outcome,
        regardless of the results.

Honor yourself each time you choose courage,
    before and after you have chosen, *regardless* of the results.

š

Courage or results: Which is primary?

Do you put your primary focus on choosing courage?
Or do you put your primary focus on getting results?
Whichever you choose as primary (again and again)
    will make *all* the difference in your life.

It's great when we have enough power and/or knowledge
    so that our actions can guarantee results we want.
      But the real power and juice of life
        is not lived in the security of what we already know for sure,
        is not lived with the assurance
          that our actions will always hit the mark,
        but always on the edge of what we don't know for sure,
        and on the precipice
          of what we cannot guarantee and control.
When we live our lives
    with a primary intention of always getting results,
    when we begin to judge ourselves
      on whether or not we got results
      (in the areas that cannot be guaranteed),
    when avoiding the fear
      of not getting results becomes primary,
    when we limit ourselves in what we're willing to go for
      because we cannot know the outcome for sure,
        then our life becomes an ever-contracting cage of avoidance.

This is the life that most people live most of the time.

On the other hand,
    when we begin to hold the choice of courage as primary,
    when we begin to see and act upon the fact that the results
      of any one choice of courage cannot be guaranteed,

when we begin to accept and even play with the fear
associated with taking the actions that may or may not
get results we want,
when we begin to choose the courage to enjoy the process,
independent of whether or not we get results,
when we begin to appreciate ourselves consistently
for choosing courage each and every time we go for it,
regardless of the results,
then our life becomes an ever-expanding panorama
of empowerment, accomplishment, and self-expression.

Why is putting the primary focus on results so disempowering?

Because if we don't get results,
we are likely to have thoughts and feelings like these:
"What's wrong with me?"
"What's wrong with them?"
"What's wrong with it?"
"Other people would get results. Why can't I?"
"I feel so embarrassed."
"Life is so hard."
"Life is unfair."
"It makes me angry."
"I'm not going to try this again."

Or more often, we end up not going for the results at all,
with likely thoughts and feelings like these:
"I probably wouldn't get the results I want anyway."
"I don't want to look foolish."
"It just feels easier to not go for it."
"I don't deserve it."
"I don't believe I can make a difference."
"What will other people think?"
"I don't want to feel rejected."

"I'm just unlucky."
"I want my life to feel safe."
"I just want to withdraw."
"Life is difficult."

Why is putting the primary focus
on choosing courage so empowering?

Because if we don't get results,
we can easily have thoughts and feelings like these:
"I feel good about myself for choosing courage."
"I enjoyed the process,
even though I didn't get results I wanted this time."
"I have learned something about how to do it next time."
"I found out the way it may not work; I'll try another way."
"I feel complete and empowered with what happened;
now I'm in a resourceful place to choose what's next."
"Feeling good about myself
helps me to feel good about others."
"Life is such an adventure!"

Because if we do get results (which is more likely over time),
we can easily have thoughts and feelings like these:
"I feel more confident in my ability to get these results again."
"Life is such a bonanza: I enjoyed the process,
I feel great about myself,
and also, as a very nice extra, I got the results!"
"Life just gets easier and easier as I continue
to put my primary focus on choosing courage."
Either way, whether you get the results you wanted or not,
you can still say,
"I feel so proud of myself for choosing courage
to create the life I want."

The fundamental and most poignant difference
    between "results" and "courage" is an issue of *access*.

Consider these basic facts:

Results are never really guaranteed.
    There is always a level of risk.
Results are almost always in the future
    (whether an immediate or more remote future).

Courage, in contrast, can always be "guaranteed"
    in that it is always *your* choice;
        to choose courage (or not) is *always* within your "control."
Courage is always in the *now*.
    Even to commit yourself to choosing courage in the future
        is a choice of courage *now*.

The reason we habitually put the primary focus on results
    (instead of on choosing courage) is because it *seems* safer.

However, counter-intuitively, *the exact opposite is true*.

To put the primary focus on results,
    instead of on choosing courage, is *more* dangerous.
To put the primary focus on choosing courage,
    instead of on getting results, is *safer*.

Notice the choice of courage it takes
    to put your primary focus on choosing courage!

Honor yourself for that choice (again and again).

৯

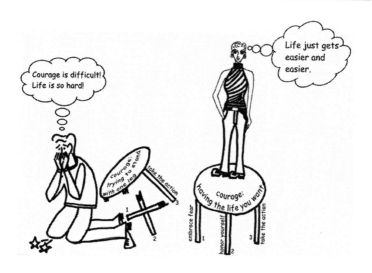

Is it hard for you to choose courage?

I consistently hear the complaint
  that choosing courage is hard.

In fact, when you fully understand the distinction of courage,
  you will find that choosing courage is easy,
  and the more you choose it, the easier it gets.

Courage must include *three* legs (three cornerstones)
  in order to qualify as full courage.
The reason we often believe choosing courage is hard
  is that we are trying to choose courage
  using only *one* of its *three* legs.

As a reminder and memory aid for the three legs,
  remember these four letters: EHAH
  (there are four letters because one leg
  is repeated twice in the process of choosing courage).

EHAH!

E = Embrace and breathe into the fear.

H = Honor and appreciate yourself
for the courage you're about to choose.

A = Act (take the action).

H = Honor and appreciate yourself for the courage you chose
(regardless of the outcome).

Let's review each of these three legs.

E = Embrace and breathe into the fear (Leg 1).

Most often, the best way to do this
is to take some very, very deep breaths
and speak/shout (as loudly as possible, given the environment)
"Boy, am I scared!"

Continue taking these deep breaths
and repeating "Boy, am I scared!"
until you can feel the energy of the fear flowing through you,
instead of blocked inside of you.

Even in a public place, you can always do the deep breathing
and say "Boy, am I scared!" under your breath.

Consider the "FOE" formula:
Fear + oxygen = energy and excitement

H = Honor and appreciate yourself
for the courage you're about to choose (Leg 2).

Most often, the best way to do this
is to consider the idea
that it is not the adult you who is frightened.
It is the five-year-old you who is frightened.
From an adult perspective,
the thing to be frightened of is *not* taking the action.
But from the five-year-old perspective,
the idea of taking the action stimulates fear.

Get in touch with that five-year-old.

Use a young picture of yourself if that is helpful.

Then say to h/im:

"I can see and feel that you are frightened.

It's okay to feel frightened.

And I *really* admire and appreciate you

for accepting and embracing the fear

and taking the action anyway."

Keep expressing this admiration and appreciation

in different ways until you can see and feel

that s/he really accepts and appreciates

your admiration, honor, and respect.

A =   Act (Leg 3).

Only *after* the first two legs of courage have been chosen

do you choose the third leg, the leg of action.

The actions of courage can take many forms.

The action may be a physical action:

picking up a package that a stranger dropped

and giving it to h/im.

The action may be a request:

asking for a salary raise or a date.

The action may be keeping silent:

not opening your mouth

to try to control something you can't control

and that you will most likely worsen

by your attempt to control.

The action may be saying "no":

declining an invitation to be with a person

you really don't want to spend time with.

The action may be sharing your thoughts or feelings:

"I *really* like you" or

"I felt automatically hurt when you said that."

H = Honor and appreciate yourself
for the courage you've just chosen (repeating Leg 2).
Again, get in touch with your five-year-old,
honoring and appreciating h/im for the courage
s/he just chose.
Do this *regardless* of the outcome.

EHAH!

Embrace, honor, act, and honor.

Each of the three legs of choosing courage is important.
Each of the three legs is essential
to making the process of choosing courage
fully effective, consistent, and *easy*.

Start experimenting today
by rigorously including *all* three legs
in each choice of courage whether that choice be big or small.

Notice how this makes choosing courage *much* easier!

❧

_____

_____

_____

_____

_____

_____

_____

_____

If you think that being ordinary is easier than being extraordinary,
you are mistaken.

—*from the movie 'Hilary and Jackie'*

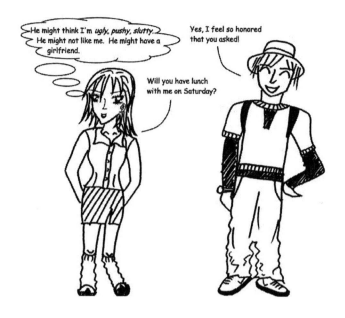

Courage may be dangerous

"Liberty is always dangerous, but it is the safest thing we have."
  —Harry Emerson Fosdick

Actually for similar reasons,
"Courage may be dangerous. But it's the safest choice we've got."
  —GoldWinde

It is dangerous to ask for a date.
  You might look foolish and your feelings may be hurt.
  But if you keep asking for dates,
    you will probably be safe from being dateless
    (and lonely and so on).

It is dangerous to go to a job interview.
  You might not get the job
    and you might feel embarrassed or disappointed.

But if you keep going to job interviews,
    you will probably be safe from being jobless
    or be safe from staying in your current joyless job.

It is dangerous to say "no" to your friend.
    S/he might feel hurt and withdraw from you.
    But if you say "no" to your friend when you need to,
        you will probably be safe
        from feeling resentment toward your friend.

It is dangerous to leave a violent husband.
    He might try to stop you and hurt you more.
    But if you actually leave him,
        you will probably be safe
        from his violence for the rest of your life.

It is dangerous to start working for yourself.
    You might fail at it and won't be able to pay the bills.
        And people might say, "Who are you to do that?"
    But if you start working for yourself,
        you will probably be safe
        from feeling like you sold out on yourself.

It is dangerous to establish and maintain good boundaries
    with your spouse.
    S/he might not accept your boundaries
        and it could precipitate a big conflict or even a divorce.
    But if you establish and maintain good boundaries,
        you will probably be safe
        from a marriage of resentment and bickering.

It is dangerous to be open and vulnerable
    about your feelings of fear, hurt, or love with a friend or lover.
    H/is response could stimulate even more fear and hurt.

But if you are open and vulnerable with your friend or lover,
   you will probably be safe
   from having a passionless and careful relationship.

It is dangerous to ask for a raise.
   You might be disappointed if your boss says "no"
      and your boss might resent you for asking.
   But if you ask for a raise,
      you will be safe from the uncertainty you would have felt
      if you had not asked for one.
      You might also be safe from earning less money.

It is dangerous to leave an unhappy marriage.
   You might regret it later.
      Or you might feel lonely.
      Or you might have financial difficulties.
      Or it might be difficult for the children.
   But if you leave an unhappy marriage,
      you will probably be safe from living a life
      of interminable resentment of your spouse,
      and you will probably also be safe from causing damage
      to your kids by not providing them
      with role models of long-suffering parents.

It is dangerous to change careers.
   How can you know if the new one
      will be financially rewarding and satisfying?
   But if you do change careers,
      you will probably be safe
      from living a life of resignation in your current career.

Courage may be dangerous, but it's the safest choice we've got.

How do you create *real* danger in your life
    by playing it safe (not choosing courage)?

Explore at least one area in your life where you do this
    and choose courage to create a safer life.

❦

_____

_____

_____

_____

_____

_____

_____

_____

_____

_____

_____

_____

_____

_____

The important thing is this: To be able at any moment to sacrifice
what we are for what we could become.

—*Charles du Bois*

Security is mostly a superstition. It does not exist in nature nor do
the children of man as a whole experience it. Avoiding danger is no
safer in the long run than outright exposure. Life is either a daring
adventure, or nothing.

—*Helen Keller (1880-1968, social reformer, writer)*

All life is a chance. So take it! The person who goes furthest is the
one who is willing to do and dare.

—*Dale Carnegie (1888-1955, author, public speaker)*

Courage here is not courage there

When I speak with my Chinese friends about courage,
    they will often respond with,
    "You don't really know the Chinese culture."
Or sometimes they will respond with,
    "Courage is easy for you; but it's something I can't do."

What my friends are missing
    (and I am forgetting when I speak with them)
    is that courage is always contextual.

What is courage for me is not courage for you.
An example:
    I'm not afraid to start my own business,
        but I'm afraid to ask for a date.
    You're not afraid to ask for a date,
        but you're afraid to start your own business.

What is courage in one culture is not courage in another culture.
An example:
    In Chinese culture, it's often a major choice of courage
        for an unmarried woman to live separately from her parents.
    In American culture, it's rarely a major choice of courage
        for an unmarried woman (after the age of 18 or 21)
            to leave her parents' home;
        it is often expected of her by her parents and society.

What is courage in one family is not courage in another family.
An example:
    In my family, when I was growing up,
    I didn't have to choose courage to follow
    my own heart and head to explore and discover my life career;
        my parents unconditionally encouraged me
        to pursue whatever interests I developed.

In many families children face a lot of pressure
    from their parents to pursue (or avoid)
        a particular career,
    thereby opening up the opportunity for the children
        to choose courage in order to follow their own interests.

What is courage for me today is not courage for me tomorrow.
An example:
    At one time, I had to choose courage
        to turn to the person standing next to me in line and ask,
        "What do you like best about standing in line?"
    Today, I have no nervousness or fear associated with doing this.

Courage is *not* measured by the size of the action.
Courage is measured by the size of the fear one embraces,
    and by honoring oneself for taking the action
        in the presence of that fear.

As such, both fear and courage
    are *totally* contextual and individual,
    only applying to you,
        with your background, with your family,
        with your culture, in this moment, in your current mood,
        in your current physical surroundings,
            as you are alone or with others,
            as you are currently speaking with and listening to others,
        with your current thoughts,
        with your current desires and commitments,
        with your current way of interpreting the world,
        and so on.

When we don't know or we forget that courage is contextual,
    we limit our power to choose it;
    we therefore restrict our ability to have the life we want.

Now that you understand that courage is contextual,
   what new opportunities for choosing courage
   do you see for yourself that you didn't see before?

Now tell yourself and/or someone else
   which of these opportunities you will embrace.

❧

_____
_____
_____
_____
_____
_____
_____
_____
_____
_____
_____
_____
_____
_____
_____
_____
_____
_____

This place where you are . . . this place where you stand . . . is where
you must start. From here you can go in any direction and to any
destination . . . and it is impossible to start from anywhere else.
—*Ron Atchison*

The dumbest risk is not taking risks, specifically those gambles that
enliven and flesh out our resonance with our core of Being.
—*Robert Augustus Masters*
(author of Truth Cannot be Rehearsed)

All virtues come from courage

Consider the idea that at the *core* of all virtues
    is the virtue of courage.
    Every other virtue,
        when clearly defined, grounded, and contextualized,
    can be reduced to the virtue of courage.

[Special note: the word "virtue" in this essay
    is *not* intended to have any good/bad
    or right/wrong connotations.
    I use it simply to denote
        those types of chosen behaviors which,
        when practiced with some consistency,
        will typically give us a life we love.]

Here are some character traits
    that are generally considered virtuous:
compassion, courage, empathy, fairness, faith, faithfulness,
fortitude, friendliness, friendship, frugality, generosity, hope,
honesty, humility, innocence, integrity, loyalty, openness, patience,
perseverance, prudence, reliability, respectfulness, responsibility,
spontaneity, unselfishness.

It is far beyond the scope of this essay
    to show how all these virtues
        (when well-defined and contextualized)
    are expressions of choosing courage.
        That is the larger purpose of this book as a whole.

Courage is the source of all virtue.
    And when we can, step by step,
        begin to discern and uncover that courage is that source,
        then, not only does it make choosing virtue much easier,
        it also begins to dissolve the seeming conflicts
        among the various virtues
        as they are practiced around the world.

Seeing that the choice of courage
    is the source of all virtues
    is often more difficult with a special class of virtues.
This class of virtues include
    perseverance, fortitude, will-power,
    self-discipline, and self-denial.
When, indeed, these virtues
    have been rigorously defined and contextualized,
    then they too can be reduced
    to the choice of courage.
At first brush, it seems that the exercise of these virtues
    does not involve facing any fear.
    It seems that it only involves facing pain and discomfort.
    Yet it is our resistance to pain and discomfort
        that underlies our fear of these experiences.

One of my agreements with myself
    is to climb the seven flights of stairs
    to my apartment in Shanghai
    every time I return from outside.
Often, I didn't feel like it, but I did it anyway,
    using perseverance, fortitude, will-power,
    self-discipline, and self-denial.
When I approached the task this way, I did it,
    but it did not get any easier.
    It continued to be difficult for me each time I did it.

More recently, however, I started experimenting
    with taking very deep breaths and saying,
    "Boy, am I scared!"
    as I began to climb the stairs.
I noticed immediately how much easier it was
    to climb the stairs and how much easier
    it was to honor myself for the courage
    I was choosing in climbing those stairs.
Little by little, I became aware of the fear
    which I had so adeptly hidden from myself,
    the fear that I have been resisting all my life.

With this new insight, a whole new domain of actions
    is getting easier and easier for me.

Try this experiment.
Choose some important action
    that normally requires perseverance, fortitude,
    will-power, self-discipline, and/or self-denial.
Then, just before stepping into that action
    (or non-action as in *not* smoking),
    take several deep breaths,
    breathe into your fear (whether you can feel it or not)
    and speak/shout many times,
    "Boy, am I scared!"
Also, take a moment to get in touch with that five-year-old within
    and honor h/im for the courage that s/he is choosing.
    Do this until you can feel that s/he gets your admiration.

Notice how this makes things *much easier*!

Enjoy!

Every courageous choice counts

Do you notice every time you choose courage?

Do you acknowledge and honor yourself
　　every time you choose or chose courage?

Probably not.

I am constantly pointing out to my friends and clients
　　how they are choosing courage
　　in instances they did not recognize as choices of courage.

Recently, a friend told me,
　　"I didn't want to go to the party.
　　But I went anyway. And I'm glad I did."

I asked, "Why didn't you want to go to the party?"

"I felt nervous about talking with people I didn't know."

"So you felt some fear in association with talking with new people.
　　You chose to accept the fear and chose the courage
　　to talk with them anyway, right? That inspires me."

"You're right. I didn't think of it that way,
　　but I was choosing courage without realizing it."

Not only do we often fail to recognize
　　the many opportunities for courage
　　that we either take or don't take throughout each day,
　　we also regularly dismiss most choices of courage
　　with comments like, "It's nothing to brag about."

This lack of awareness and dismissive attitude
    constitute two major stumbling blocks
    in establishing the choice of courage
    as an integral and powerful part of our life.

Consider all of the following
    as possible/probable expressions of courage:
    —taking your wife's hand while shopping
    —asking someone, "What do you like best about yourself?"
    —saying "no"/ "yes" to a party invitation
    —taking a minute to wash some dishes,
        rather than giving in to the internal pressure
        to skip over them for "more important" things
    —calling a friend to ask when s/he can return a book
    —calling a friend when you're in a funk
    —doing something that you've been avoiding
    —smiling at a stranger you pass on the street
    —driving more slowly
    —asking for help in a department store
    —asking for a refund
    —telling your child how much you admire h/im
    —establishing and maintaining
        an important boundary with someone
    —keeping silent instead of advising
        your son/daughter/friend/co-worker
    —saying "no" to a friend's loan request
    —throwing a party
    —initiating a conversation with someone
    —scheduling a vacation
    —sharing a feeling of hurt or loneliness
    —engaging in physical exercise
    —looking at the big picture and direction of your life
    —placing or responding to an ad on the Internet
    —trying something even though you'll probably do it poorly

—turning off the TV and calling a friend
—planning your day
—setting up a budget
—declining an invitation from someone who is attracted to you
—getting out of bed in the morning

When we create some consistency
    in recognizing and taking advantage of
    the smaller opportunities for courage,
    we create not only results,
    but also a solid sense of confidence and self-esteem.
    We further pave the road
    for making the larger opportunities for courage
    seem like real possibilities in our lives, rather than opportunities
    that we either avoid or fail to recognize.

Remember the simple adage:
    Inch by inch, life's a cinch. Yard by yard, life is hard.

By applying this simple principle
    to the most important choice in your life, the choice of courage,
    you will make more difference for yourself and others
    than with *any other* life-guiding principle.

Be vigilant for the small opportunities for courage.
Count each one that you recognize today.

Breathe into the fear. Celebrate the opportunity. Take the action.

ço

_____

_____

_____

_____

_____

Do you take on your fear
one step at a time?

We all know the old joke:
    "How do you eat a whole elephant?"
Answer: "One bite at a time."
Or do you know the aphorism:
    "Inch by inch, life's a cinch; yard by yard, life is hard"?

This simple idea becomes a profound idea
    when we apply it to the process
    of acknowledging and facing our fears.
Almost any fear that seems too big
    can, with some thought and creativity,
    be broken down into "baby steps."

Let's take, as an example, the goal of wanting to
    approach a stranger in a park to start up a conversation.

Some of us might think and feel,
    "Oh, I could never do that!
    What would they think of me?"
    It might seem like too much fear to confront.

Let's see how we might break this goal down into steps.

The nature of fear is such that,
    as you repeat over and over an action
    that initially stimulates a certain level of fear,
    the fear slowly dissipates.
    This is especially true
        if you breathe into the energy of the fear each time
        and you honor yourself each time for your courage,
        regardless of the outcome.

Step #1

During your walk in the park smile at enough people
    so that at least five people smile back at you.
Continue with this process each day
    until you feel comfortable with it.

Step #2

Smile and say "Good morning" (in a casual, friendly way)
    to enough people
    so that at least three people verbally greet you back.
Continue with this process each day
    until you feel comfortable with it.

Step #3

Approach at least three people who are sitting or standing
    and smile at them, saying, "Good morning,
    would you happen to know when the park closes today?"
Continue with this process each day
    until you feel comfortable with it.

Step #4

Approach at least three people who are sitting or standing
    and smile at them, saying, "Good morning,
    I was wondering if I might ask you something?"
    (Pause for a response.)
    "Every day, I notice how much I enjoy strolling in this park,
        listening to the birds and observing all the interesting people.
    Today, I am curious about
        what other people might enjoy about this park.
    Would you be willing to share with me
        what *you* like about this park?"

There may be a higher likelihood of rejection
    with this step than with the previous steps.
        If the person doesn't seem open to your approach,
        then back out as gracefully as possible.

But *honor yourself*
for your choice of courage to speak with h/im,
regardless of h/is response.
Remember, courage exists *regardless* of the outcome.
Continue with this process each day
until you feel comfortable with it.

Step #5
Repeat step #4, with the intention
of keeping the dance of the conversation going,
with the person who answers your initial question.
Continue with this process each day
until you're comfortable with it.

Congratulations!
You've now "eaten the elephant," one bite at a time.

The above example is just a playful exercise.
And, for some of us, it would not present much of a challenge.
But the principle of taking on your fear
step by step is a powerful one
that can be applied to *any* area or issue of your life.

Brainstorm on how you might break down your fears into steps
as they might apply to your life
in these different areas or circumstances:
—making solicitation calls for your business
—asking a man or woman for a date
—speaking in front of groups
—saying "no" to your friends, spouse, parents, or boss
—asking for a raise
—changing careers
—quitting a job
—quitting school
—starting your own business
—making a choice about marriage

—making a choice about divorce
—setting clear boundaries with others
—doing something crazy
—fully expressing your love to another
—saying "no" to deadlines or long work hours
—not rescuing someone
—taking care of yourself and being selfish
—taking a stand about something important
—stepping outside your culture

Remember,
    "Inch by inch, life's a cinch; yard by yard, life is hard."

❧

_____
_____
_____
_____
_____
_____
_____
_____
_____
_____
_____
_____
_____
_____

Courage is more exhilarating than fear and in the long run it is easier. We do not have to become heroes over night. Just a step at a time, meeting each thing that comes up, seeing it is not as dreadful as it appeared, discovering we have the strength to stare it down.
—*Eleanor Roosevelt (1884-1962,*
American author and former first lady)

Which actions are courageous?

Courage has three cornerstones:

(1) embracing your fear
      so that you can be empowered by its energy,
(2) honoring yourself for embracing the fear
      and for taking the action,
(3) and taking the action.

Taking the action, however, can assume many forms,
    some of which might not seem to be courageous.

For example, consider such actions as
    physically touching the hand of the one you're dating,
    verbally requesting a raise,
    verbally sharing an uncomfortable feeling,
    mentally deciding to think about a difficult issue.

They could be the actions of
    physically removing your hand
        from the one who has just taken your hand,
    verbally saying "no" to a request for a raise,
    mentally choosing to start a new project,
    spiritually taking a stand for your own magnificent life.

They could be the actions of
    keeping your mouth shut when you want to control things
        that you can't (or shouldn't) control,
    really listening to someone,
    allowing your mind to be present to the ecstasy of silence.

They could be the actions of
    expressing fully and completely
        how much you appreciate someone,
    expressing in rapturous sounds and words
        how you're feeling as you're making love,
    telling every person you come in contact with
        something about h/im that you appreciate.

They could be the actions of
    spending more money on something than is your habit,
    spending less money on something than is your habit,
    taking the scenic route to work,
    ironing the clothes in a "work of art" manner
        or performing the same task
            while acting foolishly and working inefficiently.

They could be the actions of
    quitting high school or college,
    leaving your wife, saying goodbye to a boyfriend,
    moving to a new country,
    quitting a job, changing careers,
    moving out of the house,
    saying goodbye to a friend.

They could be the actions of
    really choosing high school or college and making it fun,
    really choosing your wife and creating romance,
    really choosing your boyfriend and learning who he really is,
    discovering your own country,
    creating a new passion in your current job,
    making a great game out of your current career,
    discovering the people who live in the house with you,
    finding the mystery in your friend.

The opportunities for courage can express themselves in all forms
of action and non-action, of speaking and not speaking,
of thought, attitude, and intention.

What new openings for courage do you now see in your life?

Which ones will you take?
Today? Tomorrow? When?

❧

_____

_____

_____

_____

_____

_____

_____

_____

_____

_____

> Often the difference between a successful man and a failure is not
> one's better abilities or ideas, but the courage that one has to bet on
> his ideas, to take a calculated risk and to act.
>
> —*Maxwell Maltz (1895-1971,*
> *author of Psycho-Cybernetics)*

> Avoiding danger is no safer in the long run than outright exposure.
> The fearful are caught as often as the bold.
>
> —*Helen Keller (1880-1968,*
> *social reformer, writer)*

> All life is a chance. So take it! The person who goes furthest is the
> one who is willing to do and dare.
>
> —*Dale Carnegie (1888-1955,*
> *author, public speaker)*

Learn about the three types of OFCs

An OFC (opportunity for courage)
    occurs as one of three different types.

To illustrate, let's consider three different OFCs
    that someone might encounter
    in a hypothetical business context.
Let's say that Jane works in a sales office
    as an administrative manager for 43 salespeople.

The first type of OFC
    is a *forced* opportunity for courage.

Jane's boss says to her
    "Jane, our sales manager will be out sick
    for our important sales meeting on Monday,
    and I'm tied up with another obligation.
    You're the only one available
    who really knows the new data
    that we need to present to our salespeople.
    I want you to prepare a 20-minute talk
    and inspire them to take action on this new data."
Jane is really scared
    about how she will look if she doesn't give a good presentation.
Jane does have a choice.
    She could quit her job.
    She could refuse the assignment
        and deal with her boss' response to that.
    She might come up with a third alternative.
But most of us would see this as a *forced* OFC.
In preparing for and giving the presentation,
    Jane is stepping into an opportunity for courage.

Typically, forced OFCs don't present themselves often.
Some people have been inspired into a whole new life
    by responding to a forced OFC.
Nevertheless, I consider forced OFCs
    to be the least important type of OFC.

The second type of OFC
    is an *optional* opportunity for courage.
These occur much more often than forced OFCs,
    especially as you begin to look for them
    and learn to recognize them as they occur.

Jane's boss just gave her another task to finish
    before the end of the day.
Jane knows that she will have to stay overtime to finish the task
    and she will resent her boss
    if she accepts this task without speaking up.
She has two basic *options* to choose from:
    She can choose to stay overtime
        and resent her boss.
    Or she can choose to speak to her boss
        (with a partnership attitude) to work out something
        where both of them feel good about the outcome.
For Jane, choosing to speak to her boss is frightening.
The second choice is the choice of courage.

Once you begin to recognize them,
    optional OFCs will present themselves to you
    many times each day.
I consider optional OFCs to be everyday opportunities
    to keep your life exciting,
    your stress level low, and your relationships rewarding.

The third type of OFC
    is a *created* opportunity for courage.

Created OFCs occur only when you decide
to invent them and then take advantage of them.
Of the three types of OFCs,
created OFCs are potentially the most powerful
for helping you to fully realize the life that you want.

Jane is fairly satisfied, well-respected,
and well-paid as an administrative manager.
Nothing is really pushing her to consider changing her job.
Yet, if she examines more closely what turns her on the most,
what gives her the most day-to-day pleasure in her life,
she'll probably realize that she would love to be a saleswoman.
But what a risk!
She feels safe in her current position.
She knows her job well.
She has a guaranteed income.
People appreciate and respect her for what she does.
She automatically thinks to herself,
"If I move into selling,
I might not be good at it,
I will risk my guaranteed salary,
people will think I am crazy,
and I will give up the comfort I'm feeling now."
For Jane, to even consider stepping into selling,
she must step out of her everyday life
and *create* a new opportunity for courage
that would never present itself to her
in the normal course of events.
This is a *created* opportunity for courage.
Created OFCs will never present themselves to you.
You must look for them.
You must invent them.

The person who consistently looks for created OFCs,
in all domains of h/is life,

is the person who has fully embraced the risk that life is and declared h/imself a *full* participant in h/is own life.

Identify and isolate three past examples of OFCs in your life:
  one that was a forced OFC,
  one that was an optional OFC,
  one that was a created OFC.

Now invent a newly created OFC for your future
  and step into it.

❧

_____

_____

_____

_____

_____

_____

_____

_____

_____

_____

_____

_____

Opportunity is often difficult to recognize; we usually expect it to beckon us with beepers and billboards.

—*William Arthur Ward*

I shall be telling this with a sigh
Somewhere ages and ages hence:
Two roads diverged in a wood, and I—
I took the one less traveled by,
And that has made all the difference.

—*Robert Frost (1874-1963, American poet)*

Learn "the five Cs"

Do you
    choose
    courage,
    creativity,
    curiosity, and
    context?

Of these, choosing courage is the foundation,
    because it is often required
    in order to choose creativity, curiosity, and context.

Creativity

Most of us are familiar with the process of brainstorming
    to facilitate group creativity.
This is a powerful process with a well-documented ability
    to create breakthrough results.
Yet, when we are stuck, when we have a real problem,
    how often do we think of and initiate
    a brainstorming session?
This would be a choice of courage on several fronts.

Or, even more simply,
    when we are faced with a seemingly lose-lose situation,
    how often do we ask ourselves the simple question,
    "How might I use my creativity
        to create a more winning result?"
Look deeply and you may see
    that the choice of creativity is also a choice of courage.

Curiosity

Curiosity is the forerunner of creativity.
Curiosity is the natural birthright of children.
> We never have to teach children to be curious.
It is only when we begin to acquire and resist our fear of discovery
> (when it becomes important to us to avoid looking foolish
>> or to feel like we have it all together)
> that we begin to lose our curiosity.

For example, how many of us,
> when we feel stuck or stopped,
> ask ourselves the questions:
> "What is the benefit of feeling this way?"
> "How might I change my attitude right now?"
> "What resources might I use to get unstuck?"
Just when we need it most,
> our curiosity is the least available to us.
Especially in these types of circumstances,
> the choice of curiosity is a choice of courage.

Context

It could be argued that choosing *context*
> is more powerful and more important
> than choosing courage.
However, to choose a more empowering context
> is almost always a choice of courage.
No matter the cost and the pain incurred,
> the old contexts and interpretations we grew up with,
> the ones that permeate our language and our culture,
> have their own comfort and feeling of rightness.

If my wife expresses jealousy
    because I enjoyed talking with another woman at a party,
    my automatic response might be one of defensiveness,
    created out of the context and interpretation
    that she is attacking me and wants me to feel hurt.
I could switch my context and consider
    that her response is an expression of her deep love for me.
She would not feel jealous if she did not love me.
Choosing this new context would likely involve
    choosing the courage of vulnerability.
If I really embraced this new interpretation,
    then my defensiveness would likely disappear.

My wife and I are getting a divorce
    and my automatic context and interpretation
    is that we have failed in our marriage
    and that somebody and something is to blame.
I could choose a new context,
    a context that holds divorce as something to celebrate,
    as something to learn from,
    as a valuable process in the continuing discovery
    of how to live my life to the fullest.
Choosing this new context, this new interpretation,
    however, is often a major choice of courage.

I have just been fired.
The automatic context and interpretation is
        that I have suffered a major setback
    and anticipate that my life will not be as good as before.
I could choose a new context,
    a context that *everything* in life that happens to me is a gift,
    especially in cases where
    something occurs that seems
    to be the opposite of a gift (like getting fired).

To assume that getting fired is a gift,
 to keep looking for that gift,
 to keep creating that gift,
 is a choice of courage.

Remember the five Cs:

Choose courage, creativity, curiosity, and context.

∽

_____

_____

_____

_____

_____

_____

_____

_____

_____

_____

_____

_____

_____

To live a creative life, we must lose our fear of being wrong.
         —*Joseph Chilton Pearce*
       (author of The Crack In the Cosmic Egg)

Creativity is allowing yourself to make mistakes. Art is knowing which ones to keep.

               —*unknown*

Curiosity is a willing, a proud, an eager confession of ignorance.
      —*S. Leonard Rubinstein (professor of English)*

What are the
"Three Cornerstones of Courage"?

Courage, to be fully exercised and empowered,
    includes three interwoven, yet distinct, expressions.

Resistance to fear is automatic for all of us.
Therefore the first expression of courage
    is choosing to embrace and embody our fear.
    One of the best ways to embrace fear is to
    first, consciously, take several very deep breaths,
        visualizing the fear flowing through you without resistance;
    then, while continuing to breathe very deeply,
        shout, speak, or whisper several times
        (as loudly as the situation allows),
        "Boy, am I scared!"

Many of us exercise courage,
    yet, in omitting this first expression of courage,
    we have adopted the stiff-upper-lip approach to courage.

Without embracing the fear,
    we disempower ourselves by using our resources
    to fight our fear rather than tapping into its energy
    to vitalize our commitments and deepest desires.

Choosing to embrace your fear is the first cornerstone of courage.

The second expression of courage
    is choosing to honor yourself for choosing courage
    before *and* after each act of courage.

This is most easily done (right after you have embraced your fear),
by getting in touch with your "five-year-old" within.
Consider the idea that it's not your adult who is frightened.
It's your five-year-old who is frightened.

After getting in touch with your five-year-old,
(use a picture of yourself from that age, if helpful),
say to h/im,
"I can see and feel that you are frightened."
"It's okay to feel frightened."
"I really appreciate and admire you
for your choice to feel your fear and to take this action
while feeling your fear."

Express this to your child until you can feel
that s/he feels admired and appreciated by you, the adult.

But that's only half of this second expression.
After you have taken the action, *regardless* of the outcome,
get back in touch with your five-year-old child
and again express your appreciation and admiration
for the courage s/he has just finished exercising.

Remember that courage exists *independent* of the outcome.
In becoming so attached to the outcome,
we disempower ourselves and reduce our chance of actually
getting the outcome we desire!

Most of us let our "courage muscles" wither and weaken
by not consistently honoring ourselves
each time that we exercise courage.

Choosing to honor yourself for exercising courage
is the second cornerstone of courage.

The third expression of courage,
>   the one we usually associate with courage,
>   is choosing to act (or not act)
>   in service to our commitments and deepest desires
>   in the face of fear.

Choosing to act in the face of your fear
>   is the third cornerstone of courage.

If you will look for opportunities to choose courage each day,
if you will practice courage daily,
>   including all three of its expressions,
then you will transform your relationship to fear (and to yourself),
>   within a month!

❧

_____

_____

_____

_____

_____

_____

_____

_____

Knowing is not enough; we must apply. Willing is not enough; we must do.

>   —*Johann Wolfgang von Goethe*
>   *(1749-1832, German poet, novelist)*

Courage is being scared to death and saddling up anyway.
>   —*John Wayne (1907-1979, American actor)*

Life shrinks or expands in proportion to one's courage.
>   —*Anaïs Nin (1903-1977,*
>   *French-born American novelist, dancer)*

Choose the courage to think

How many areas of our lives
    have we declared off limits
    for further examination?

How many of us avoid looking at and thinking about
    —the direction of our lives?
    —the day-to-day satisfaction and joy in our lives?
    —where our marriage is and where it's taking us?
    —our full expression of passion and lust?
    —the extent and method of our indebtedness?
    —the corners and boxes
       we have somehow managed to put ourselves into?
    —whether we have the romance we want in our life?
    —where we're likely to end up
       if we continue the way we're headed?
    —our feeling of completeness with our parents?
    —our feeling of completeness and wholeness with our children?
    —our feeling of completeness with all prior relationships?
    —our friendship with all parts of ourselves?

Try out this simple exercise.
Repeat aloud
    the beginning of the following sentence stem,
    adding the first ending that comes to mind.
Don't worry about whether the ending is true or false.
    Just complete the sentence quickly.
Then repeat the sentence stem again,
    spontaneously adding a different ending.
Keep up this process until you've created
    at least 10 endings to the sentence.

Here is the sentence stem:

"One of the things
     I might be avoiding
     to think about or look at is . . ."

Repeat this sentence stem at least 10 times,
     creating a new ending for the sentence each time.

What did you come up with?
What did you discover that you are avoiding thinking about?

Did you realize that you are frightened of your own mind
     and resisting that fear?

In some sense,
     all choices of courage begin with the courage to think
     and ask questions we have not asked before,
     to think outside the boxes and boundaries
     we have retreated into and behind,
     often pulling the blinds behind us
     so that we even hide the evidence
     of our own retreat.

Choose an area that you've avoided thinking about.
Take some deep breaths and say, "Boy, am I scared!"
Honor the five-year-old within
     for the courage s/he is about to choose.
Then start asking some questions
     that will put you in contact with your fear.

Enjoy! Here lies the real opportunity of your life.

"Love, Love, love.
All you need is love." Hogwash!

"Love, Love, love. All you need is love."

This refrain from the old Beatles' song
    is a reflection from a thousand sources.
    From the minister in your church.
    From your mother and father.
    From yourself,
    and so on.
We are continually reaffirming our love
    as if we could create it through our speaking alone.

Love is absolutely great!
But love is what spontaneously arises
    when there is nothing to block it,
    when there is no resisted fear.

Love, as a spontaneous feeling and expression,
    is not something that can be created
    on top of resisted fear with the words,
    "I love you."
Love is not something that can be chosen directly.

The experience of love springs forth
    as the direct result of choosing courage.
When we choose courage, our self-esteem improves.
When we feel good about ourselves,
    it follows naturally that we love others.

When you choose courage to speak up,
    instead of feeling resentment,
    then you create an opening for love.

When you choose courage to ask for a raise,
    instead of complaining to yourself,
    then you feel better
    about yourself, your boss, *and* others around you.

When you choose courage to say "no" to a friend,
    instead of giving in to feelings of obligation,
    then you keep the relationship clean and bright.

When you choose courage to ask a spouse
    about an unspoken problem s/he seems to have,
    instead of leaving it to fester,
    then you provide a space for love to blossom.

When you choose courage to establish and maintain
    good boundaries with others,
    then you create a garden where love can grow.

When you choose courage to consistently pursue
    a life that inspires you,
    then you will automatically feel good will and love
    for the fellow travelers who share the journey with you.

We cannot directly choose love.
    But we can directly choose courage.

When you choose courage,
    the experience of love is one of its by-products.

Choose courage three times today
    and notice that, each time you do so,
    how your experience of love (for yourself and others) grows.

❧

Will you choose the courage not to rescue others?

Often our biggest opportunity to choose courage
    is choosing not to rescue others.

Choosing *not* to rescue or protect others (especially loved ones)
    from the consequences of their actions (or lack of actions)
    or from the realities of life
    is often the most fearful choice of courage we can make.

In the name of love, in the name of caring,
    (or in the name of avoiding guilt),
    we often rescue or protect others
    in a way that prevents them
        from discovering their own power
    and protects them from the opportunity
        to choose their own courage.

To be willing to empathize with their pain and fear,
    to be supportive *without* rescuing,
    is often a supreme choice of courage.

We want so much to relieve the fear and discomfort
    of those we care about
    and thereby relieve ourselves
    of *our* fear for them.
The list is endless.
    Whether it's trying to protect somebody
        from a broken heart
    or trying to protect them
        from the financial realities of earning a living
        (or spending less than their income),
    rescuing is often seen as a caring thing.

Yet, in our caring, how much do we truly disempower
those we care most about?

To say "no" to the ones we care about
is often the supreme choice of courage *and* caring.

Find at least one example in your life
where you are avoiding the opportunity to choose courage
by rescuing or protecting someone you love.

Honor yourself for choosing the courage
to *stop* rescuing h/im.

❧

_____

_____

_____

_____

_____

_____

_____

_____

_____

_____

You can't get rid of poverty by giving people money.
—P.J. O'Rourke (1947-, political satirist)

Love is not love until love's vulnerable.
—Theodore Roethke (1908-1963, American poet)

Love comes when manipulation stops; when you think more about
the other person than about his or her reactions to you. When you
dare to reveal yourself fully. When you dare to be vulnerable.
—Joyce Brothers (1927-, American psychologist,
television and radio personality)

The courage to keep your mouth shut

I have often spoken of the courage
    to express your feelings and thoughts,
    to say "no" when you need to say no,
    and to make requests.

But there is often a different expression of courage,
    an expression that is not as obviously courageous:
        the courage to remain silent,
        the courage to keep our mouth shut,
        the courage to just listen.

Sometimes we talk too much or talk when we shouldn't talk
    because we're trying to control the situation
    or control how others perceive us,
    trying to control that which we have no control over.
    And, in the process, we end up damaging
        whatever influence or results we might have achieved
        had we remained silent.
    When we stop talking and remain silent and embrace our fear,
        this is a choice of courage.

Sometimes we talk
    because we are impatient with listening,
    or have a certain fear of *really* listening
    and thus losing control of the conversation.
    In fact, if we *really* listen,
        we are much more likely to influence
        what we would like to influence.
    When we stop talking and *really* listen, we embrace our fear
        and this is a choice of courage.

Sometimes we talk
in order to ensure that others see us,
that others appreciate us, that others understand us.
However, in doing so,
we often create the opposite result,
preventing others from
seeing us, appreciating us, and understanding us.
When we stop talking and *really* listen we embrace our fear
and this is a choice of courage.

Sometimes we talk
because we *have to* get something off our chest,
to really tell someone how we feel,
or to just be ourselves.
However, in doing so,
we can damage important relationships
and cause unnecessary problems.
Holding your tongue
can be a choice of courage,
especially if you embrace the fear and pain
that you want to get off your chest,
expressing it, instead, in a private, non-destructive way.
(It is *very* important to get it out; just don't do it publicly).
When we hold our tongue and really listen we embrace our fear
and this is a choice of courage.

Think of three recent times where you had an opportunity
to choose courage by remaining silent.
Did you choose courage each time?

What might be the next opportunity
to choose the courage of silence?

Lighten up your life with foolishness

We normally think of foolishness as something to avoid.
But a certain type of foolishness can invigorate us,
    can stretch our courage muscles,
    especially if we embrace the fear
    that we might appear foolish to someone.

In most cases, our dislike of appearing foolish
    is simply a fear that someone might judge us as foolish.

Let me give you an example of an exercise in foolishness:
As I was walking down the street near my apartment,
    I began smiling at people
    and saying "Ni hao" ("hello" in Chinese).
My intention in saying "Ni hao"
    was to give them a feeling
    of a fresh connection to life and people.
Many people smiled and said "Ni hao" back.
But some just blankly looked at me or ignored me altogether,
    as they might a beggar asking for money.
When this happened, I found myself automatically thinking,
    "Oh, I'm looking foolish!"
I then took a deep breath to move the fear through myself,
    and then honored myself
    for choosing the courage to feel the fear of looking foolish.

How might you stretch your courage muscles today
    by taking on some foolishness?

Have some fun with this one!

❧

Are you resisting your fear?

Fear is an automatic mental-emotional response,
    putting the mind and body on alert
    that something is (perceived as) a threat
    to the (perceived) integrity
    of the mind-body-spirit system.

Fear, like every other emotion, has two components:
    bodily sensations and
    automatic thoughts.

For simple, *un-resisted* fear,
    the bodily sensations are normally
    an increased heart rate
    and an added feeling of alertness.
For simple, *un-resisted* fear,
    the automatic thought is typically,
    "How can I address this threat?"

Fear, however, is rarely *un-resisted*.
    We have all been taught, from a very early age,
        to resist our fear, to push it down, to argue it away,
        to make ourselves wrong for having it,
        and to hide it from others, and even from ourselves.
    What we call "fear" is *not* simply fear;
        it is almost always *resisted* fear.

For resisted fear,
    the bodily sensations may include any of the following:
    tightness in the chest, stomach, or other parts of the body,
    dry mouth and/or tight throat,
    sweaty palms,
    cold feet or coldness in other parts of the body,
    a feeling of weakness in the limbs and body,

drowsiness or dizziness,
headache,
quivering,
a shaking body or chattering teeth,
and so on.

For resisted fear
the automatic thoughts may include the following:
"I can't do this."
"This is too much."
"What will happen if I fail?"
"I don't deserve to be treated this way."
"I don't deserve to get a raise anyway."
"She'll think I'm a fool for asking her out."
"What will people think?"
"It's not going to work anyway."
"This is not the right way to do things."
"Why can't life be easier?"
"What does it matter?"
"Why can't s/he just know what is right?"
"Things can't really be any different."
"I don't want to look at this."
"It just doesn't feel comfortable to me."
"I don't think I'm ready yet."
"I'll do it some other time."
"I just feel like giving up."
"I'm confused."
"I don't know which way to go,"
and so on *ad infinitum.*

Fear will be your friend if you will treat it as such.

Identify some resisted fear right now
(check out the symptoms above).

Take several deep breaths,

breathing into the energy of that fear,
saying as loudly as you can or are willing to,
"Boy, am I scared!"

Notice the difference this makes
in your feeling of resourcefulness
and in your experience of the fear,
as it changes from resisted fear into fear you can work with.

൙

_____
_____
_____
_____
_____
_____
_____
_____
_____
_____
_____

We gain strength, and courage, and confidence by each experience
in which we really stop to look fear in the face . . . we must do that
which we think we cannot.
—*Eleanor Roosevelt (1884-1962,*
American author and former first lady)

Courage is doing what you're afraid to do. There can be no courage
unless you're scared.
—*Eddie Richenbacker (1890-1973,*
World War I aerial hero)

Taking a new step, uttering a new word is what people fear most.
—*Fyodor Dostoyevsky (1821-1881,*
Russian novelist, journalist, short-story writer)

Every fear is an opportunity to choose courage

Do you make it a daily practice
> to seek out new opportunities to choose courage?

Are you consistently asking yourself,
> "What might be the opportunity
> > for choosing courage right now?"

If we intend to make friends with our fear,
> so that its energy becomes our ally rather than our enemy,
> we will need to, step by step,
> train ourselves to see and experience fear
> as an opportunity to choose courage.

Fear is *always* an opportunity for courage.

And, within that opportunity are three sub-opportunities:
> (1) the opportunity to embrace
> > and "breathe into" the energy of the fear,
> (2) the opportunity to express appreciation
> > to yourself and to your five-year-old within,
> > for embracing the fear *and* for taking the action,
> > regardless of the outcome,
> (3) the opportunity to take action.
> > (In some circumstances, there is no new action to take;
> > the courage consists simply of embracing the fear
> > and honoring yourself for doing that.)

Sometimes resisted fear presents itself as partially visible,
> as in the expressions of:
> > anxiety, worry, shyness, embarrassment,
> > jealousy, and/or feeling foolish.

But more often, resisted fear hides behind a heavy cloak,
    as in the expressions of:
        resentment, complaining, blaming others,
        guilt and blaming ourselves,
        thinking that something is wrong,
        trying to make the right decision,
        trying to do it the right way, working hard,
        stress and tension, perfectionism, depression,
        cynicism, hatred, laziness, low self-esteem,
        feeling overwhelmed, indecisiveness, procrastination,
        shame, feeling betrayed, over-controlling, lying,
        boredom, crankiness, resignation, impatience,
        defensiveness, over-protectiveness, obsessiveness,
        stubbornness, inflexibility, self-consciousness,
        animosity, ingratitude, arrogance, showing disrespect,
        envy, petulance, righteousness, hostility, rebelliousness,
        rudeness, whining, and/or always keeping busy.

Take a few moments to ask yourself
    how each of these expressions involves a resistance to fear.

There are so many opportunities for courage!
There are so many opportunities for self-discovery!

Identify at least three opportunities for courage each day.

And then use them!

                            ஐ

_____

_____

_____

_____

_____

_____

_____

Is your fear really fear?

Fear has long been portrayed as the enemy, as the spoiler.

From a very early age, we have been taught
>to hide it, to avoid it,
>to deny it, to resist it,
>to make it wrong, and to make ourselves wrong for having it.

Even people who typically regard themselves as enlightened
>see fear as something to be belittled, resisted, or argued away
>(For example, some New Age people characterize fear as
>"false experiences appearing real.")

Fundamentally, fear is just energy,
>energy that can be used to serve our desires and commitments.

When animals are frightened,
>they are in their *most* resourceful state.
>They can fight or flee very effectively.

When humans are frightened, however,
>we are often in our *least* resourceful state.

Why?

Because it is not simple fear we are feeling.
>It is fear that we are resisting.
>It is the "resisting" part that makes us unresourceful,
>>not the fear itself.

We treat fear as an enemy.

And as long as we treat it as an enemy,
    as long as we resist it,
    as long as we deny it and hide it,
    as long as we make ourselves wrong for having it,
    as long as we avoid it,
        it *will be* our enemy.
        It becomes *us* against *ourselves.*

However, if we embrace our fear,
    if we breathe into it, if we tap into its energy,
    allowing it to flow through us, our fear *can be* our friend.

We can use the energy of the fear
    to serve our desires and commitments.

You may have heard the phrase: "What you resist, persists."

This is especially true of fear.
    When we resist our fear,
    our fear resists us as well
    and all our energy gets tied up in an internal knot,
    making us feel weak and ineffective.

What we normally call fear is *not* fear; it is resisted fear.
The knot in your stomach is not fear; it is resisted fear.
The tension in your body is not fear; it is resisted fear.
Your sweaty palms are not fear; they are resisted fear.
Your headache is not fear; it is resisted fear.
Your thought "I can't do this" is not fear; it is resisted fear.

When we embrace our fear,
    when we breathe deeply into its energies,
    then it doesn't feel much like fear anymore.

As I said, what we call fear is, most often, resisted fear.

Once we embrace our fear,
    then it feels much more like energy,
    energy we can use and work with.

Experiment with breathing into your fear
    at least three times today.

❧

_____

_____

_____

_____

_____

_____

_____

_____

_____

_____

_____

_____

We spend our time searching for security and hate it when we get it.

>—*John Steinbeck (1902-1968,*
American novelist)

Fear is the main source of superstition, and one of the main sources of cruelty. To conquer fear is the beginning of wisdom.

>—*Bertrand Russell (1872-1970,*
British philosopher, mathematician and social critic)

The thing I fear most is fear.

>—*Michel Eyquem De Montaigne (1533-1592,*
French philosopher, essayist)

Do you know the five types of fear?

Fear is not just fear.

There are five basic types of fear; these can be distinguished
    only through curiosity and discernment.

There are:
    validated fears,
    paper-tiger fears,
    red-herring fears,
    non-specific fears,
    and hidden fears.
Most often, a particular fear will be a combination
    of two or more of these five types of fear.

With every fear, whether validated (see below) or not,
    we must learn to embrace and breathe into that fear,
    allowing ourselves to use and align with its vital energies.
With every fear, whether valid or not,
    we must honor ourselves for the courage,
    not only to embrace and feel that fear,
    but also for taking appropriate action, if any is necessary.

Validated fears
Most of us, most of the time,
    act as if *all* our fears are validated fears.
However, most of our fears
    have little, if any, basis in fact.
Here are some examples of validated fears:

"If I drive drunk,
    I am much more likely to have an accident."
"If I continue to smoke,
    there is a good chance I will significantly degrade
    the quality of my 'golden years'
    and die several years younger than otherwise."
"If I continue to scream at my employee,
    she is likely to quit."

Paper-tiger fears
A paper-tiger fear is a fear that disappears
    when the fear is examined up close
    and/or when the fear is confronted and found to be illusory.
Here are some likely examples of paper-tiger fears:
    "If I ask her out on a date,
        she'll think I'm foolish and tell everybody else."
    "If I ask for a raise at work,
        my boss will dislike me."
    "If I take a trip when the stars aren't right,
        something bad will happen."
    "If I say 'no' to my friends,
        they won't be my friends anymore."

Red-herring fears
A red-herring fear is a specific fear
    that draws our attention away from the main fear.
    The main fear is usually a fear of disapproval
    or a fear of not looking good.
Here are some likely examples of red-herring fears:
"I'm frightened that I won't be able to do a good job."
    (Meaning: "I'm frightened that they will disapprove
    of my performance.")

"I'm frightened that I don't have credentials."
(Meaning: "I frightened that they will think less of me
because I don't have credentials.")
"I'm frightened I won't say the right thing
if I stand up and share my thoughts with the class."
(Meaning: "I'm frightened that they will think
I am stupid and/or foolish.")

Non-specific fears
A non-specific fear is a feeling of fear or general anxiety
that seems unrelated to any specific event or condition.

Hidden Fears
Most fears are hidden fears.
Since almost all of our fears are resisted fears,
they end up going underground,
causing major damage to the quality of our lives.
Here are some examples of hidden fears:
"I don't feel comfortable taking on this project."
(Hidden fear: "I'm frightened I won't succeed
and will then be criticized by others.")
"I resent her for talking so much."
(Hidden fear: "I am frightened to speak up
in a way that might change the situation.")
"I feel guilty that I forgot your birthday."
(Hidden fear: "I'm frightened that you will blame me
for forgetting your birthday if I don't beat myself up first.")

Many common feelings and behaviors
can be full or partial expressions of resisted and hidden fears.

It is often an interesting and productive challenge
to search for the hidden fears
inside these feelings and behaviors.

See if you can find the hidden fears inside
    abusiveness, anger, arrogance, bitterness, blame, boredom,
    crankiness, cynicism, defensiveness, depression, envy, guilt,
    hate, hope/hopelessness, hostility, impatience, indecisiveness,
    inflexibility, ingratitude, insensitivity, intolerance, jealousy,
    lack of self-confidence, laziness, low self-esteem, malevolence,
    obsessiveness, perfectionism, petulance, procrastination, racism,
    rebellion, resentfulness, resignation, righteousness, rudeness,
    self-consciousness, self-suppression, shame, stubbornness,
    submissiveness.

Look also for the fears hidden within
    complaining, controlling, being critical, being busy,
    dominating others, lying, nagging, trying, whining,
    showing disrespect, feeling betrayed, dispirited, foolish,
    overwhelmed, uncomfortable, feeling like a victim.

Get curious about your fears.

Whenever you experience a fear
    or whenever you experience what might be a hidden fear,
    breathe into the energy of the fear,
    honoring yourself for the courage
    to examine it and feel it fully.

Your fears can be fascinating
    if you begin to make friends with them
    with the intention of understanding them more fully.

                          ॐ

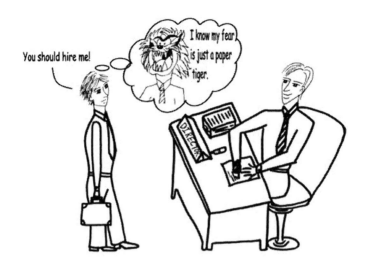

Is your fear a paper tiger?

Occasionally, we choose courage
    in the face of a possible/probable cost.

For example,
    if you make a significant investment
    in an entrepreneurial project,
    then your choice of courage
    will probably include the valid fear
    that you may lose
    part—or all—of your investment.
If you choose to have open heart surgery,
    then your choice of courage
    will probably include the valid fear
    that you will not only need to endure a lot of pain,
    but also risk the worsening of your condition
    and even death.

If, in service to your highest commitments,
    you choose a major at the university
    against your parents' wishes,
    then you may face a valid fear
    of their disapproval and criticism,
    as well as the loss of their financial support.

These are examples
    in which choosing courage
    embraces a fear of likely costs
    associated with the choice of courage.

Most opportunities for courage, however,
    if executed with some planning and sensitivity,
    include little, if any, likelihood of cost,
    regardless of whether or not
    the desired outcome is achieved.

For example,
    if you choose courage
    to ask a man or woman for a date,
    then you will most likely be no worse off
    if s/he declines than you were before you asked.
If you choose courage
    to start a conversation with the person beside you
    in the line at the bank or supermarket,
    then you will most likely be no worse off
    if s/he ignores you
    than you were before you opened your mouth.
If you choose courage
    in calling a prospective client to make h/im an offer,
    then you will most likely be no worse off
    if s/he says "no"
    than you were before you picked up the telephone.

If you choose courage
> in gently but clearly letting a friend know
> that you felt hurt by h/is showing up late,
> then, even if the friend doesn't change h/is behavior,
> you will most likely be no worse off
> than if you had kept your mouth shut.

If you choose courage
> in expressing a commitment to your friendship with another
> by saying "no" and *not* lending h/im money,
> then you will most likely be no worse off
> than if you had lent h/im the money
> (incurring the unnecessary risk
> of damaging your relationship with h/im).

If you choose courage
> to express your desires openly and without demand
> in making a request of a friend,
> then, even if s/he should say "no,"
> you will most likely be no worse off
> than if you had not made the request.

If you choose courage
> in vulnerably expressing to another how you feel about h/im,
> then, even if s/he is not responsive to your expression,
> you will most likely be no worse off
> than if you kept your feelings to yourself.

In the last seven examples,
> the *real* cost,
> the *real* danger,
> the *real* risk
> is that you will *not* choose courage.

The *actual* risk is exactly the *opposite*
> of what you *feel* is the risk.

Identify an opportunity for courage
    that's available to you now, where
    the *real* cost,
    the *real* danger,
    the *real* risk
    is in *not* choosing courage.

Are you willing to choose that courage now?

∿

_____

_____

_____

_____

_____

_____

_____

_____

_____

_____

Fear is met and destroyed with courage.
> —*James F. Bell (1923-1999, American educator)*

There is no terror in the bang, only in the anticipation of it.
> —*Alfred Hitchcock (1899-1980, British film maker)*

Existential Courage
Consider that there's a certain type of fear, where you know that once you've chosen to face that fear, you'll see that, all along, there was nothing to fear. Prior to choosing, however, that knowledge makes little difference. It's still frightening to make that choice. To choose to step through this fear into the serenity that's waiting for you on the other side is an existential act of courage.
> —*GoldWinde*

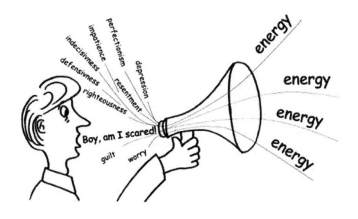

Turn your fear into your friend

Fear will never stop you.
It is your *resistance* to fear that stops you.
Most of what we call "fear" is resisted fear.

Fear doesn't have very good PR, does it?
    Both you and I have been taught from a very early age
    to resist our fear, to push it down,
    to hide it from others, and even from ourselves.

We treat fear as an enemy.
    And when we treat fear as our enemy, it will be our enemy.
    When we resist our fear, then our fear resists us.
    All of our energy, all of our resourcefulness
        gets tied up in an internal knot.

Battling your fear becomes a war of you against yourself!
Place the palms
    of your two hands together right now,
    pressing them against each other as hard as you can.
    This is what you do with your fear.
    You have no energy, no resourcefulness
        left over after fighting with yourself.

When we treat fear as a friend, however,
    then fear becomes our friend.

Fear is just energy.
Animals, who have no capacity to resist their fear,
    are generally very resourceful when they are frightened.
They can fight or flee very effectively.

Humans, on the other hand,
    have the ability to resist their own internal processing.

When you embrace your fear,
    when you take deep breaths
    and say to yourself,
    "Boy, am I scared!" many times,
    then you can tap into the energy of your fear,
    opening up the possibility of using its energy
    to serve your vitality, and to serve your commitments.

The first step in acknowledging your fear
    is to distinguish your fear from your resistance to your fear.

For example,
    if you notice that you are worrying,
    then you are definitely resisting your fear.
Worry is an attempt to do away with fear.
Worry is a resistance to fear.
In most cases, stress is a resistance to fear.

It is a choice of courage to find the fear
 that you are resisting inside your stress.

Although it is beyond the scope of this essay
 to explain why all of the following
 are often, either fully or partially,
 the symptomatic results of resisted fear,
 I suggest that you experiment with the idea that they are.

  feeling betrayed, depression, cynicism, guilt, resentment,
  hatred, laziness, low self-esteem, lack of self-confidence,
  feeling overwhelmed, indecisiveness, procrastination,
  worry, anxiety, shame, bitterness, blaming others, stress,
  over-controlling, lying, lack of self-expression, boredom,
  complaining, crankiness, resignation, feeling dispirited,
  impatience, defensiveness, over-protectiveness,
  ingratitude, perfectionism, obsessiveness, petulance,
  stubbornness, inflexibility, self-consciousness, righteousness,
  animosity, callousness, criticism of others, self-criticism,
  arrogance, feeling foolish, nagging, bitchiness, rebelliousness,
  showing disrespect, rudeness, jealousy, envy

Once you've identified a suspected symptom of resisted fear,
 regardless of whether or not
 you can feel it as fear, the second step is
 to breathe deeply and relax into the fear,
 speaking/shouting as loudly as possible
 (given the immediate environment),
 "Boy, am I scared!"

 By doing this, you will begin to align with your energy
  (so that you can use it),
  rather than continuing to resist the energy of your fear.
 Notice how, in doing this,
  the symptoms (worry, guilt, resentment, etc.)
  lessen or disappear!

I invite you to find at least five occasions today
where you are resisting your fear.

Then breathe!

❧

_____
_____
_____
_____
_____
_____
_____
_____
_____
_____
_____
_____
_____
_____
_____
_____
_____
_____
_____
_____

Confront your fears, list them, get to know them, and only then
will you be able to put them aside and move ahead.
—Jerry Gillies (American author, speaker)

Feel the fear and do it anyway.
—Susan Jeffers (American author, speaker)

People always make the wolf more formidable than he is.
—French proverb

How frightened are you of their fear?

"I cannot ask him for a date;
    what if he doesn't know how to say 'no'?"
"I cannot ask her for a favor;
    she might not choose the courage to respond honestly."
"I cannot say 'no' to my friend's request;
    it would hurt his ego too much."
"I cannot tell my parents that I don't want to live with them;
    it would make them upset with me."
"I cannot move to another country;
    it would make my family and friends worry about me."
"I cannot refuse my 23-year-old's request for money;
    it would be too difficult for him without a car."
"I cannot quit the job I am unhappy with and get one that I love;
    it would frighten my wife too much."

Often, our own desire to feel safe and comfortable
    is disguised by our desire for others to feel safe and comfortable.

We have little tolerance for their fear.
Their resisted fear stimulates us to resist our fear.
At the core of the problem, however,
    is the resistance to our *own* fear.

Often, our willingness to choose courage seems stronger
    if no one else is frightened in the process.
For us to choose the courage that allows others
    the opportunity to choose courage
    often includes letting go of
    our largest and most foreboding fear:
    the fear of another's fear.

Perhaps the most effective and loving way
    to support those we care about
    is to create opportunities,
    through the expression of our own
    deepest desires and commitments
    (through our requests and refusals),
    for them to choose courage in their own lives.

Are we willing to support our children and/or parents
    in the development of their growth, creativity, and character
    by providing them with the opportunities to choose courage,
    while at the same time giving them examples
    of our own expression of courage with them?

Are we willing to support our boss, colleagues, or employees
    in a fuller expression of their lives
    by providing them with the opportunities to choose courage
    through our own "unreasonable" requests and refusals
    (which are our own choices of courage)?

Are we willing to challenge our friends
    to embrace the fear in their lives
    through our own expression of courage
    when we're with them?

I've had more than one friend who has told me,
    "I feel safer with you than
        I've ever felt with any other person in my life."
        (By this she meant that she felt
        safer from feeling judged or criticized
        for anything she might say or do).

Moreover, in the same breath, she said,
"You scare me more than any other person in my life."
(By this she meant that I presented her
with significant opportunities to choose courage,
because of my own requests and refusals.)

How might you be hiding from challenges in your own life
under the guise of protecting others?
In doing so, what opportunities
for choosing courage and creativity
might you have stolen from them?

Select and act upon one choice of courage today and every day
that may present another
with the opportunity to choose courage.

❧

_____

_____

_____

_____

_____

_____

_____

_____

_____

_____

_____

_____

_____

The Last Hurdle
The last hurdle in transformation is letting go of being a victim of
other people's being a victim.

—GoldWinde

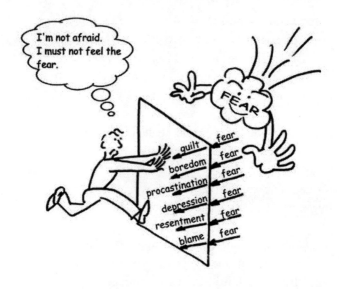

How deeply is your fear buried?

I was once working with a client
    who brought up an interesting issue.

My client John said to me,
    "Dwight, I would like a little extra money.
    I have this opportunity to sell a product.
    It's a good product.
    I know enough about the product,
    I know enough about myself,
    I know enough about the prospects
        on the list of names I have to call to know that
        if I would just get on the phone and make the calls,
        I would earn about $300 per hour."

"But I'm having trouble getting myself
to sit down and make these calls
and I don't know why!
I *know* that I am *not* afraid."

If any of you ever met John,
you would probably agree with him that he was not afraid.
John is one of the most charismatic, outwardly self-confident men
I have ever met.
In fact, his job takes him all over the world,
leading workshops for high-level managers and executives.

I asked John this question,
"Imagine, John, that somehow you were able to *guarantee*
that *every* person you telephoned
would respond to you by saying,
'John, I am so glad you called to tell me about this product!
How soon can it be delivered?'"
"If somehow we were able to guarantee this,
would you have any reluctance to sitting down, right now,
and making those calls?"

John laughed and said,
"No, I would not!"

It was only then that he could see that he *was* frightened,
frightened of rejection, frightened of what people might think,
frightened of . . .

Once he could see that it was only fear,
then he could see that he had a clear choice:
he could choose courage
(and the probability of getting the results that he wanted)
or he could choose to feel safe and comfortable in the moment.

John chose courage and got the results.

Most of the resisted fear we have
    is hidden away inside of us where we cannot feel it.

As a rule of thumb,
    every time you feel stopped in some way,
    then you are resisting (and hiding from)
    your fear (even if you can't feel it).

As a rule of thumb,
    guilt and self-blame are resisted fear,
    resentment is resisted fear, depression is resisted fear,
    resignation is resisted fear, hostility is resisted fear,
    righteousness is resisted fear, lethargy/laziness is resisted fear,
    hatred is resisted fear, overwhelm is resisted fear,
    stress is resisted fear, procrastination is resisted fear,
    perfectionism is resisted fear, blaming others is resisted fear,
    defensiveness is resisted fear, discouragement is resisted fear,
    nagging is resisted fear, worry is resisted fear, and so on.

The next time you feel any of these,
    the next time you feel stopped in any way
        (even if you can't feel the fear),
    take five very deep breaths,
    and then, as you continue with the deep breathing,
    say to yourself (out loud, if possible),
    "Boy, am I scared!"
Repeat "Boy, am I scared!" at least five times,
    continuing with the deep breathing
    and allowing the fear to flow through you
    so that you begin to align with the energy of your fear
    instead of resisting it.

After doing this,
> take a moment to get back in touch
> with the original feeling (e.g., guilt)
> and notice the difference.

You may be quite surprised.

ॐ

_____

_____

_____

_____

_____

_____

_____

_____

_____

_____

Everything in Nature contains all the powers of Nature. Everything is made of hidden stuff.

> —*Ralph Waldo Emerson (1802-1882,*
> *American poet, essayist)*

The diversity of the phenomena of nature is so great, and the treasures hidden in the heavens so rich, precisely in order that the human mind shall never be lacking in fresh nourishment.

> —*Johannes Keppler (1571-1601,*
> *German astronomer)*

Each problem has hidden in it an opportunity so powerful that it literally dwarfs the problem. The greatest success stories were created by people who recognized a problem and turned it into an opportunity.

> —*Joseph Sugarman (American businessman)*

Choose courage
not to use the word "coward"

Using the word "coward" (or "cowardice" or "wimp")
    to characterize either yourself or another
    involves a resistance to fear
    and misses an opportunity for choosing courage.

Let me explain.
The *American Heritage Dictionary* defines cowardice as
    "ignoble fear in the face of danger or pain."

Both from our everyday feeling
    about the words "coward" and "cowardice"
    and from the above definition,
    we know that whoever we might call a coward
    (either ourselves or another)
    is engaging in a blameworthy and dishonorable action.

To act cowardly then is, in some measure,
    to engage in a wrong, bad, immoral,
    sinful, evil, or unprincipled act.

Yet, if we strip away the judgmental connotations
    of the word "coward,"
    what is left of the denotative meaning?
    "Cowardice" then is only the choice to feel safe
        (not necessarily *be* safe) in the moment
        at the expense of not going for what we really want
        and/or are committed to.

When we use the word "coward" (or wimp), however,
    we are not interested in communicating
    this simple denotative meaning.

What we are interested in is expressing
  our make-wrong, blaming attitude toward
  a particular human (whether ourselves or another).
As such, *our action of placing blame* by using the word "coward"
  is in *itself* a resistance to fear
  (fear of acknowledging and embracing our own or another's
    desire to feel safe and comfortable in the moment;
    fear of what will happen if we don't try to change the
    "coward's" behavior by blaming h/im)
  and misses an important opportunity for choosing courage.

As such, coward is a toxic word
  and, for the most part, it's useful to avoid using it.

I have coined a new term called "coverage."
  Coverage is the antonym of courage.
  Coverage is the choice to *feel* safe and comfortable
    (not necessarily to *be* safe) in the moment
    at the expense of not going for what
    we really want and/or are committed to.
  There is nothing wrong with choosing coverage.
  We will accrue certain costs and benefits
    from choosing coverage.
  We will accrue different costs and benefits
    from choosing courage.
  Most often coverage provides the benefit
    of *feeling* safe and comfortable in the moment
    at the expense of longer-range safety and results.

Explore the opportunities for choosing courage.

&

Do you complain about the complainers?

Do you hate it when others complain and whine?
Do you complain about those who complain about you?
Are you the long-suffering good guy
    in your relationship with others?
Are you negative about other people's negativity?
Do you complain about yourself
    when you find yourself complaining?

If so, then you are a victim of the victims.

Being a victim is the most sought-after position on earth
    (although almost no one would see it that way)!
In any transaction that involves discomfort, fear, or pain,
    we yearn to be the good guy,
        and find someone else (occasionally, a part of ourselves)
    to be the bad guy.
Many of us,
    recognizing that something is amiss in being a victim,
    have made being a victim wrong,
    thereby perpetuating our entrapment inside the victim box!
    We have become sophisticated victims,
        limiting our indulgence as victims
        to our complaint about others
        who are more obviously gluttonous
        in their status as victims.

Show me righteousness and I will show you victimhood.
Show me a good guy and I will show you victimhood.
Show me resentment and I will show you victimhood.
Show me rebelliousness and I will show you victimhood.
Show me guilt and I will show you victimhood.

Show me blame and I will show you victimhood.
Show me a feeling of betrayal and I will show you victimhood.
Show me complaining and I will show you victimhood.
Show me resignation and I will show you victimhood.
Show me nagging and I will show you victimhood.

Choosing courage is always the antidote to victimhood.

What actions are you not taking?
What requests are you not making?
How are you trying to control that which cannot be controlled?
What boundaries are you not setting and maintaining?
What stands for yourself have you not made?

❧

_____
_____
_____
_____
_____
_____
_____
_____

People are always blaming their circumstances for what they are.
The people who get on in this world are they who get up and look
for the circumstances they want, and, if they can't find them, make
them.

—*George Bernard Shaw (1856-1950,*
Irish dramatist, literary critic)

Accept fate, and move on. Don't yield to the seductive pull of self-
pity. Acting like a victim threatens your future.

—*unknown*

You will always be afraid

Most of us are hoping for the day
    when we won't be afraid anymore.
Most of us imagine that there are some people
    who have attained a fearlessness.
Living without fear has even become a Holy Grail,
    immortalized by Nike's "No Fear" slogan.

Having had the privilege of working (as a life coach)
    with thousands of people on a very intimate level,
    I can tell you unequivocally
    that *everyone is frightened.*
And almost everyone *resists* their fear,
    arguing against it, pushing it down,
    denying it, camouflaging it,
    contracting against it, hiding it from others,
    if not from themselves.
The number one thing we don't want others to know about us
    is how frightened we are,
    especially how frightened we are
    of how we will appear to them.
As a result, many of us become masters at appearing fearless,
    at least to others,
    and, sometimes, even to ourselves.

Certainly, as you consistently choose courage
    for one action in your life,
    the fear will, step by step, disappear
    for that action.

In the Chinese movie *Crouching Tiger, Hidden Dragon*
    I found it interesting that the main male and female characters
    were fearless in the domain of physical danger
        (perhaps foolishly so),
    but timidly resisted their fear
    when it came to expressing their love for each other.

To the extent that you accept and embrace
    the three following ideas,
    the freer and more powerful you will be.

First, there will always be a new level of fear
    that will confront you or that you may choose to confront.
    There will always be opportunities for courage.
Second, there is no "should" involved in
    choosing courage in the face of fear.
    It is simply a choice.
        Choosing courage
            takes you along one path.
        Choosing to feel safe and comfortable in the moment
            takes you along another path.
        There is no right or wrong
            about choosing courage.
        There is no right or wrong
            about choosing to feel safer in the moment.
    Choose: each path has its costs and benefits.
And third, the good news is
    that, fundamentally, fear is only energy,
    energy that you can use
    once you breathe into it and embrace it.
    As you begin to treat fear as your friend,
        it *will* be your friend.

The only reason you have experienced fear
    (or more accurately, resisted fear)
    as your foe,
    is that you have been treating it as your foe
        (by resisting it).

Will you let go of your resistance
    to the fear that fear will always be with you
    (or just around the corner)?
Will you honor yourself when you choose courage
    and will you have compassion for yourself
        when you choose to feel safer
        and more comfortable in the moment?
Will you start playing with your resisted fear,
    breathing into it and experimenting with treating it
    as your friend instead of your foe?

**For more essay(s) on different ways to look at courage,
see www.GoldWinde.com/Cbook/More/Cdistinction.**

It all changed when I realized I'm not the only one on the planet who's scared. Everyone else is, too. I started asking people, "Are you scared, too?" "You bet your sweet life I am." "Aha, so that's the way it is for you, too." We were all in the same boat. That's probably what is so effective at our workshops. When I ask, "Who else feels like this?" the whole room of hands goes up. People realize they are not the only one who feels that way.

                                    —*Stan Dale*

The only thing we have to fear is the lack of fear itself.

                           —*Lawrence Summers*
        (former deputy secretary of the United States Treasury)

How to make friends with your fear and pain

When we are very small children we urinate and defecate whenever and wherever the urge arises. Early on, however, we learn to control these basic urges and limit their expression to a private place (the toilet room). And, for the most part, this limitation does not seriously hamper our elimination or our health.

Can you imagine, however, what would happen if we were somehow "suppressed" in urinating and defecating under *any* circumstances, private or not? What if we were given the messages that something was wrong with us if we had to "express ourselves" in this way? What if we were given the messages that others would not like us, would not love us, would not respect us if we didn't somehow "keep it in," or, at worst, keep it as a dirty secret that we needed to express ourselves in this way?

Of course, it is obvious that "keeping it in" would be impossible. "It" will come out one way or another. But, given our desire to be liked, loved, and respected, we would go to great lengths to pretend that we don't need to pee or "take a dump."

Can you imagine a society in which there were no public or private toilets, no acceptable and official place to take a dump (shades of the movie *Pleasantville!*)—and somehow we had to pretend that we didn't need to "do that"? Can you begin to imagine all the obscure, circuitous, and damaging effects that this would have on each and every moment of our lives?

I submit that, in large measure, regarding our mental/emotional/spiritual life, we essentially do what we would never think of doing regarding the natural process of defecation: we suppress and hold in what we need to express and let out.

Young children typically express any and all feelings immediately in sound, with nothing held back. This applies equally to feelings of joy, excitement, anger, fear, and pain. Yet, slowly but surely, children accept the thousands of subtle and not-so-subtle messages that say, "If you want to be liked, loved, and respected, you will not express certain feelings so spontaneously, especially those of fear, anger, and pain." *And,* we are *not* provided with any method or approach to express these feelings privately where they will not cause damage to others or to how others see us.

It could be argued that the defining difference between a child and an adult is that an adult has learned to censor the expression of thoughts and feelings. This learning process typically starts around the age of four and is usually well established by the age of eight. I am not going to suggest that we go back to being "uncensored children," even if it were possible. But just because we learn to censor and edit what gets verbally expressed doesn't mean that we still don't have the need (in order to remain happy and joyous) for the regular self-expression that a young child spontaneously exudes. When it comes to taking a dump, we acknowledge and recognize that physical need and we provide the ongoing acceptance and encouragement for handling it. However, in the arena of "taking a dump" with our emotions, for the most part, we have not acknowledged that this need continues throughout adulthood.

As a result, to a lesser or greater degree, emotional constipation is a chronic condition afflicting almost every human being above the age of five. And, for the most part, since it is a condition that everyone shares, no one recognizes it as an aberration.

The four processes in this section are designed to assist in the execution of the first cornerstone of choosing courage, embracing the energy of one's fear (and pain) and making friends with that fear.

The first process, **Making friends with your fear and pain,** can be used in any and all situations to quickly eliminate the resistance to your fear and tap into its vital energies for your own use. Look for opportunities to use this process many times every day.

The second process, **EnChanting™,** takes a deeper cut at de-repressing and expressing pent-up feelings. Unlike the first process, it generally should be done when no one else is around. If you want to really keep the feelings well expressed, do this at least 30 minutes a day (you can probably find a way to do it concurrently with some other task such as driving).

The third process, **Create quickly a "deep awakening renewal,"** is the most powerful of all these processes. Thirty minutes alone with this process will transform any mood, attitude, or feeling. This is another process that requires privacy. Take on this process at least once a week to create a deep feeling of energized serenity in your life.

The fourth process, **Create a "whine list" for whining,** is the only process that is not done alone. It has its own unique power in helping you move through feelings of depression, resignation, anger, etc. This process should be done anytime you feel stuck. Choose the courage to call someone on your "whine list" and then really whine!

Although the space allotted to the description of these processes is a relatively small percentage of this total book, perhaps 50% of the power of this book is encapsulated within these pages.

❧

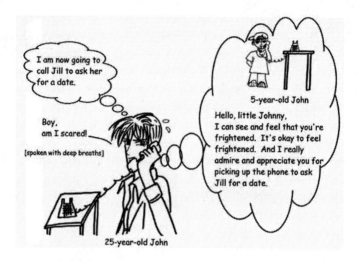

Making friends with your fear and pain

Fundamentally, fear is just energy,
    energy we can use
    to serve our desires and commitments.

When animals are frightened,
    they are usually in their most resourceful state;
    they can fight or flee very effectively.

When humans are frightened, however,
    we are often in our least resourceful state.

Why?

Because, unlike animals, we are able
    to resist our fear, to push it down.
    We are able to do this through the mechanism of language,
        which animals don't have.
Fear doesn't have good PR, does it?
    You and I have been taught from a very early age,
        both implicitly and explicitly,
      to not be frightened,
      to hide our fear from others, and even from ourselves.
We treat fear like an enemy.
    And when we treat fear like an enemy,
    it becomes our enemy.
    When we resist our fear, our fear resists us
      and all our energy, all our resourcefulness
      gets tied up in an internal knot.
However, when we treat fear as a friend,
    when we breathe into its energy,
    when we tap into its vitality,
    then it becomes our friend,
    giving us the fuel and excitement
    to live our life and fulfill our commitments.

But how do we become friends with our fear—
    especially since we have treated it as our enemy for so long?

Here is a simple process you can use anytime and anywhere
    to make friends with your fear.
    This process is the first of three legs of choosing courage.
Because our resistance to our fear has become automatic,
    we have to become proactive
    in order to make friends with our fear
    and tap into its energy.

Here are the steps to this process.

(1) Be present to your fear.

Mentally create those circumstances
    that you associate with your fear.
    Visualize the details of the circumstances.
    Hear the sounds.
    Be present to your bodily sensations and feelings.
Notice the bodily sensations associated with your fear.
    Describe these sensations (out loud if possible)
        either to yourself or to another.
    Is there tightness in your shoulders or back?
    Is there a knot in your stomach?
    Is your stomach queasy?
    Do you feel weakness in your legs?
    Do you experience your body as small and powerless?
    Are your hands cold or clammy?
    Do you have a headache?
    Do you feel sleepy or numb?
    Is your breathing shallow?
    Describe specifically to yourself the sensations in your body
        that you associate with your fear.
Now notice the automatic thoughts associated with your fear.
    Describe these thoughts to yourself or another.
    Listen to the automatic thoughts
        that you associate with your fear.
    Here are some possibilities:
    "There's no reason to be frightened."
    "Why am I worrying?"
    "They are just going to say 'no'."
    "What will I think of myself if I mess this one up?"
    "What will I feel if it doesn't go right?"
    "What if I make a fool of myself?"

"I don't think I can do this."

"Who am I to think that things could be different?"

(2) Embrace the fear in your mind.

Visualize a mountain brook with the water bouncing
　　from rock to rock and flowing energetically downstream.
　　Begin to see and feel your fear as this flowing water,
　　　　allowing the fear to flow through you,
　　　　　　to pass through you, without resistance.
　　See and feel the energy and power of your fear
　　　　flowing through you without resistance.
Begin to know that you are bigger than your fear.
　　Know that fear is your friend.
　　Now you can begin to experience the fear,
　　　　knowing that it is no threat to you.
　　You only resist those things that you think
　　　　are larger than you are.
　　When you have truly learned that you are bigger than your fear,
　　　　bigger than your circumstances,
　　　　　　then there's no longer a need for resistance.
　　When you have learned that your fear is your friend,
　　　　you will begin to embrace your fear,
　　　　　　loving, using, and blessing its energy.
　　You will allow your fear to be present,
　　　　to pass easily and naturally through you, without resistance,
　　　　and you will be able to tap into its energy and vitality.

(3) Embrace the fear in your breathing.

Know that the air you breathe
　　holds the life-giving energy of your fear.

Begin to take very, very deep breaths
    into the depths of your abdomen,
    breathing that energy into yourself,
    allowing yourself to accept that energy,
    relaxing into your fear,
    embracing your fear as your friend,
    allowing your fear to pass easily and naturally
    through you, without resistance.
Take each breath deeply, in and out.
Take each breath easily, in and out.
Take each breath, allowing the fear
    to flow in and through you, without resistance.
Continue to breathe deeply, embracing and accepting the fear,
    knowing that you are bigger than the fear
    and accepting the fear as your friend.

(4) Embrace the fear in your speaking.

After you have taken 5-12 deep breaths, move on to this next step.

As you continue to take the very deep breaths,
    on your next exhalation, shout,
    "Boy, am I scared!" as loudly as you can
    (as loudly as is appropriate in your current surroundings).
    Allow yourself to fully express the energy
        of your fear in your voice.
    Again, "Boy, am I scared!"
    Really trail the "boy" out, as in, "Boooooooyyy, am I scared!"
    Again, "Boooooooyyy, am I scared!"
Continue breathing and deeply expressing,
    "Boooooooyyy, am I scared!!!"
    until you feel the energy of the fear flowing freely
    and vitally in and through your body and your mind.

Know that you are bigger than your fear.
Know that your fear is your friend.
Allow yourself to tap into the energy and power
    of this fear to serve your commitments, your passions,
    your confidence, your vitality, and your joy!

(5) Being present to your fear again (the test).

Now get back in touch with your fear as you did at the beginning.
Notice the sensations in your body associated with your fear.
How are they different than before?
    Do your hands feel different?
    Does your stomach feel different?
    Does your head feel different?
    Are you breathing more naturally and fully?
    Can you feel a new level of relaxation in your body?
    Do you feel more awake?
    Do you have an added feeling of energy?
Notice the thoughts that you *now* associate with your fear.
    Have they changed at all from before?
    Have any of the previous thoughts
        lessened in intensity or disappeared?
    Have the internal voices become softer or less intrusive?
    Is there an added sense of relaxed self-confidence?
    Is there an added sense of self-acceptance?

Have you ever heard the expression:
    "What you resist persists?"
    This is especially true with fear.
    If you resist it, it remains in place.
    If you embrace it, the dam is broken
        and the fear can flow through you
        and dissipate in your expressions and actions.

Actually, when you were describing your fear
at the beginning of this exercise,
you were *not* describing fear;
you were describing *resisted* fear.
Only after you had fully embraced your fear
could you begin to experience
it without the *added* resistance.

Special note: Although specifically designed
to deal with resisted fear,
this process can also be used to address
issues of resisted pain (as distinct from fear).
Just substitute, "Boy, do I feel hurt!"

Take a moment now to honor and appreciate yourself
(that is, honor and appreciate the five-year-old child within)
for choosing the courage to engage in this process.

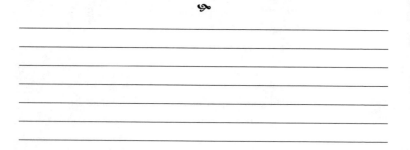

If you can find a courageous man who has no fear, then how will
you call him courageous? He will be a machine, not a man. Only
machines don't have fear. But you don't call machines courageous.
How can you call a machine courageous? Courage simply means
that something is happening in spite of the fear. The fear is there,
the trembling is there, but it is not stopping you, you are not being
blocked by it. You use it as a stepping-stone. Shaking, trembling,
but still you go into the unknown.

—*Osho (1931-1990, Indian mystic, writer)*

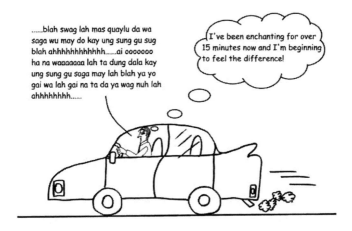

.....blah swag lah mas quaylu da wa saga wu may do kay ung sung gu sug blah ahhhhhhhhhhhh......ai ooooooo ha na waaaaaaa lah ta dung dala kay ung sung gu saga may lah blah ya yo gai wa lah gai na ta da ya wag nuh lah ahhhhhhhh......

I've been enchanting for over 15 minutes now and I'm beginning to feel the difference!

EnChanting™

Here's how to change any feeling or mood!

Do you ever get stuck in feelings of
   animosity, anxiety, arrogance, bitchiness, bitterness, boredom,
   callousness, crankiness, cynicism, defensiveness, depression,
   envy, guilt, hatred, impatience, indecisiveness, inflexibility,
   ingratitude, jealousy, laziness, obsessiveness, overwhelm,
   perfectionism, petulance, procrastination, rebelliousness,
   resentment, resignation, righteousness, rudeness,
   self-consciousness, shame, stress, stubbornness?

Do you find yourself stuck being
   over-protective or over-controlling,
   being too critical of yourself or others,
   blaming others, complaining, feeling betrayed,
   feeling dispirited, feeling disrespected, feeling foolish,

feeling like a victim, feeling unloved, showing disrespect,
lacking self-confidence or self-esteem, lying,
nagging, suppressing yourself, or worrying?

Most of us get stuck
in one or more of these feelings, moods,
or thought/behavior patterns fairly often.

Sometimes, they pass quickly.
Sometimes, they stick around much longer than we'd like,
even becoming a chronic part of our life.

I have discovered a *simple, easy* technique
that will help you dissolve
most unwanted feelings or moods.
I call this technique "EnChanting."

Let me tell you how I discovered it.
(If you want to go straight to the description of the technique,
feel free to skip over the following example.)

On Valentine's Day 1994,
I was lying on my bed at 2:30 in the afternoon.
I was depressed.
I had been depressed for over two months.
I was barely getting by in my work.
(I worked at home and for myself,
so it was easier for me to hide my condition
than it would be for most people.)
The only things I wanted to do were eat, watch TV, and sleep.
Everything else occurred to me as an overwhelming burden.
Every time I would think of something I needed to do,
the automatic response in my mind was,
"So what? It's all pointless anyway."

I had had periodic bouts of depression before,
    but never one as long or severe as this one.
    I was beginning to get seriously concerned.
I started praying to God
    to show me something I was willing to do
    that would move me out of my depression.
Then, from my intuition,
    I started "EnChanting" (see explanation below).
    I EnChanted for three hours straight:
    the first hour while lying in my bed,
the second and third hours
    while walking along the canal bank (in Phoenix, Arizona).
    I would tone it down when I would pass people
        so they wouldn't think I was crazy.

At the end of the three hours
    I was on cloud nine.
    I was feeling great!
    My mood was great!
The circumstances of my life were exactly as before.
    But, instead of feeling burdened and overwhelmed,
        I felt fully resourceful and excited
        about my life and its possibilities!

Since that day, I have had no significant bouts of depression.
    Whenever I begin to feel depression
    (or any other undesired feeling),
    I try a little EnChanting.
I have also shared this technique with hundreds of clients.
    The feedback reports range from
    "It's a very powerful stress releaser" to
    "The results were miraculous!"

Here's a description of the EnChanting process.

EnChanting is a means of gently focusing
   on the deep mood and feelings of a particular moment,
   allowing these feelings to resonate and bubble out
   into extemporaneous sounds/chanting.
These sounds are spontaneous,
   nonsensical, and non-conceptual.
   The wrong way to do this is to try to do it right.
   There are no right sounds.
   The experience is one of ease and effortlessness,
      although you may feel a bit embarrassed or silly.
   Allow your feelings to lead the chanting.

Where do I EnChant?
EnChanting is done privately.
   For many people, the best place is their car,
   where they can allow themselves to really belt it out.
   Other good places are your house or apartment.
   EnChant for as long as possible. An hour or more is very good.
   EnChant until your mood or feeling changes.

What can I expect from EnChanting?
At the very least, EnChanting provides
   an immediate release of tension.
Fundamentally, EnChanting is a generic de-repressor,
   dissolving our resistance to ourselves and to our lives,
   allowing our true joy and aliveness
      (which is always underneath the calcified shell of our
      protection)
   to bubble forth.
The more you EnChant, the more you will wake up.
   Use your judgment in deciding how fast you want to wake up.

Why does EnChanting work?

Consider this question:

 As a group, who are the most joyous,
   energetic, alive, present, creative,
   and curious people on earth?

 Young children.

And what do young children (typically those under six years old)
 consistently do that we adults don't do?

Children freely and immediately express in sounds
 (often non-verbal sounds), with no censorship
 and with nothing held back,
  exactly what they are feeling when they are feeling it.

When a child cries for a long time, the child does not think,
 "My mother might not love me or take care of me
  if I continue to cry."

When a child squeals and/or babbles with delight,
 sometimes for hours, the child does not think,
 "They might decide I'm not a serious person if I'm too happy."

But at a certain point a child starts to become an adult,
 and that is the point when the child begins to learn
  that certain verbal expressions are not acceptable.

 In fact, one way to make a child act like an adult faster
  is to give the child strong, consistent messages
  that certain verbal expressions
  of pain, fear, anger, joy, and/or pleasure
  will not be tolerated and/or will be frowned upon.

As adults we have *no* outlet to verbally express our feelings
 in any way that begins to approximate
 the outlet that children have.

 Even so-called outlets such as singing do not fit the bill,
  since when we sing, we have to do it "the right way."

 Imagine the effects of trying
  to get a child to squeal "the right way."

EnChanting offers
the first easy-to-do methodology to express our feelings
(without having to put words to them).
It can usually be tailored to require no additional time.
For most of us, it can be combined with other activities
such as walking, jogging, housecleaning, driving, etc.
Unlike meditation mantras or Buddhist chants,
it allows/includes full flexibility and encouragement
for the emanating sounds to flow freely
and to be full expressions of the feelings/moods of the moment,
just as the sounds that a child makes
are full, unedited expressions of that child.

How is EnChanting distinct
from other change-your-attitude techniques?
Has the average happy child learned how
to focus h/is mind and think positively?
No.
Does the average joyous child hear and/or read
uplifting stories to inspire h/im during a bad day?
No.
Does the average happy child meditate
or engage in stress reduction techniques?
No.
Does the average creative child spend hours in front of the TV
to distract h/imself from life's concerns?
No.
Most of the ancient and modern-day
techniques and approaches that adults use
to attempt to manage our feelings
(over the top of our calcified protections) are just that:
an attempt at management *on top of* a calcification
that prevents us from experiencing
our innate joy, energy, and happiness.

EnChanting dissolves the years of calcification,
    allowing us to spontaneously express
    our birthright of joy, energy,
    happiness, aliveness, and creativity.

Here are some words that suggest
    the full range and expression of EnChanting:

baaing, babbling, bantering, barking, baying, bellowing, bewailing, bleating, booing, bubbling, cackling, chanting, cheeping, cheering, clucking, cooing, croaking, crooning, crying, displaying, exclaiming, expressing, groaning, growling, grumbling, gurgling, harping, heehawing, hissing, honking, hooting, howling, humming, intoning, jabbering, laughing, mewing, moaning, murmuring, muttering, neighing, non-conceptual verbalizing, making nonsense sounds, parroting, peeping, prattling, praying, preaching, purring, quacking, ranting, raving, razzing, resonating, rhyming, roaring, sassing, scolding, screaming, screeching, shouting, shrieking, singing, snarling, sobbing, sounding, speaking, squawking, squealing, stammering, stuttering, susurrating, talking, taunting, teasing, telling, toning, tweeting, ululating, uttering, verbalizing, voicing, vowing, wailing, warbling, whimpering, whining, whispering, yakking, yelling, yelping, yodeling, yowling.

Think of the maxim,
    "If I can't, then EnChant"
    to remind you of this powerful tool.

For many, it is a choice of courage to EnChant.

Honor yourself for that choice.

෨

Create quickly a
"deep awakening renewal"

Use the following process to instantly dissolve
    fear, stress, worry, resentment,
      anger, depression, resignation, etc.
Use this process to create
    a quick, deep, and profound renewal.

Setting:
Set aside 30 uninterrupted minutes for this process.
Make sure you are alone or at least have some modicum of privacy.
Find a comfortable place to lie on your back.
Place a pillow at your side.
Find a countdown timer or other alarm device.
Dim the lights and/or have some blinders to shade your eyes.
Make sure you have some tissues handy.
It's helpful to have a tranquil, relaxing CD/cassette ready to play
    to bring you out of the process during the last five minutes.

The Process
Set the timer on 25 minutes and press "start."

Sub-Process 1:

Lying on your back,
    with your arms at your sides,
      make loose fists with both of your hands.
Start to breathe as deeply as you can,
    filling up both your chest and your stomach,
      as you would fill two balloons.
Pull each breath in as deeply as you can.
Then release each breath
    without forcing the air out.

Breathe at a rate of 20-22 breaths per minute,
    or one breath every three seconds.
As you take each breath,
    open one finger of your hand,
    so that you're counting the breaths
    as you open the fingers on your hands.
When you have opened all 10 fingers,
    then you will have taken 10 breaths.
After the first 10 breaths,
    make two fists again,
    repeating the counting process.
As you continue with this process
    you will probably notice an increasing sense
    of discomfort and tension in your body.
Allow the tension to build,
    taking no fewer than 20 breaths
    and no more than 50 breaths
    (2-5 sets of "fist openings").

Sub-Process 2:

Discontinue the deep breathing.
Take the pillow and press it tightly
    over your face/mouth.
Scream as loudly as you can into the pillow!
Scream at the top of your lungs!
You can just scream spontaneous sounds or you can scream words.
You can choose your own words.
I also suggest that you experiment
    with screaming the words listed below
    to see which phrases work for you.
Create your own variations.
And *listen* to what you are saying.
The listed order of these phrases is not significant.
For examples with instructions in parentheses,
    substitute the appropriate word.

"You've been asleep for (your age minus 5) years!
It's time to wake up now!"

"You've been dead for (your age minus 5) years!
Wake up! Wake up!"

"For everything that's worth living for, wake up!
Wake up now, (your name)!"

"Wake up now! Live now! It's time!
Not later! Not later! Now! Now! Now!"

"Get out of my mind!"

"Get out of my body!"

"Get out of my life!"

"This is my life!"

"Wake up!"

"Wake up, (your name)!"

"It's time to wake up!"

"It's time to wake up, (your name)!"

"It's time for *real* life, *now*!"

"You've been asleep long enough!"

"God, let me live my life fully!"

"This is *my* life!"

"This life is *my* playground!"

"Give in to your power!"

"God, let me accept your power in me!"

"Give in to love!"

"God, let me feel *all* of my love!"

"Give in to peace!"

"God, let me feel the *depth* of your peace!"

"Wake up to the ecstasy of life!"

"Give in to the ecstasy of life!"

"Give in to the lightness of being!"

"God, grant me the lightness of being!"

"For the sake of life, wake up!"

"For the sake of God, wake up into life!"

"For the sake of all people, wake up!"

"For the sake of all men, wake up!"

"For the sake of all women, wake up!"
"For the sake of all children, wake up!"
"For the sake of all creatures, wake up!"
"For the love of your mother, wake up!"
"For the love of your father, wake up!"
"For the love of your children, wake up!"
"For the love of your brother, wake up!"
"For the love of your sister, wake up!"
"For the love of your friends, wake up!"
"Wake up into your sensuality!"
"Wake up into your sexuality!"
"Listen to what you're saying, (your name)!"
"Let in what you're saying, (your name)!"
"Wake up to *now!*"
"Wake up to this moment!"
"Wake up!"
"Wake up, (your name)!"
"Wake up now!"
"Wake up now, (your name)!"
"Celebrate *now* every moment of *now!*"
"Let your body wake up now!"
"Let your mind wake up now!"
"Let your spirit fly now!"
"Let go of every guilt!"
"Let go of all regret!"
"Let go of the past!"
"Wake up to life now!"
Scream until you're all screamed out,
    until there's nothing more to scream.
Then remove the pillow from your face.
If you need to spit anything out,
    use a tissue.
Then return to Sub-Process 1 (the breathing process).
    Repeat Sub-Process 1 and Sub-Process 2
    until the timer beeps.

Then start the relaxing music
and allow the peace of the universe
to flow through your body, mind and spirit.

Try this out today
and see what you notice.

Honor yourself for the courage
to do this.

❧

_____
_____
_____
_____
_____
_____
_____
_____
_____
_____
_____
_____

The best way to make your dreams come true is to wake up.

—*J.M. Power*

When you bury feelings, you don't bury them dead. You bury them alive.

—*Donna Fried*

Anger is a symptom, a way of cloaking and expressing feelings too awful to experience directly—hurt, bitterness, grief and, most of all, fear.

—*Joan Rivers*

I don't want to do anything.

...

What's the meaning of life?

...

It's one of those days.

...

I lost my job.

...

What's the use?...

I've felt that way, too.

...

It seems meaningless, doesn't it?

...

Maybe you shouldn't have gotten out of bed.

...

That's terrible.

...

It seems hopeless, doesn't it?...

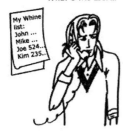

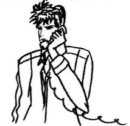

Create a "whine list" for whining

Do you ever get in one of those moods
    where nothing seems right,
    where your mind is fidgety,
    where you can't figure out what to do,
    where you don't want to do anything,
    where you have no energy for no reason,
    where your mind seems in a turmoil or a muddle,
    where you want to avoid life,
    or where there is no answer to the question "so what"?

Most all of us pass through
    this type of mood sooner or later,
    for shorter or for longer periods of time.
There is a solution.
    I call it your "Whine List."

Whining, complaining, groaning and moaning, bitching.

We grant no space to ourselves
    or to others for these behaviors.
It's okay to be optimistic, to be cheerful, to be happy.
    But don't whine.
    Or, if you do, keep it to yourself!

Whining is like fear in this way.
Fear doesn't have good PR,
    and we all pretend to ourselves and others
    that we don't have much of it.
    Whining may even have worse PR than fear.

Who wants to be around a whiner and complainer?

Consider what might happen
    if we gave ourselves full permission
    to whine, moan, groan, complain, and bitch.
Let me suggest that you enlist
    some special friends in your life
    (I would recommend a minimum of five)
    to be on your Whine List.
        For most of us making this request
        will be a choice of courage!
These special friends will make themselves
    available to you to be on call as needed or wanted
    for whining sessions.
You could offer to do the same for them.

During these whining sessions,
    your listener will be there for you
        (either on the telephone or face to face)
    to *really listen* to how things
    occur for you in your world.

Your listener will desire to see (and even feel) your world
    as you see it and feel it,
    to understand
    what your automatic thoughts and feelings
    are about yourself, about others,
    and about the circumstances of your life.
Your listener will give you the non-judgmental space
    for you to speak about how bad it is for you in your world,
    without any need for sugar-coating
    and without any need to look good.

Your listener will *not* try to cheer you up,
    will *not* try to fix things,
    will *not* try to coach you,
    will *not* give you any advice.
S/he will only *listen*,
    inviting you to tell h/im more
    so that you can express it *all*
    and s/he can fully understand how things
    occur for you in your world.
Your listener may say things with empathy like,
    "Please tell me more,"
    "I'm so sorry,"
    "It's hard to keep going, isn't it?"
    "Life is really tough,"
    "Thank you for telling me how you feel,"
    "It's not fair,"
    "It really seems hopeless, doesn't it?"
Whereas, you, as the speaker,
    will choose the courage
    to give yourself *full* permission
    to whine, moan, groan, complain, and bitch,
    with nothing held back and with no sugar-coating,
    even giving yourself permission to exaggerate
        in expressing how bad it is.

It's actually quite amazing what happens out of this process.
When we choose the courage to whine (in the above context)
  and we have a great listener who is encouraging us to whine
  (and who is *not* resisting our whining in any way),
  then a new clearing almost miraculously appears
  for something fresh to show up.
When we keep our whining inside and suppress it
  (which includes thinking we shouldn't feel this way),
  we keep ourselves stuck.

I have never experienced a whining session yet,
  where I was either the speaker or the listener,
  that lasted longer than 30 minutes
  before a shift occurred.
One time, I started whining
  with a person who was on my Whine List
  (after feeling stuck for two days),
  and I was out of my mood within two minutes!

See if you can get at least five friends on your Whine List!
Then overuse them.
To really get the value out of this new practice,
  you'll have to overdo it,
  since all your life
  you've blamed yourself and others for whining.
  Enjoy!
The importance of having at least five friends on your list
  is so that you'll be able to easily reach someone
  when you need to whine.

It will probably be a choice of courage
  to invite each friend to be on your Whine List.

It will also be another choice of courage
  to call one of your listeners

when you're not in the mood
to ask h/im if s/he is available for a whining session.

Honor yourself for this courage.

֍

_____
_____
_____
_____
_____
_____
_____
_____
_____
_____
_____
_____
_____
_____
_____
_____
_____

The tears I shed yesterday have become rain.
—*Thich Nhat Hanh*

Shared joy is double joy and shared sorrow is half-sorrow.
—*Swedish proverb*

I imagine one of the reasons people cling to their hates so stubbornly
is because they sense, once hate is gone, they will be forced to deal
with pain.
—*Sydney J. Harris*

How to Encourage Your Courage

Since choosing courage is the source of everything else we want or may want in our lives, it becomes extremely important to do whatever we can to "encourage our courage." I provide two distinct methods for doing this.

The first process **Courage: The Child's Choice** is a quick, simple, powerful technique. Make the process an integral part of your distinction of courage so that courage becomes a "friendly virus" that begins to multiply itself throughout your life.

The second is the **Partner Acknowledgment Process.** Create an ongoing partnership with one or more of your colleagues or friends for the purpose of mutual acknowledgment. Acknowledge each other both for the courage you have chosen and the courage you intend to choose.

❧

_____

_____

_____

_____

_____

_____

_____

_____

_____

_____

_____

_____

_____

_____

_____

_____

Encourage your courage

The three cornerstones for expressing full courage are:
 (1) embracing and tapping into the energy of the fear,
 (2) honoring ourselves for choosing the courage
   (before *and* after the action), and
 (3) taking the action in the face of the fear.

Even if we focus on
 the first and third cornerstones of courage,
 most of us pay little or no attention
 to the *second* cornerstone of courage.
In fact, out of habit, we often do the opposite:
 we discourage ourselves from choosing courage.
Instead of honoring ourselves for choosing courage,
 we often dishonor ourselves by saying to ourselves,
 "I should have done that sooner," or
 "It was no big deal; such a small thing," or
 "Why am I such a baby about these things?" or
 "I shouldn't have been afraid of that."
These dishonoring comments undermine our ability
 to choose courage again in the future!

A quick and simple way
 to honor and appreciate ourselves
 for choosing courage is to express
 quick acknowledgments to ourselves like,
 "Good job, Jamie!" or
 "What courage, Pat!"

However, a much more powerful and effective method
 of encouraging courage is to take yourself through
 the "Courage: the Child's Choice" process.

In this process, I also explain
   the other two cornerstones of courage,
   but the main focus is on encouraging courage.

Courage: The Child's Choice

(1) Recognize your *resisted* fear
   (resisted fear = fear that is disempowering).
   Sometimes you'll be aware that you're frightened.
      Other times you won't.
   Here are some possible indicators of resisted fear:
      something seems difficult to you, you're procrastinating,
      you're resentful, you're critical of others (blaming),
      you're critical of yourself (guilt), you're withdrawn,
      you're depressed, you're putting up with something,
      you're resigned, you have no energy,
      you're confused, you feel like a victim,
      you're angry, you're defensive,
      you're compulsive and/or perfectionistic,
      you're overeating, you're watching a lot of TV,
      etc.

(2) Embrace your resisted fear
   (the FOE formula: fear + oxygen = energy).
   Even if you can't feel the fear,
      take a few very deep breaths.
   Speak as loudly and as drawn-out as possible,
      "Boy, am I scared!"
      Do this 5-15 times.
      Breathe deeply into the fear.
      Allow the fear to flow through your body.
      Begin to know that you are bigger than the fear.

(3) Connect with your child
(child + adult = aliveness + power).
Get in touch with your five-year-old child within.
Listen to and speak with your child
until you're really in touch with h/im.
(Use a picture of yourself around the age of five
to help you feel the realness of your child within.)
Say to your child:
"I can see and feel that you're feeling frightened."
"It's okay that you're feeling frightened."
"I admire and appreciate you so much
for your willingness to fully feel this fear."
"I admire and appreciate you so much
for choosing courage while experiencing this fear."
Listen to and speak with your child
until you feel that your child fully experiences
your admiration and appreciation.

(4) Act to serve your commitment
(courage = empowerment).
Fully nurture and empower your child
to take the actions associated with the fear
that accompanies a choice of courage.

(5) Connect with your child again
(being the best parent for your child).
Once the action is over,
reconnect with your five-year-old child again.
Listen to and speak with your child
until you are really in touch with h/im.
Say to your child:
"I can see the results of your actions."
"Let's acknowledge and accept those results together."

If the result was disappointing, say to your child,
  "It's okay to feel disappointed."
If the result was a success, say to your child,
  "Congratulations on your success!"
Regardless of the outcome, say to your child,
  "I admire and appreciate you so much
    for your willingness to fully feel your fear."
  "I admire and appreciate you so much
    for the courage you chose
    to take the actions you just took."

Listen to and speak with your child
  until you feel that s/he fully experiences your admiration.

How might you support yourself
  in consistently looking for opportunities
  to encourage your courage?

_____

_____

_____

_____

We never grow up, we only learn how to act in public.
  —*Bryan White*

Adults are obsolete children.
  —*Dr. Seuss (1904-1991, humorist, illustrator, author)*

There is no comparison between that which is lost by not succeeding
and that which is lost by not trying.
  —*Francis Bacon*

Partner Acknowledgment Process

Skyrocket your courage with this process.

Two distinct ways exist to encourage your courage.

The first is by using the process detailed in the previous essay,
    which I call "Courage: the Child's Choice."

This process is always available to you,
    since it relies on no one outside of you
    and you can always use it immediately,
    regardless of your circumstances.

However, soliciting and accepting
    appreciation, admiration, acknowledgment,
        and/or just *listening* from another
        for your choices of courage can be an important addition
        to "strengthening your courage muscles."

This can be done informally
    or you can create a structure of support
    to ensure regular use of this
    "Partner Acknowledgment Process."

Let me explain how I use the informal method in my life today.
Often, when I meet with a friend
    or talk with h/im for any length on the telephone,
    I ask h/im the following, "Please tell me a story about
        how you chose courage since we last talked."
    Then I listen, ask some questions,
        and express my admiration and appreciation
        for h/is choices of courage.

Then I ask h/im, "Please share with me about some courage
   you intend to choose in the near future."
   I then express my admiration and appreciation
      for h/is intended choice of courage.
Then I say, "Please let me share my experiences
   regarding my choices of courage
   (both completed and intended)."
   After my sharing, s/he expresses
      h/is admiration and appreciation of me
      for both the courage that I chose
      and the courage that intend to choose.

Now let's look at a more formalized version
   of the "Partner Acknowledgment Process."
   Using this, you can receive regular acknowledgment
      from others for the courage that you have chosen
      and that you intend to choose,
   in addition to being inspired by another's choices of courage.

Although this method could make use of any form
   of regular communication, I will use email in this example.

Set up an agreement and structure with one or more friends.
   Create an email template with the following contents:

(1)   Here's how I appreciate and admire you
      for the courage that you have chosen:
         . . . .
      Tell me another choice (or other choices) of courage
      that you have taken
      that you would like acknowledgment for.

(2)   Here's how I appreciate and admire you
      for the courage that you intend to choose:
         . . . .

Tell me the choice(s) of courage that you intend to take that you would like acknowledgment for.

(3) Please express appreciation and admiration for me
for the following choice(s) of courage
that I have already taken:

. . . .

(4) Please express appreciation and admiration for me
for the following choice(s) of courage that I intend to take:

. . . .

(5) Please share with me an opportunity for courage
that you *did not* choose.

. . . .

For example, here is an email I received from Jessica:

(1) Please appreciate me for having called Beverly
to see if we might have lunch together.
I would really like her as a friend and
I was automatically frightened of her possible rejection.
She said "yes!"

(2) Tomorrow I will start working on my taxes.
I notice that I want to avoid finding out
how much money I may owe the IRS.

(3) That's really great, Dwight, that you told your friend
that you needed to have some private space.
You inspire me with your willingness
to keep good boundaries with others.

(4) I'm excited to hear what happens in your promise
to ask that famous author to provide a testimonial
for your book. Wow! Your courage encourages me.

(5) One of my friends was smoking in my home and I did not
ask them to stop.

And then my email back to Jessica might say:

(1)   I know that cultivating Beverly as your friend
        is important to you. Keep me posted.
        I really admire you for this!

(2)   I can relate to wanting to avoid doing your taxes.
        That definitely is a choice of courage! Bravo!

(3)   Yesterday I made a promise to eat only raw foods
        until 5 PM. I was scared of the craving I would have
        for other things. To make the promise and keep it
        was definitely a choice of courage for me.

(4)   Later today I will call an old friend
        with whom I feel awkward and have a conversation
        to make sure everything is okay.

(5)   Yesterday I was feeling unresourceful. I didn't choose
        courage by calling someone to get help with that.
        Instead I just indulged.

Keep this email going back and forth, at least on a daily basis.
    If one of you drops it out,
        the other can just pick it up and start it again.
    If you find that your Acknowledgment Partner
        is unreliable or non-responsive, then choose the courage
        to enroll another Acknowledgment Partner.

A note of caution.
    Make sure that your partner can give
        h/is genuine appreciation and admiration for the types
        of courageous actions that you are up for in your life.
    It might be helpful to have different
        Acknowledgment Partners for different areas of your life.
    Regardless, you may want to have
        two or more Acknowledgment Partners.

Choose the courage now to contact someone
to be your first Acknowledgment Partner.

સ

How to bring the power of courage into every part of your life

If you don't already have a broad glimpse of it, by the time you finish this section (consisting of 128 essays), you will know, both panoramically and profoundly, how the opportunities for courage exist everywhere and at every time.

This section is divided into 31 subsections.

For the most part, it does not matter which essays you read first. These essays could have been arranged either randomly or alphabetically with perhaps as good an effect. Many of the essays do fall rather easily into one category or another, while others might often be placed into more than one category. For example, many of the essays in the category of "Listening" could arguably be categorized under "Partnership" or "Intimacy and romance."

Also, some categories clearly encompass only specific essays. But others, like "Benefits of the negative," "The lure of feeling secure," or "Empowerment through context" could also include many essays that were categorized otherwise.

When dealing with subjects as broad as life and courage, any categorization system is likely to be more a work of art than one of science.

Enjoy!

❦

How do you use and abuse time?

Before the beginning was the time before time.
And in this time before time,
    in this world of timeless change
    everything flowed ever new and fresh.
There was no past to regret or justify;
    there was no future to fear or anticipate.
There was no waiting and no postponing;
    only the glorious and incomparable new and now.

In this time before time, only the *now* spoke to us
    in words of brilliant sight, instant sound,
        and spontaneous expression.
The *past* was unborn. The *future* was undiscovered.
    Everything lived in this timeless and eternal *now*.
In this time before time
    we were never waiting for things to get better,
    we were never wasting a single moment of our lives,
    we had no guilt, no regret, no worries,
        no wishing we had a different life.

But after the beginning came the time after time.
    The *past* arose in our wake.
    The *future* appeared at our bow.
We began to discover the power of time,
    the power to direct, to control, to predict,
    the power to become unique and distinct.

We relished this power of time,
    grasping more and more of it each day
    living more and more in the house of time,
    living more and more in the house of language,
        the keeper and creator of time.

Yet, as we began to use time,
    we also began to abuse time.
We began to abuse time
    by waiting for it to move into the *past*.
We began to abuse time
    by hoping for a better *future*.
We began to abuse time
    by using it to resist *what is now*.

Time became our great guardian,
    protecting us from being present to
    the way it is *right now*,
    protecting us from the fear that *this is it*.

Before the beginning was the time before time.
And then after the beginning came the time after time.
Can there be another time?
    A time of time and timeless together?
    A time of exquisite paradox and wonder?
    A time when time paints itself again and again
        upon the tapestry of the timeless?
    A time of unspeakable and eternal bliss
        cradling the joys, pains, and dramas
        of our time-filled lives?

I invite you to live inside these questions.
 I invite your moment-by-moment vigilance
   of the timeless and eternal now.
 I invite your choice of existential courage
   in embracing and allowing
   an eternal timelessness,
   to transform your life.

∽

_____

_____

_____

_____

_____

_____

_____

_____

_____

_____

_____

_____

_____

_____

_____

_____

_____

_____

_____

_____

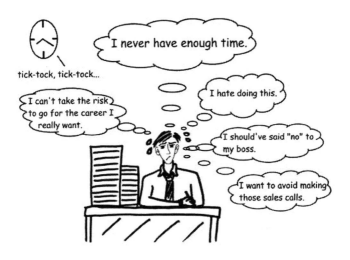

Do you have enough time?

"I don't have enough time"
  is perhaps the most frequent of all complaints.
Yet I have found that this complaint
  is *rarely* of the James-Bond type,
    where, if the bomb isn't defused in the next 23 seconds,
    it's "Goodbye, Earth!"

The real problem most often is not an issue of quantity of time
  but an issue of quality of time.

Next time you're feeling that you don't have enough time,
  ask yourself,
    "Am I enjoying the *process* of what I am doing?"
    "Am I savoring the journey itself?"
    "Am I being present to the eternal now of this moment?"

Next time you're feeling that you don't have enough time,
  ask yourself,
    "Am I choosing courage to design my life
    by saying 'no' to what I need to say 'no' to
    so that I can 'smell the roses' along the way?"

Next time you're feeling that you don't have enough time,
  ask yourself,
    "Am I choosing courage to go for what I *really* want,
    rather than playing my life
    in the half-shadows of safety and security?"

Next time you're feeling that you don't have enough time,
  ask yourself,
    "What might I be avoiding that, if faced,
    would provide a new level of freedom and self-expression
    in my life?"

Consider that the next time you're thinking or saying
  you don't have enough time,
    it is likely a smoke screen for the real issue(s).
Use the above questions to help you uncover the *real* issue(s)
  so that you can address it powerfully.

Do you feel that you have enough time?
  If not, then slowly and deeply ask yourself
  each of the questions above.

❧

_____

_____

_____

_____

_____

_____

Enough time is not the problem

All we have is time.
    We have time and more time
    —until we die.

So why do we often feel
    that we don't have enough time?

Why do we set our lives up
    so that we feel
    that we don't have enough time?

I believe that not having enough time
    is rarely the real problem.

Perhaps the real problem
    is that you're trying to prove something
    by accomplishing more than you can accomplish
    in the time frame allowed.
Perhaps the real problem
    is that you're trying to control things
    that you really can't control
    in order to try to feel safer.
Perhaps the real problem
    is that you're making your life so busy
    that you will not have to face the emptiness of it
    should you slow down.
Perhaps the real problem
    is that you want approval from others
    and want to avoid their disapproval
    by accomplishing so much.

Perhaps the real problem
 is that you're unwilling to choose courage
 to say "no" to others.
Perhaps the real problem
 is that you want to avoid the feeling of guilt
 you would feel if you began to enjoy
 the process of your life.
Perhaps the real problem
 is that you haven't designed the process of your life
 so that you enjoy "doing"
 and, as a result, you procrastinate on doing things
 in a timely manner.

Consider the idea
 that 99 percent of the reason
 for doing anything or for going after a goal or destination
 is to *enjoy the process!*

What if the primary focus was on enjoying the process
 and the secondary focus was on getting the result?

Would you still feel that you didn't have enough time?

If not, which of the above problems
 might apply to you?

Consider that having access
 to enough time
 is a choice of courage.

      &ptstsc;

_____

_____

_____

_____

_____

Are you an accomplishment machine?

"I don't have enough money."
"I don't have enough time."

Most often, the complaint "I don't have enough time,"
    whether expressed out loud or kept within one's own mind,
    is the more insidious and chronic
    of these two virtually universal complaints.

When a problem (e.g., "I don't have enough time"),
    remains fundamentally unsolved,
    it's a very strong indication that the problem, as identified,
    is *not* the problem at all.
Its current and mistaken identification
    is what keeps us from finding the solution.

Most of us realize that if
    we were magically granted a 36-hour day,
    it would not be very long
    before we again had the problem of "not enough time."

I say the *real* problem is *not*
    that we don't have enough time;
    the *real* problem is that we have chosen *accomplishment*
        (usually by cultural default and pressure)
    to be the "lead horse" or primary theme of our life.

For almost all of us,
    the "lead horse" of our life is *accomplishment.*
    Accomplishment! Accomplishment! Accomplishment!
    The more, the better.
    Whom do we admire? Who inspires us?

The person who accomplishes *so* much.
The person who works *so* hard.

Study hard. Get the best grades. Take the most classes.
Work hard. Hold down two jobs. Take on another project.
Do everything for the kids.
Have the cleanest house. Cook the best meals.
The focus is always
      on more *accomplishment* and *working hard.*
The success of our life is measured by our accomplishments.

So *time* becomes a problem.
      Let's do this more efficiently so I can get to that.
      I must hurry up with this so I won't be late for that.
      Where can I find time for exercise
            when I don't have enough time for sleep?

Time will always be a problem
      as long as accomplishment is the lead horse.

To solve the problem of time,
      you must follow a *new* lead horse.
This new lead horse is
      the continuing process and dance
      of creating and expressing your moment-by-moment,
            hour-by-hour, day-by-day, year-by-year
      life and living as a *work of art,*
            a work of art that really inspires you,
            that really appeals to you,
            that's *so good* you would wish it on your best friend!

Certainly, accomplishment will still be
      an important part of your life.
But it will *not* be the lead horse.

It will be a "following horse" that is guided by the lead horse
of creating and living your life *now,* moment to moment,
as a work of art.

Accomplishment will owe its primary reason for being
to how well it serves the process
of creating and expressing your life
as an enriching, fascinating, and dynamic *work of art.*

As a side note, for those rare individuals who have too much time,
the issue is still the same:
how to use accomplishment and goals
to serve the expression of your life as a work of art.

There is a benefit
of having accomplishment be our primary focus in life:
it helps us to feel safer and more in control.
It also gets us a lot of good PR
and helps us look good to others.

Most of us will need to continually
choose courage, step by step,
in order to create and express our life
as a work of art,
and maintain that work of art as the primary focus
in the design and expression of our life.

What would be the first choice of courage
needed to create your life
as the work of art you've always wanted?

༄

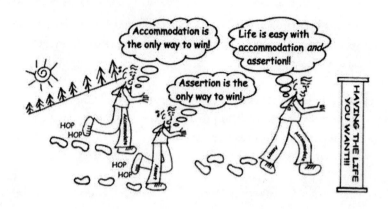

Are you an asserter or an accommodator?

An "asserter" (from the word "assert"),
   is, in essence, someone who speaks and/or takes actions
   to express or fulfill h/is own desires or commitments
   with little or no concern and/or awareness
   of the fears, desires, and commitments of others.
A good way to get an idea of a "pure asserter"
   is to think of the behavior of a typical one-year-old child.

An "accommodator" (from the word "accommodate"),
   is, in essence, someone who speaks and/or takes actions
   in such a way as to always ensure
   that everyone else's fears, desires, and commitments
   are included as primary considerations in h/is decisions.

A good way to get an idea of a "pure accommodator"
    is to think of a person who is good,
    who is always giving to others,
    who wouldn't hurt a flea,
    who is always thinking about the feelings of others,
    and who always puts h/imself last on the list.

Many adults have learned to manage an uneasy balance
    between the asserter and the accommodator
        in their personalities,
    but not really feeling truly comfortable with either one.
    However, real power and satisfaction
        come from balance and synchronicity
        between these two modes.

Often, we will favor one mode over the other,
    especially in a given area of life
    or in a relationship with a particular person.
For example, in a marriage, often one spouse will be an asserter
    and the other will be an accommodator.

It is common to be attracted to our lover or spouse
    because s/he expresses in some way
    what we have disowned in ourselves.
In my relationship with my ex-wife (when we were married),
    she was the asserter and I was the accommodator—
    until I became an asserter and said, "goodbye!"

It is often a choice of courage
    for an asserter to be an accommodator,
    and it is often a choice of courage.
    for an accommodator to be an asserter.

True power and freedom come from consistently exercising
    both the left leg of accommodation
    and the right leg of assertion,
    as well as being able to choose appropriately
    between the two according to the situation.

In what areas or situations in your life
    might you choose the courage
    to exercise your "leg of accommodation"?
In what areas or situations in your life
    might you choose the courage
    to exercise your "leg of assertion"?

∝

_____

_____

_____

_____

_____

_____

_____

_____

_____

A successful social technique consists perhaps in finding
unobjectionable means for individual self-assertion.
    —*Eric Hoffer (1903-1983, American author, philosopher)*

"Love" is an expression and assertion of self-esteem, a response to
one's own values in the person of another. One gains a profoundly
personal, selfish joy from the mere existence of the person one
loves. It is one's own personal, selfish happiness that one seeks,
earns, and derives from love.
    —*Ayn Rand (1905-1982, writer, philosopher)*

There are only two sources
of ALL problems

Every issue, *every* problem, *every* conflict
    lives inside one or both of two fundamental balances:

    Me or you
        and
    now or later.

I challenge you to find *any* issue or problem
    that is not fundamentally based in
    a perceived conflict between *me* and *you*
    or between *now* and *later.*

For the most part, in the *me or you* conflict,
    you gets almost all the good PR.

    The ideals of altruism, unselfishness, giving, charity,
        thinking of others first, duty, obligation, loyalty,
        sacrifice, giving to your country, and so on
    are ingrained deep within the hearts
        (whether acted upon or rebelled against)
    of every human within every culture
    on the face of this earth.

    The evils of greed, selfishness, egoism, conceit,
        personal desire, and so on
    are branded upon the souls
        (whether avoided or indulged)
    of every human within every culture
    on the face of this earth.

For the most part, in the conflict between now and later,
    later gets almost all the good PR.

    The ideals of perseverance, self-discipline, goal-setting,
           eating a healthy diet, waiting for your reward in heaven,
           avoiding your punishment in hell, not procrastinating,
           getting organized, keeping things neat, working hard,
           persistence, planning and saving for the future, and so on
    are what every "good" person is made of.
    We have been taught these ideals by countless sources—
        from the *The Little Engine That Could*
        to Christianity to Nike ads.

    The evils of self-indulgence, gluttony,
           drugs, alcohol, smoking, sex, passion, laziness,
           lack of self-discipline, anger,
           in general, anything that focuses on pleasure *now*
           (or reducing pain *now*)
    have most often been demonized, if not criminalized.

The sad history of our world has been
    defined by wars—
        within ourselves,
        within our families,
        between friends and neighbors,
        within and between businesses,
        between philosophies and religions,
        and between nations—
    that have been the direct expressions
    of the perceived conflicts
    between *you* and *me*
    and between *now* and *later*.

It is time to build a new alliance,
    a new friendship, new structures,
    new viewpoints and paradigms,
    where *you* and *me* both win,
    where *now* and *later* can *both* be served.

The next time you encounter a perceived conflict
    between *you* and *me* or
    between *now* and *later*,
    explore how making the choice of courage
    may offer you the opportunity
    for *both* (or all four) to win.

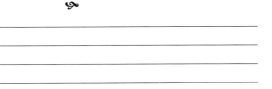

I conceive that pleasures are to be avoided if greater pains be the consequence, and pains to be coveted that will terminate in greater pleasures.

—*Michel Eyquem De Montaigne (1533-1592, French philosopher, essayist)*

We've been warned about not trying to fool Mother Nature. But I say that most progress has come from doing a good job of fooling Mother Nature so that she gives us the benefits of what we want without a lot of the previously associated costs.

—*GoldWinde*

Remember, anything you want that's valuable requires that you break through some short-term pain in order to gain long-term pleasure.

—*Anthony Robbins in Awaken the Giant Within*

What is your first focus?
Safety? Or passion?

We all want peace, security, stability, safety.
>   These are essential to our lives.

We sell out on life,
>   however, when we make these protective values
>   the primary basis of our decisions.

It's great to have a good, stable income;
>   but have you made your income more important
>   than following a passionate career?

It's great to have a reliable (life) partner;
>   but have you made having that reliability more important
>   than having a partner who inspires you?

It's great if you're a good person
>   who takes care of your aging parents;
>   but have you made being good more important
>   than caring for your parents out of love?

Deciding what you will hold as primary
>   and what you will hold as secondary
>   is fundamental to creating a life of joy,
>   self-expression, and passion.

Notice that it is a choice of courage,
>   again and again,
>   to make joy, self-expression, and passion
>   the primary focus of your life.

❧

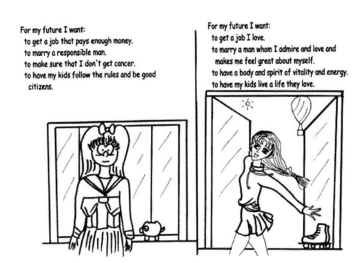

For my future I want:
to get a job that pays enough money.
to marry a responsible man.
to make sure that I don't get cancer.
to have my kids follow the rules and be good
citizens.

For my future I want:
to get a job I love.
to marry a man whom I admire and love and
makes me feel great about myself.
to have a body and spirit of vitality and energy.
to have my kids live a life they love.

Are you living a life of inspiration
or a life of avoidance?

Do you view your life as an expression of ever expanding
possibilities, opportunities, and inspirations?

Or do you view your life as a continuous and problematic
set of roadblocks and contractions,
with fewer and fewer possibilities?

If you are present to the former,
then your life orientation is primarily one of going for
"what you *really* want."
You are *inspiration* oriented.

If you are present to the latter,
then your life orientation is primarily one of trying to avoid
what you really don't want.
You are *avoidance* or *security* oriented.

It's fine to want to avoid certain things in life.
   I definitely recommend avoiding certain things!

However, if avoidance—"playing it safe"—
   has become your *primary* orientation in life,
   then you have already embraced the process
   of shutting down your life.

Sometimes we are avoidance oriented
   in one area of our life (e.g., love and romance),
   while remaining inspiration oriented
   in another area (e.g., work).

Can you find any area
   of your life in which you are avoidance oriented
   instead of inspiration oriented?
Can you identify an area
   in which you would like to be
   more inspiration oriented?

What specific acts of courage might you choose
   to begin to shift this area of your life
   from avoidance to inspiration?

∾

_____

_____

_____

_____

_____

_____

_____

_____

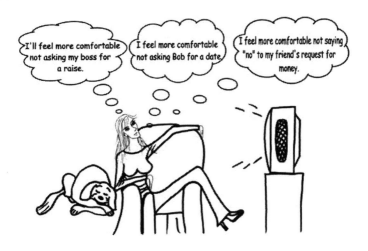

Comfort now or passion later?

I like comfort.
I think we all like comfort.

However, many times when we say,
 "I don't feel comfortable doing that,"
what we *really* mean is,
 "I'd rather choose the feeling of safety
 over the choice of courage
 in going for what I *really* want."

Next time you use the word
 "comfort," "comfortable," or "uncomfortable,"
ask yourself,
 "Am I missing an opportunity for courage here?"
 "What opportunities am I missing
  for getting what I *really* want?"

There's nothing wrong with comfort.
There's nothing wrong with a feeling of safety
    (although very often it does not mean *real* safety).

The question is,
    what possibilities,
    what life,
    what self-expression,
    what love,
    what accomplishment
are you sacrificing
    in order to feel safe and comfortable in the moment!?

Ask yourself,
    "How am I currently trading comfort
      in exchange for what I *really* want?
        In my job?
        In my career?
        In my family?
        In my love life?
        In my friendships?
        In my lifestyle?"

Is this trade acceptable to you?
    Do you think you are getting great value
      in exchange for the safety or relief
      you occasionally feel from time to time?
    Really?

∾

_____

_____

_____

_____

_____

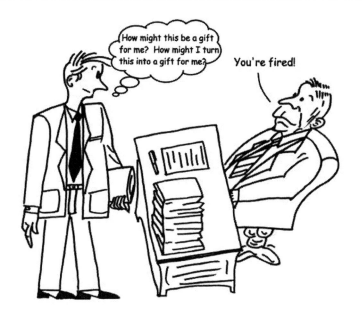

Is everything a gift?

I believe that everything in life is a gift.
There are two types of gifts:
    immediately obvious gifts, and
    immediately un-obvious gifts
        (the things you're complaining about or putting up with—
        either out loud or silently to yourself).

Consider the empowerment and openings that you'd experience
    if, whenever you encountered an un-obvious gift,
    you took it as an opportunity to discover and/or create it
    as an obvious gift.

Consider the degree to which your life would change
    if you believed that *everything* could be a gift.

You cannot prove that everything in your life *is* a gift.
You cannot prove that anything in your life is *not* a gift.
However, if you begin to believe
    that everything in your life is a gift,
    your life will be magnificent.

Choose something in your life
    that currently doesn't look like a gift.

Notice the courage it takes to keep asking yourself the questions,
    "How might this be a gift for me?"
    "How might I create this as a gift for me?"

❧

_____

_____

_____

_____

_____

_____

_____

_____

_____

_____

_____

Nothing vast enters the life of mortals without a curse.

—*Sophocles*

What I'm looking for is a blessing that's not in disguise.

—*Kitty O'Neill Collins*

Out of every crisis comes the chance to be reborn.

—*Nina O'Neill*

Do you get upset with God's plans?

My client was upset today.
> He had plans, *important* things to do.
> But God messed up his plans.
> His computer broke down
>> and he had to deal with God's plans
>> instead of following his own.

Do you get upset with God's plans?

It's important to have your own plans.
But despite the best of planning,
> the best of preparation,
> sometimes God has plans
> that are different from yours.
And She won't let you know about them
> until the last minute.
> God is the master of the *fait accompli*.

But what is our typical response
> when God interrupts our plans?
> We get upset with ourselves,
>> we get upset with others,
>> we get upset with God or the universe.

Why do we get upset
> when God substitutes Her plans for ours?
Because it frightens us
> and we don't want to feel the fear.
Because it gives us pain
> and we don't want to embrace the pain.

But what if you were willing
    to breathe deeply into your fear and pain,
    to honor and appreciate it
    as an expression of your love and commitment?
You would not feel fear,
      you would not feel pain
      if you didn't love and you didn't care.

But what if you were willing
    to become interested in God's plans?
What if you asked yourself,
    "What is She trying to do for me?"
    "How might She be providing
      a gift to me in this breakdown?"
    "How might I create a gift
      out of this breakdown?"
    "What really valuable lesson
      might I learn out of these circumstances?"
    "How might I begin to see God's plans
      as preferable over the plans
      that I had that She interrupted?"

Can you feel how letting go
    of trying to control God's plans
    is a choice of courage?

Breathe into the fear
    and honor yourself for choosing that courage.

❦

_____

_____

_____

_____

_____

_____

Why don't we feel more gratitude?

Let me clarify what I mean by gratitude.
    Gratitude may *include* a feeling,
        but it does not *start* with a feeling.
    It starts with an intention, a choice
        to "wear the glasses" of gratitude.
    Gratitude builds by simply
        focusing our attention on being grateful.

Given the infinite number of things
    we could be grateful for in any moment,
    we might wonder why we're not all basking in gratitude.

The reason we're not all basking in gratitude
    is that gratitude is risky;
        feeling grateful is often a choice of courage.

If we're too grateful,
    we might not stand up for our rights and for what we need.
If we're too grateful,
    we might get disappointed or hurt later
        if what we're grateful for is taken away from us.
If we're too grateful,
    others might take advantage of us.
If we're too grateful,
    we might not be able to resist the pain and fear in our life.
If we're too grateful,
    we will be like an innocent child,
        vulnerable to disillusionment.
If we're too grateful,
    we might let go of our ability to be in control.

Yes, gratitude is a risky business.
It's much safer
    to depreciate our lives
    to feel ungrateful
    to avoid celebration
    to harbor resentment
    to look for imperfections
    to blind ourselves to miracles.

Take one minute each hour
    to create deep gratitude
    for something in your life.

Honor yourself for this choice of courage.

෨

_____

_____

_____

_____

_____

_____

_____

_____

I have learnt silence from the talkative, toleration from the intolerant, and kindness from the unkind; yet strange, I am ungrateful to these teachers.

    —Kahlil Gibran (1883-1931, mystic, poet, artist)

Gratitude unlocks the fullness of life. It turns what we have into enough, and more. It turns denial into acceptance, chaos to order, confusion to clarity. It can turn a meal into a feast, a house into a home, a stranger into a friend. Gratitude makes sense of our past, brings peace for today, and creates a vision for tomorrow.

    —Melody Beattie (American author)

How often do you give appreciation?

We all hunger for appreciation,
　　while not wanting to admit our hunger
　　to ourselves or to others.

Yet, out of habit and our resistance to fear,
　　most of us are not consistent
　　in noticing and expressing our appreciation
　　to those we love and care about in a way
　　that both consistently and pleasurably impacts them.

The "Appreciation Process" is a proactive and intensive process
　　that will change this habit,
　　creating new learning in ourselves that
　　supports and nourishes both us and those around us.
Although you can do this process quickly
　　with just one or two appreciations each time,
　　I recommend setting aside a minimum of 10 minutes
　　　　(or perhaps three appreciations each time)
　　for this process.

Start by noticing something you like about the other person:
　　h/is body, h/is clothes,
　　how s/he presents h/imself to the world,
　　what s/he provides or has provided to you,
　　who s/he is for you, h/is personality or character,
　　how s/he makes you feel, how s/he inspires you,
　　what s/he provides or what s/he is for others,
　　h/is essence, what you see in h/im for h/is future,
　　and so on.

Then, express to h/im the first thing you notice
    with the intention that s/he will experience it in a way
    that creates acceptance and pleasure for h/im.

After you have expressed your appreciation to h/im
        about what you've noticed,
    s/he then shares with you the automatic thoughts and feelings
    s/he had in response to your expression of appreciation.
    In letting you know how s/he experienced
        your expression of appreciation,
    you can begin to discover
        how your appreciations are received by h/im.

You may then take the opportunity
    to re-express your appreciation to h/im
    so that it is received the way you intended.

Remember, the meaning of the communication
    is the response that you get.
Don't get caught up in
        whether or not your partner understood
        what you *really* meant.
    You give away your power with this attitude.

Once you have expressed an appreciation
    and s/he has shared h/is response, then switch,
    so that s/he expresses an appreciation to you
    and you share your automatic response
    to the expression of h/is appreciation.

Continue back and forth for a minimum of 10 minutes
    or three appreciations each.
You can keep going for as long as you like or as time allows.

For couples in romantic/marriage relationships,
    I recommend doing this process a *minimum* of once each day.

Choose someone *today*
    to explain and do
    the Appreciation Process with.
Then notice how it changes how you feel
    about your relationship with h/im.
Notice also the courage you chose
    in initiating and following through on this process.
    Honor yourself for that courage.

                                        ೲ

_____

_____

_____

_____

_____

_____

_____

Once in a century a man may be ruined or made insufferable by praise. But surely once in a minute something generous dies for want of it.

                                       —John Masefield.

The greatest need of every human being is the need for appreciation.

                                       —unknown

You have it easily in your power to increase the sum total of this world's happiness now. How? By giving a few words of sincere appreciation to someone who is lonely or discouraged. Perhaps you will forget tomorrow the kind words you say today, but the recipient may cherish them over a lifetime.

                                     —Dale Carnegie

The Meaning of the Communication is the Response that you Get.

                               —NLP (Neuro-Linguistic Programming) axiom

Are you feeling blessed
in your life now?

Are you out of touch with how great your life is?

Then take yourself through the following process.

Telephone or visit a friend, family member, or colleague.
   Set aside 15 to 30 uninterrupted minutes.
The person with the lowest voice goes first.
Take 10 to 30 seconds each,
   and take turns answering quickly (without thinking too much),
   each of the following questions, starting with the first:

   —What do I like about myself?
   —What's great about my life?
   —What's great about today?
   —How am I blessed?
   —What miracles have I experienced in my life?
   —Who do I love?
   —Who loves me?

After the first person answers
   one of these questions in 15 to 30 seconds,
   then the other person does the same.
Take turns answering the questions for 15 to 30 minutes.
Keep it moving. Enjoy!

Call a friend right now and do this process with them!

Honor yourself for the choice of courage
   to initiate and follow through with this process.

ശ

Is your past past?

For most young children, there is little or no past.
The child anticipates h/is future with peace, excitement,
    and a natural joy that comes from living in the moment.

But for most adults, the past is a reminder
    of guilt, of regret, of blame, of mistakes that we made,
    of unfulfilled dreams,
        of what we didn't do and what others did to us.
For most adults, the past is remembered as a minefield,
    keeping us constantly aware
        of what we must avoid in our present and in our future.

We remain incomplete and disempowered by our past.
We treat our past as if somehow we could change it.
The past is *entirely* past.
    Your past of one minute ago is as unalterable
    as the assassination of Julius Caesar twenty centuries ago.

The only things you can alter about your past (and your present)
    are how you interpret it
    and what new insights you can learn from it
    that will empower you into your future.

I once worked with a woman who experienced her divorce
    as a tragedy in which she blamed both herself
    and her ex-husband.
Her experience tainted her everyday feelings about herself
    and also clouded the possibilities
    for her relationships with men.

I invited her to explore the questions,
 "What were the gifts of my divorce?"
 And "What gifts might I create out of my divorce?"
At first, she resisted the questions, saying,
 "There were *no* gifts in my divorce."
But slowly she began to discover
 gift after gift that came out of her divorce,
 gifts that she would in no way give up today,
 even in exchange for not having gone through the divorce!

We have *only* the present, *now* and *now* and *now*.
We can ask of ourselves *only* what can we do *now*.

The good news is that what we can do *now*,
 both in action and in interpretation,
 can completely alter both our experience of the past
 and our experience for the future,
 thereby altering our experience of *now*!

Is your past past?
Do you anticipate your future
 so that you are empowered by your past
 rather than disempowered by your past?

What aspects of your past do you experience
 as bad or damaging?
What gifts might you discover or create
 out of these experiences?
What new interpretations might you explore
 that would empower you?

Use your courage and creativity to live in the present.

◦∾

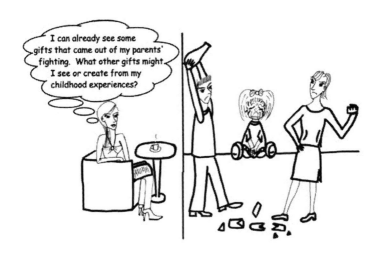

How can your past be a present to you?

How can your past be a gift to you?

When my new Chinese friends ask about the women in my past,
    I often respond with, "I've been happily married
        and happily divorced twice."

However, in saying this I am not being completely accurate.
    There were many rough times in my marriages.
But I realize that I would never
    have grown and developed into the person I am today,
    if it had not been for the contribution my wives
        and my marriages made to my life.

My father and I had a difficult time with each other
    when I was a child and a teenager.
But the gifts that my father
    gave to my life are incalculable!

Some of the schools I attended and some of the teachers I had
   were of very poor quality (and absolutely boring).
But I can see now that they were the perfect stimulus
   to help me become the person I am today.

It is often an inconvenience that I am borderline hypoglycemic.
But this condition has motivated me
   to eat more healthfully than most people.
      Partly for that reason, I am one of the most
      energetic and vital 59-year-olds I know.

If you experience any part of your past
   as a *goft* (a word I created that means the opposite of *gift*),
   then your lifeblood is being drained by your past,
   sapping your energy, your courage, and your spirit,
   and blocking your ability to live life to its fullest.

Do you think of any part of your past as a *goft* instead of a *gift*?

If so, begin to play with the following questions:
   "How might that have been a gift?" and/or
   "How might I create that as a gift?"
   Notice the choice of courage involved
      in exploring these questions.

Keep asking yourself these questions
   until you begin to discover and create more and more gifts
   from the past circumstances of your life.

സ

_____

_____

_____

_____

_____

_____

Will your unspoken appreciation of others die with you?

Consider as a fact that many times each day
    you do *not* speak words of appreciation
        (thanks, admiration, inspiration, etc.)
    that you are already feeling and thinking
    to those around you.

Somehow, usually without awareness,
    we imagine that those around us,
    those who are important in our lives,
    already know and already feel
    our appreciation, saving us the effort
    (and perhaps the courage)
    of expressing the difference (however big or small)
    these people are making for us.

And, in particular, we rarely *genuinely*
    express our appreciation to those *most* dear to us.

Let me give you an example
    of how I expressed my appreciation to my mother.
Here is what I mailed to her
    and to some other friends in July 2000.

Sometimes, Mama, I imagine
    what I will say about you at your funeral
    (hopefully many, many happy years away from now).
I can always feel the depth of my love for you
    and gratitude to you,
    for what you've done for me, and, especially,
    for who you were and are for me.

But you are the number one person
    whom I want to hear what I would say about you.
I have decided to write a eulogy now,
        not only so that I can share it with my other friends,
        but *mainly* so that I can share it with you.
Every day you are happily alive, I am grateful.
May you have many, many more years of enjoyment in your life.

For my mother, Dorothy,
    78 years old now, living in the beautiful mountains of Tennessee.

I remember
. . . after walking a mile and a half home from grammar school,
        you would have pan-fried potatoes
        (with a bottle of catsup) waiting for me.
        We would sit and talk together as I ate my potatoes
        (my favorite dish then, next to hamburgers).
. . . lying on the bed, with you in the middle,
        my sister on one side and me on the other.
        We would be propped up on our elbows
        and you would read to us for an hour at a time:
        Little Men, Little Women, Old Yellar,
        How the Leopard Got Its Spots,
        articles from the *Reader's Digest,* etc.
. . . having long, enjoyable conversations with you
        about the meaning of life, God, psychology, etc.
. . . you calling me in from playing in the backyard
        to let me know that my favorite radio show was on,
        either *The Shadow Knows* or *Yukon King.*
. . . building a fire with you
        and canning vegetables together in the backyard.

. . . how you would express appreciation and admiration
      for my crazy projects like
      digging tunnels all through the backyard,
      blood typing all the neighbors,
      preparing and conducting the yearly "great leaf party,"
      planning and conducting the egg-fight contest,
      building various tree houses, snow sleds, and go-carts,
      trying to enroll neighbors and students
          into my libertarian political philosophy.
. . . always knowing and feeling that,
      whatever troubles I had in school or with my peers,
      you were always there for me.
. . . how you would wake me up in the morning for school
      with a cheerful "Rise and shine!"
. . . how I always felt that you treated me,
      my brother, and my sister fairly.
. . . how I always knew and felt
      that you loved me, liked me, respected me, and honored me.
. . . how I always felt listened to by you
      and how you made me feel special.
. . . how you always made me feel smart and kind.
. . . how you gave me the message
      that being selfish was okay (we're all selfish).
. . . how you managed to let me grow up
      without my having to worry about the "adult problems"
      you had with my father and with the finances.
. . . you telling me that I had the power
      and the freedom to become anything I wanted to become.
. . . you telling me that I should always think for myself.
. . . you telling me that I should look both ways
      before crossing the street.

. . . thinking that your life and the way you led your life
    was greater and more magnificent
    than any of the lives of great people I had read about,
    and that I had the privilege
    of being the son of this great person.
. . . so many of the aphorisms or thoughts that you would repeat
    (with help from my sister Karen in remembering
    some of these and apologies for any paraphrasing):

"Act the way you want to be,
    and soon you'll be the way you act."
"People residing in glass houses
    should refrain from throwing hard obstacles."
    (It took me a while to understand this one).
"It's the purpose of teenagers to rebel."
"Children should be seen *and* heard."
"When parents say to their children, 'Act your age,'
    they don't see that the children *are* acting their age."
"We're all here to leave the world
    a little bit better place than we found it."
"The world doesn't owe us a living."
"Don't be an iconoclast."
    (I was rather argumentative as a child and young teenager).
"Politeness is the grease that helps us get along better."
"You can be dead right or dead wrong.
    But both ways you're dead,"
    (usually spoken with regard to driving a car).
"Remember, there's over a million dollars in this car,"
    (emphasizing love for us
    and the need for safety when we went driving).
"I am captain of my fate, I am the master of my soul;
    and I thank what Gods may be for my unconquerable soul."

"To thine own self be true,
    and it must follow as night follows day,
    thou then cannot be false to any man."
"Let us then be up and doing with a heart for any fate;
    still achieving, still pursuing, learn to labor and to wait."
"Oh joy! Oh rapture! Unforeseen!"
"When the sun in the morning peeps over the hill
    and kisses the roses on my windowsill . . ."
    (singing).
"Whatever things are lovely, think on these things."
"A person is about as happy as they make up their mind to be."
"People make their own good luck."
"Wherever you go, you can find friends."
"Strangers are just friends you haven't met yet."
"By and large, people are decent."

But one gift, Mama, stands out above all the rest,
    a gift, not of what you gave me or did for me,
    but a gift of who you were and are for me.
I always knew that you loved your life
    and were glad to be born into this world.
Your greatest gift to me was your own happiness.
Whenever I felt a little depressed or resigned,
    you were always there as a first-hand example
    that joy in life was always open to me.

Also, you never made me feel "responsible" for your happiness.
    I always knew and know that you love me, think about me,
    are glad to hear from me.
But you were and are not waiting around for me to "fill your life."
Whenever I call you from Tokyo
    (where I was living when I wrote this),
    I have to call you two or three times
    before I can catch you home.

You're out busy having a great time
　　playing bridge or partying with your friends,
　　volunteering for the hospital or park service,
　　tending your flower garden, reading a book,
　　or walking through your beloved woods.
You're *my* mom!

Ask yourself throughout your day,
　　"How might I express appreciation now?"

Have you ever *really* expressed
　　to your mother, to your father,
　　to your child, to your brother or sister,
　　to your wife or husband,
　　to anyone really important in your life,
　　the incredible difference s/he has made for you?

Do it now.

Isn't it interesting that expressing appreciation
　　is often a choice of courage?

**For more essay(s) on courage and gratitude,
　　see www.GoldWinde.com/Cbook/More/Gratitude.**

The bitterest tears shed over graves are for words left unsaid and
deeds left undone.
　　　　—Harriet Beecher Stowe (1811-1896, American writer)

What is the difference between power and empowerment?

Knowing and living the difference
  between power (control) and empowerment
  is perhaps the most important distinction in creating a life
  of genuine self-expression and accomplishment.

Power is fairly simple and straightforward.
  If we ask ourselves directly and honestly,
  we know where we have power.
For example, under normal conditions,
  we all have the power
  to brush our teeth,
  to pick up the telephone and dial a number,
  to open our mouth and say "yes" or "no,"
  to write or speak a request,
  to show up for an appointment on time.

We can acquire and develop
  knowledge, tools, and relationships
  that can increase the number and type of events
  we have power over.
Almost all of education (unfortunately)
  is focused *only* on how to acquire more power.
  Empowerment is usually treated as if it did not exist
  or was not centrally relevant to one's life and education.

We all want power.
We all need power.
It helps us to predict and control outcomes
  and to feel safer and act more safely.

However, our single-minded focus
>on power and control disempowers us.
We neglect the domain of empowerment,
>the domain in which we have no guarantee
>our actions will cause the results we want.

Consider again the examples given above.
We have the power to brush our teeth;
>but we cannot guarantee our teeth will be cavity-free.
We have the power to dial a number;
>but we cannot guarantee
>the person we want to speak with will be there.
We have the power to say "no"
>to a request from a friend to borrow money;
>but we cannot guarantee
>our friend will take our refusal in the spirit of friendship.
We have the power to request that we be hired for a job;
>but we cannot guarantee that we will get the job.
We have the power to show up for an appointment on time;
>but we cannot guarantee
>the other person will show up on time or even at all.

We have power and control over a million things.
But there are ten billion other things that we can't control.

Becoming more and more aware
>of where we have control and where we don't
>is a choice of courage, again and again.

Courage is the *key* to empowerment.

If we always insist on power and control,
  we disempower ourselves,
  missing the countless opportunities for courageous action
  —courageous action that will bring joy and results to our lives
  that power and control alone can *never* do.

Continually ask yourself,
  "Where do I have power?"
  "Where do I have control?"
And most importantly,
  "Where do I lack power but could empower myself
    through the choice of courage?"

**For more essay(s) on courage and control vs. influence,
  see www.GoldWinde.com/Cbook/More/Con-vs-Inf.**

_____

_____

_____

Most of us will trade anything we have for a good false sense of control.
—*Brad Blanton in Radical Honesty*

There is a time to let things happen and a time to make things happen.
—*Hugh Prather*

If we are not responsible for the thoughts that pass our doors, we
are at least responsible for those we admit and entertain.
—*Charles Newcomb (screenwriter and director)*

Nearly all men can stand adversity, but if you want to test a man's
character, give him power.
—*Abraham Lincoln (1809-1865, U.S. President)*

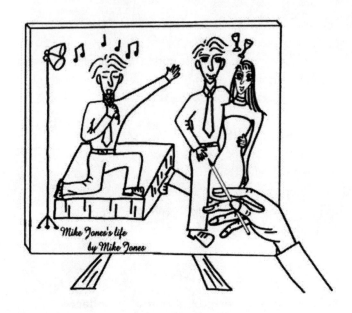

Mike Jones's life
by Mike Jones

Create your life as a work of art

By default, most of us design our lives
　　with accomplishment as the primary focus.

Accomplishment!
　　Accomplishment!
　　　　Accomplishment!

We think more accomplishment is always better.
We are driven toward accomplishment
　　both by our desire for approval from others
　　　　(and from ourselves)
　　and by a compelling desire to feel safe and secure.

This life paradigm, however, is ultimately bankrupt.

When accomplishment is the *primary* focus of our lives,
    then accomplishment is a bottomless bucket,
    always beckoning us forth
    like a proverbial carrot on a stick, always promising,
    but never really delivering the satisfaction
    that we have done enough, and that our life is great.

Instead, how might we experience our lives
    if we began to live and design them as a work of art,
    a work of art that inspires us,
    that gets us up in the morning,
    a life that we would wish on our best friend
    —not only into our future, but moment by moment,
    minute by minute, and hour by hour?

Choose courage now to start creating the grand design
    for *your* life as a work of art,
    a work of art that continuously renews your passion for life.

In each moment, ask yourself,
    "How might I bring
        beauty, drama, artistry, and fun
        to this moment,
        to this hour,
        to this day?"

"No pain, no gain?"
"More pleasure, more gain!"

Did you ever wonder,
    "What if Mother Nature forgot to make sex pleasurable?"
Imagine for a moment,
      what it would be like if sex was *not* pleasurable,
        either for men or women.
Imagine that, if a man and woman wanted to have a baby,
    they would have to think to themselves,
          "We want a baby. We want to tie ourselves down
          for at least 18 years. We want to spend at least $150,000
          that we don't currently have. We want to worry
          about our child's safety and how s/he will turn out.
          We want the woman to go through nine months
          of discomfort, not to mention the pain of childbirth.
          Why don't we do this 'messy thing' called sex
          that is required to get the woman pregnant
          so we can have a baby?"
How many babies do you think would be born
    if Nature forgot to make sex *really* pleasurable?
    Not very many.
But Nature decided that having babies
    was essential to the survival of the species.
So she made sex so pleasurable for both men and women,
    at least long enough to get the woman pregnant,
    that we don't have to worry
    about people having enough babies.
If fact, it could be said that we have the opposite problem!
    China, with its one-child policy,
    uses the strong force of government
    to try to prevent its citizens
    from having too many babies.

What if we took a lesson from Mother Nature
    in designing pleasure and fun
    into what we consider to be important?

What if we could somehow attach
    fun and pleasure
    to other important things we need or want to get done?

Exercise. Studying. Doing our job. Keeping our desk clean.
What are you doing that you don't enjoy doing?
What do you need to do that you're not doing?
Or, what do you need to stop doing that you're not stopping?

If you used your creativity (and the choice of courage)
    to design ways to make fun and pleasurable
    those things that you need to do,
    imagine the difference that would make for you!
If you used your creativity (and the choice of courage)
    to design ways to make fun and pleasurable
    not doing those things which would be better left undone,
    imagine the difference that would make for you!

Let me give you an example from my own life.
I was living in Phoenix, Arizona in 1995.
I was not exercising, even though I knew the value of exercise,
    because it seemed boring and uncomfortable to me.
I asked myself, "How can I make exercise fun?"

Then, I created a solution:
About four times per week, a different friend of mine
    would show up at my apartment at 6:30 in the morning.
We would drive 10 minutes away
    to Camelback Mountain or Squaw Peak Mountain.

Together, we would climb the mountain,
    adjusting our climb for a one-hour workout,
    talking and having great conversations
    all the way up and all the way down.

I had no problem getting good exercise this way.
And, in fact, I received many more benefits
    than I would have obtained through
    a non-creative exercise approach.

You can create fun and pleasure in almost anything.

I invite you to choose something you have not been doing
        that you need to do
    and create a way to make it fun and pleasurable,
    so that you can *hardly wait to do it!*

Even though it might not be obvious,
    choosing to be creative and proactive in this way
    is also a choice of courage.

    Honor yourself for choosing this courage.

✎

_____

_____

_____

_____

_____

_____

_____

It is not doing the thing we like to do, but liking the thing we have
to do that makes life blessed.
        —*Johann Wolfgang von Goethe (1749-1832,*
            German lyric poet, novelist, dramatist)

Don't waste your patience by waiting

One of the best definitions of patience I have ever heard is:
"Patience is finding something else
interesting to do while you are waiting."

Let me share with you how I have applied
this definition in my own life.

When I am standing in line at the bank or the supermarket,
I turn to the person behind me or in front of me and ask,
"What do you like best about standing in line?"
This question usually gives me the opportunity
to enjoy some very good conversation.

If I'm riding in a taxi and it looks like
I will be late for my appointment,
I ask myself the question,
"How might I benefit from being late?"
I also practice embracing the fear associated with being late.

If I am going someplace where I might need to wait in line
or if I know I'll be riding in a taxi or train for a while,
I take along a good book.

If I need to do something I don't usually enjoy
or wish that I had finished,
I ask myself the question,
"How might I use my creativity
to bring enjoyment, interest, or curiosity
to my current circumstances?"

If I am not really listening to someone
    and I am waiting for them to finish what they are saying,
I ask myself the question,
        "How might I use my creativity and my courage
        to focus my attention
        to enjoy, to learn, to contribute to this person
        through my listening?"

Under what circumstances
    do you find yourself feeling impatient?

How might you bring your creativity and courage
    to these circumstances and/or
    find something else interesting to do
    while you are waiting?

Notice that creating patience in this new way
    often involves a choice of courage.

☙

_____

_____

_____

_____

_____

_____

_____

_____

_____

A truly happy person is one who can enjoy the scenery on a detour.
                                    —*unknown*

Who ever is out of patience is out of possession of their soul.
                        —*Francis Bacon (1561-1626,*
                        British philosopher, essayist, statesman)

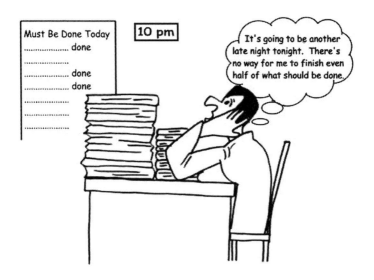

Are you a do-aholic?

"I've got to do that."

"I must do this."

"I cannot go to bed before this is complete."

"There's not enough time in the day."

"I'm so tired."

"There's never an end to it all."

"I never feel complete at the end of my day."

"Where does the day go?"

"What's it all for anyway?"

Does any of this sound familiar?

Many of us are do-aholics ("aholic" as in alcoholic).

We are task-aholics. We are do-more-more-more-aholics.

For ourselves, we are like the poor manager
    whose idea of management
    is to expect and demand far more of the employee
    than can possibly be achieved—or than can possibly
    be achieved with any grace and enjoyment.
And then, at the end of the day,
    we berate the employee for not getting it all done.

For ourselves, for our own life,
    we must fulfill at least two separate roles:
    the *doer* and the *manager*.

Most of us do a very poor job of managing our own life,
    often thinking that good management
    consists of making interminable and un-doable
    (for the time available) lists of things that must be done.

Let me suggest that the *primary* job of the manager
    is to set the week up, to set the day up
    so that the doer can win at least 95 percent of the time.
And, by winning, I mean that, at the end of the day,
    you can look back (as the doer) and say,
    "I got everything done on the list
    and even did a few extra items!"

The job of the manager
    is to *realistically* look at
    how long it will likely take
    to accomplish the different tasks,
    and to include in the planning
        enough buffer for breakdowns
    and even make room to take advantage
        of currently unseen opportunities
        that may arise.

The manager will most likely need to choose courage to say,
    "No, I will *not* do this today" or
    "No, I will *not* include this in my life."

For every *yes* you say, you must say *no*
        (to yourself and/or to others)
    a thousand times (either implicitly or explicitly).
When you are not willing to say *no*,
    then you sabotage the *yes* you have previously said
        (and the *yes* that may arise in response to a new
        opportunity).

Again, the job of the manager is to set things up
    so that the doer can win!

Do you consistently set aside time for your "manager"
    to set up your year, to set up your week, to set up your day
    so that your "doer" can win?

If not, put a structure in place to do that now.

Honor yourself for the courage that you choose
    to say *no* to yourself and others
    so that you and the "doer" can win.

                     ข

_____
_____
_____
_____
_____
_____
_____
_____
_____
_____

Do you get overwhelmed?

Most of us get overwhelmed sometimes.
Some of us live in a constant state of overwhelm.

Overwhelm usually has two aspects that need to be addressed.

First, overwhelm is a form of fear.
We are frightened of what will happen
    if we don't get everything done.

Because our deep habit is to resist our fear,
    what we are feeling is not simply fear,
    it is resisted fear.
Therefore, the first step in dealing with overwhelm
    is to embrace our fear by taking deep breaths,
    breathing into our fear and saying to ourselves
        (out loud, if possible),
    "Boy, am I scared!" several times.
By doing this,
    we can begin to align with the energy of our fear
    so that we can tap into that energy
    and use it for good purposes.
Often, this exercise alone will provide us
    with the sense of resourcefulness
    needed to dispel the overwhelm and get the job done.

However, there is often a second aspect of overwhelm.

Our overwhelm, our fear is trying to tell us that something is off,
    that the design of our life and our choices are not working.

This occurs most often when,
    instead of focusing on creating our life
        so that we can enjoy the process
        of getting to wherever we are going,
    we create our life (either by default or by design)
    as a series of tasks and goals,
        in which the primary focus is just getting things done.
This also occurs when we live out of the idea
    that "we can do it/have it all."
    We can *never* "do it all."
    For every "yes" we choose, we must choose a thousand "no's."

To begin to redesign our life,
    to choose to do things we love,
    to cancel old choices,
    to say "no" to what we put on our plate,
    to renegotiate our agreements,
    to say "no" to others and even to ourselves,
    often requires a choice of courage.
Our unwillingness to say "no" to others is most often
    driven by a fear of disapproval
    or a desperate desire for approval.
Our unwillingness to put more focus on enjoying the process
    is most often driven by our fear that we won't survive
    if we let go of trying to tightly control the outcomes of our life.

Take a moment to examine how your overwhelm
    may be related to your prior unwillingness to choose courage.

How might you choose courage now
    to address overwhelm in your life?

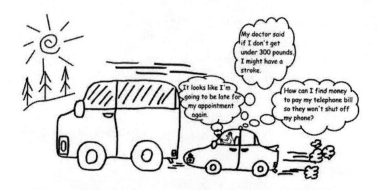

Life without buffers will kill you

Do you know what the world's safest form of transportation is
    (based upon deaths per passenger mile)?

Airplanes? Bicycles? Walking?

The answer is elevators.
    Per passenger mile traveled, elevators win the safety award
    over every other form of transportation.

Why?
One of the reasons is because
    the safety factor (the buffer) is so great.
We've all noticed those signs in the elevator that say,
    "Maximum capacity 15."
Passenger elevators are actually built
    to handle 20 times this weight
    without breaking!
A large safety buffer!

The amount of breakdown and difficulty in our lives
    is often a direct result of our failure
      to create and maintain buffers.

Consider the following questions and try to discover areas
    where your buffers are dangerously thin.

Do you maintain a low level of stress,
    so that it's difficult to push you over the edge?
Do you have extra friends you can call upon,
    so that an emotional crisis is more easily weathered?
Do you drive far enough behind the car in front of you,
    so that a quick stop doesn't result in an accident?
Do you keep your regular expenses well below your regular income
    so that you have plenty of room for unforeseen expenses
    or for taking advantage of new opportunities
        (like moving to Shanghai)?
Do you let people know (in the spirit of partnership)
    when something they do is annoying or upsetting you,
    so that you don't build up resentment
    and then either withdraw from them or blow your top,
    thereby permanently damaging the relationship?
Do you allow enough extra time and resources
    in the planning of a project so that it's no big deal
    if it takes longer than expected to complete?
Do you practice Lombardi Time
    (after Vince Lombardi, the great football coach)
    by showing up ten minutes early to your appointments?

Not only does a life with buffers
    allow greater progress and smoother sailing, it also allows us
    to derive more pleasure from the journey as well.

Ask yourself, "In what areas of my life do I lack buffers?
What does this cost me?"

Even though it may not be immediately obvious,
people often live their lives *without* buffers
because they are resisting some fear or fears.

Choose an area of your life where you consistently lack buffers
and ask yourself,
"What fear might I feel if I chose to create buffers in this area?"

Can you feel how creating buffers in your life
would be a choice of courage for you?

&

_____

_____

_____

_____

_____

_____

_____

_____

_____

_____

Next week there can't be any crisis. My schedule is already full.
—*Henry Kissenger (former U.S. Secretary of State)*

Good luck is with the man who doesn't include it in his plan.
—*Graffiti*

The time and effort required to complete a project are always more
than you expect, even when you take into account Hofstadter's
Law.

—*Hofstadter's Law*

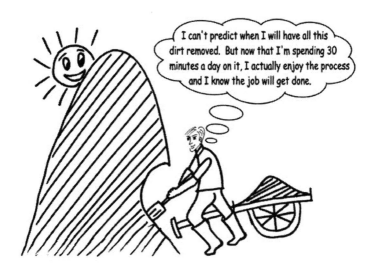

To smell the roses, get rid of some goals

Many of us are very goal oriented or think we should be.

We say to ourselves or others,
"I will finish writing my book in 40 days."
"I promise myself I will do that by the 10th."
"I will be making $6,000 per month by February 1."
"I will have a new job in six weeks."

Goals are important.
Sometimes we must "box ourselves in" and declare that
"By this date, I will have that result!"

But it may be a bad idea
to set as many goals as most of us do,
especially goals in which the result
is difficult to control or predict within a certain time frame.

In setting up goals,
> with the intention of making progress in our lives,
> we often set ourselves up for unnecessary disappointment
> *and* we create pressures in our lives
> that make it difficult to "smell the roses"
> and enjoy the journey.

Consider the idea that it may often be
> a better idea to set up a "destination,"
> rather than a goal.

A destination says,
> "I will get a certain result
> and I will be in consistent action to get that result,
> until it is achieved."

A destination does not have a deadline.

A destination moves us consistently toward our outcome,
> while allowing the flexibility
> to adjust powerfully to life's changing circumstances
> and to smell the roses along the way.

For example,
> I could set a destination of earning $10,000 per month.

To be a valid destination, however,
> it must also include some structures of support
> > and some ways to enjoy the consistent actions
> that will move me closer
> to my destination until it has been attained.

The focus is, more importantly, on the process,
> rather than the result "by a certain date."

What goals do you have in your life
> that might be more appropriately set up as destinations?
> Choose one of these and design it as a destination.

What goals have you been avoiding,
    which, when re-framed as destinations,
    now seem like something
    you'd like to do and would be willing to do?
    Set one of these up as a destination.

Notice how it may be a choice of courage
    to relinquish "control" of a goal
    and take a risk with the "flow" of a destination.

☙

It is good to have an end to journey toward; but it is the journey that matters, in the end.

    —*Ursula K. Le Guin (1929-, American writer)*

Establishing goals is all right if you don't let them deprive you of interesting detours.

    —*Doug Larson*

Plenty of people miss their share of happiness, not because they didn't find it, but because they didn't stop to enjoy it.

    —*Edward Postel*

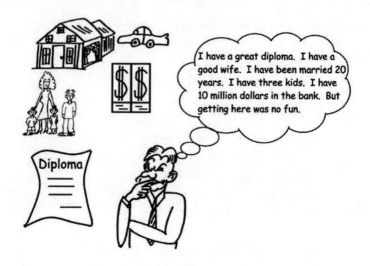

If you didn't enjoy the journey, so what?

If you're about to die and your life is over,
  but you haven't lived a life
  that you'd wish on your best friend,
    so what?

If you've stayed married to the same person
  for 30 years (or 15 or five or one),
  but you haven't loved and been loved
  with feelings of passion or tenderness
  or excitement or specialness,
    so what?

If you've made $10,000,000,
  but you haven't enjoyed and relished
  the process of doing so,
    so what?

If you've earned your degree
    and you've passed all the tests,
      but you haven't enjoyed the process of learning,
        so what?

If you've raised three kids,
    but you haven't felt blessed
    by their presence in your life,
        so what?

If you've worked hard and completed the job,
    but you haven't enjoyed the process,
        so what?

If the last hour did not bring you
    adventure, peace, love, passion,
    curiosity, excitement, or pleasure,
        so what?

Beware of the reward at the end of the tunnel!
    Let it be *only* the icing on the cake.
    Create the "journey through each tunnel"
        as the cake itself.

Choose the courage
    of context, creativity, and curiosity (the five Cs)
    to create each and every moment of your life
    as a work of art, a work of art so magnificent
    that you'd wish it on your best friend.

**For more essay(s) on courage and your life as a work of art,
see www.GoldWinde.com/Cbook/More/WorkofArt.**

Are you taking care of NOW?

"This above all: to thine own self be true,
    and it must follow, as the night the day,
    thou canst not then be false to any man."
    —from William Shakespeare's *Hamlet*

Consider as a possible corollary to this maxim:
    "If you *really* take care of *this* moment,
    then your future will take care of itself."

If you act with integrity in this moment,
    then your future will take care of itself.
If you act with courage in this moment,
    then your future will take care of itself.
If you are present in this moment,
    then it is possible to be present
        in every moment of your future.
If you are grateful for this moment,
    then it is possible to be grateful
        in every moment of your future.

In some real sense, there is *no* future.
It is always *now*. It is always this *moment*.
The future is an interesting and valuable invention
    to add intrigue, adventure, and possibility to the quality of *now*.

Welcome to the future. It is now.

Are you taking care of *now*?
It is a choice of courage to take care of *now*.

৵

The future AND the now

Almost all the people I know don't have enough time.
　　Time for what?
Almost all the people I know think their lives will be better
　　when they have . . . .
　　But what about now?
Almost all the people I know are sacrificing their present
　　for the sake of their future.

I agree that we need a future; we need things to work toward.
　　This adds aliveness and zest to our present.
However, if we have not chosen a future that excites us
　　and we have not designed a process of getting there
　　　　that is energizing and enjoyable
　　and we have not created a balance in our lives
　　　　whereby we can "smell the roses" along the way,
　　then we are sacrificing the present in the name of the future.

And once the future we have sacrificed for
　　finally arrives and becomes the new present,
　　we will continue to sacrifice our present
　　　　(because it is our habit and it feels safer at the moment)
　　on the altar of our future.
In this way, we avoid really living our whole life,
　　because it never comes, it never arrives;
　　it's always getting pushed off into our future.

Ask yourself, "Can I rejoice in *this* moment?"
What courage, focus, or creativity might be required
　　to rejoice in *this* moment?

What is SO valuable that it's NOT worth waiting for?

Some things are worth waiting for.
But the *most* valuable thing in life is *not* worth waiting for:
 savoring the process of whatever you're doing.

For example, it's worth waiting for the moment
 when you've finally created the wealth you want.
But it is more valuable to savor the process
 of creating the wealth you want.
  You can choose the courage and creativity
   to savor that process *right now*.

It's worth waiting for the moment
 when you've finally built your business step by step.
But it is more valuable to savor the process
 of building your business.
  You can choose the courage and creativity
   to savor that process *right now*.

It's worth waiting for the moment
 when you finally found that special person in your life.
But it is more valuable to savor the process
 of finding and attracting that person.
  You can choose the courage and creativity
   to savor that process *right now*.

It's worth waiting for the moment
 when your body is finally in great shape.
But it is more valuable to savor the process
 of getting your body in great shape.
  You can choose the courage and creativity
   to savor that process *right now*.

It's worth waiting for the moment
  when your marriage is finally the way you want it.
But it is more valuable to savor the process
  of making your marriage the way you want it.
  You can choose the courage and creativity
    to savor that process *right now.*

It's worth waiting for the moment
  when you can finally experience your life
    as a fantastic work of art.
But it is more valuable to savor the process
  of creating your life as a fantastic work of art.
  You can choose the courage and creativity
    to savor that process *right now.*

Are there areas of your life where you have too much patience?
Are you waiting to choose courage and creativity
  to savor the process of whatever you're doing?

Remember that your life is forever happening in the now.

Choose the courage to savor the process of life *right now.*

ͽ

_____
_____
_____
_____
_____
_____
_____
_____

Enjoy the journey, enjoy every moment, and quit worrying about
winning and losing.
  —*Matt Biondi (1965-, American swimmer)*

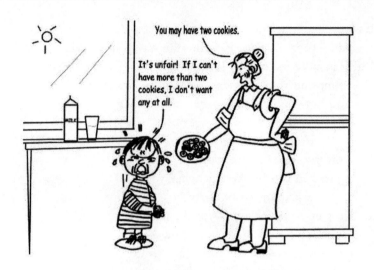

Do you cry over the cookies
you don't have?

As a child I spent summer vacations with my grandparents
    in the mountains of Tennessee, and my grandmother would
    often make batches of oatmeal cookies.
    I *loved* oatmeal cookies!

I remember the following drama (repeated many times)
    with Boog, my grandfather, and Beebe, my grandmother.

"Beebe, may I have some oatmeal cookies?" I asked.
"Sure, you may have two before dinner," she replied.
After quickly devouring the two cookies, I would ask,
    "May I have some more cookies?"
She would reply, "You may have more after dinner."
I would then start to argue with her
    and I would end up crying when she persisted in saying "no."

At this point, Boog would chime in and say,
    "You're crying because you *had* cookies!"
At the time, I did not appreciate the wisdom of his response.
    In fact, it was so infuriatingly logical that it annoyed me.

But how often do we cut off our noses to spite our faces
    by "crying because we had cookies"?
Or, in an even more common scenario,
    how often do we miss out in life
    by not taking the cookies we could have
    because we focus on other cookies that we can't have?

Have you ever *not* started a project
    because you couldn't do your *best* at it?

Have you ever *not* invited a girl or boy out
    because they were not your *first* choice?

Have you ever *not* gone for a better job
    because it wasn't your *real* passion?

Have you ever *not* spoken up about your feelings
    because you couldn't express them *perfectly*?

Have you ever *not* started a great relationship
    because you knew it would not be *forever*?

Have you ever *not* started a great relationship
    because you knew you would not be the *only* one s/he loved?

Have you ever *not* been fully present with someone
    because you're waiting to be with someone else *better*?

Our insistence
    on perfection,
    on having everything we want,
    on maintaining our standards,
    on following our rules,
    on making sure things are fair,
diminishes our aliveness,
    clogs up the momentum of our lives,
    and generally makes us rigid and inflexible.

Consider that
    waiting on perfection,
    insisting on having everything you want,
    maintaining your standards,
    always following your rules, and
    making sure things are fair
are just different ways
    of trying to feel safe and more comfortable.

To take a risk with what we could have,
    to put all our heart into what is before us,
    to live our life *now*,
this is a choice of courage,
    again and again and again.

❧

_____

_____

_____

_____

_____

_____

_____

_____

_____

Discover your life inspirations

Once you have discovered and uncovered
   your essential life inspirations,
   you will clearly make choices in your life
   that you are satisfied with and inspired by.

When we are unclear about our inspirations,
   life occurs more as a game of avoidance,
   rather than one of full self-expression.

What is a life inspiration?

If you have identified a valid life inspiration for yourself,
   then,
      when your life is filled with that particular expression of life,
   you are alive, you are self-expressed, you are free,
      you are yourself.

How do you discover your life inspirations?

First, let's consider some examples.
Here are my life inspirations:
   playfulness, interpersonal adventure,
   one-on-one connection with others,
   innocence, romance.

Let me suggest just a few other possible life inspirations:
   beauty, family, accomplishment,
   connection with God or spirit,
   camaraderie, teamwork, community,
   simplicity, passion, serenity, learning, nature,
   service to others, curiosity, leadership.

There are hundreds, perhaps thousands,
 of possible life inspirations.

Here are some guidelines for discovering your life inspirations:

Come up with at least two inspirations, but not more than five.
Imagine yourself in a culture where anything and everything
 is honored as a valid expression.
Think back upon times where you *really* felt alive,
 self-expressed, and fully yourself.
 What background feelings did you experience at that time?
When you are present to your inspirations,
 then *nothing* is missing from your life.
 What inspirations would need to be present for you
 to experience the *fullness* of your life?

If an inspiration is designed primarily
 to fix something or prevent something,
 then it is *not* a valid inspiration.
To know if you've uncovered *all* your inspirations,
 ask yourself the question,
 "If I experienced all these inspirations at the *same* time,
 would *anything* be missing from my life at that moment?"
Keep up the process
 of uncovering and refining your life inspirations.

Now that you have some idea of your life inspirations,
 how can you bring these more fully into your life?

Life inspirations are implemented in two complimentary ways:
 in the *immediate moment* and in your *life design*.

In every immediate moment, you can ask yourself the question,
    "How can I bring one or more of my inspirations
        into this moment,
    applying it to my situation and whatever I am doing?"

For example, let's imagine I am ironing my clothes,
    something I might *not* normally associate
    with playfulness, connection,
        adventure, innocence, or romance.
Yet I know I can bring the spirit of playfulness to ironing.
Or I can get in touch with how ironing clothes
    will assist me in connecting with others
    in the domains of connection, adventure, and/or romance.
I can bring the spirit of these inspirations to ironing clothes,
    or to any other activity of my life.

In regularly taking time to design
    your life, your year, your month, your week, your day,
    ask yourself the question,
    "What lifestyle, freedoms, environments, structures,
        projects, practices, people might I choose or create in my life
        that would allow me to more fully express my inspirations?"

For example,
    by living in Japan, by moving to Shanghai,
    by life-coaching over the telephone, by working for myself,
    by setting aside three hours per day for daily interpersonal
        adventures,
    by choosing the courage to speak openly
        with both old friends and new people I meet,
    I am including the lifestyle, freedoms, environments, structures,
        projects, practices, and people that support my inspirations
        of playfulness, interpersonal connection, adventure,
        innocence, and romance.

I invite you to ask yourself the questions that will
    uncover your life inspirations
    and apply these inspirations to your life,
        on both the immediate level and the design level!

Honor yourself for choosing the courage
    to do this.

{Special note: see page 29 for an expression of my life inspirations.}

❧

_____

_____

_____

_____

_____

_____

_____

_____

I've always wanted to be somebody, but I see now I should have
been more specific.

—*Lily Tomlin (1939-,*
American actress, producer and writer)

We act as though comfort and luxury were the chief requirements
of life, when all that we need to make us really happy is something
to be enthusiastic about.

—*Charles Kingsley (1819-1875,*
English author and clergyman)

Each of us has an inner dream that we can unfold if we will just
have the courage to admit what it is. And the faith to trust our own
admission. The admitting is often very difficult.

—*Julia Cameron (artist and writer)*

Who is the final judge?

Do you let your doctor decide,
    against your own judgment,
    on a course of action about your health?
If you do, then *you* are deciding
    that your doctor knows better than you in this regard.

Do you let your teacher decide,
    against your own judgment,
    some course of study?
If you do, then you are deciding
    that your teacher knows better than you in this regard.

Do you accept the recommendations,
    against your own judgment,
    of your friends and/or parents on how to live your life?
If you do, then you are deciding
    that your friends and/or parents know better than you do
    about the best life for you.

Do you accept the words in the Bible or in the Koran,
    against your own judgment,
    as the absolute way to live your life?
If you do, then you are deciding
    that the Bible or the Koran
    (or some other generally accepted religious authority)
    knows better than you do about how to live
    the best possible life for you.

Do you accept the traditions and customs of your society,
    against your own judgment,
    as the best guide for your life?
If you do, then you are deciding
    that the traditions and customs of society
    are better guides than your own judgment
    in providing the best life for you.

No matter what the decision,
    no matter what the choice,
    no matter what the judgment,
there is *no way* you can avoid the fact
    that ultimately it is *your* decision,
    your choice, *your* judgment.

To accept this fact
    and thereby embrace your own freedom
    is the ultimate existential act of courage.

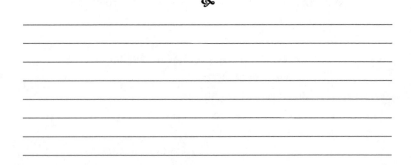

Any person who recognizes this greatest power . . . the power to choose begins to realize that he is the one that is doing the choosing and that friends, although they mean well, cannot do his choosing for him, nor can his relatives. Consequently, he develops real self-confidence based upon his own ability, upon his own action, and upon his own initiative.

—*J. Martin Kohe (American publisher, author)*

Do you know who YOU are?

Are you a case of mistaken identity?

Maybe someone else has you believing that your voice is h/is voice.
And perhaps believing that your voice is h/is voice
    is actually h/is voice also!

Do you ever think,
    "I am so stupid."
    "Don't ask for that. You'll just be rejected."
    "What's the use anyway?"
    "It's just too difficult to do."
    "Life is just so hard."
    "You can't upset them."

Do you ever have thoughts that don't empower you,
    thoughts that actually disempower you?

Consider the idea that these thoughts are *not your* thoughts.

Do you have any choice about thinking these thoughts?
I think not!
These thoughts are completely automatic.
You have no immediate or direct control over them.
How can you even say that they are *your* thoughts,
    just because they appear to emanate from inside of you?

Consider the idea that these thoughts
    are spoken to you by "Mr. Green Man,"
        who sits just inside your right ear and is able to make his words
        sound just like your thoughts.

Consider the idea that Mr. Green Man
  (or Ms. Green Woman, if you prefer)
  loves to fool you into thinking that what he speaks to you
  are *your* thoughts and you *must pay attention* to these thoughts.
S/he's got you well fooled, hasn't s/he?

But it doesn't empower you, it doesn't enliven you
  to listen to these thoughts as if they were your own.

May I suggest a new practice.
Start to notice every time Mr. Green Man
  says something to you
  that doesn't empower you or enliven you.
When he does this, say back to him
  (silently is best if you're around other people!),
  "Thank you for expressing your opinion, Mr. Green Man.
    Right now, I am going to entertain, instead, another
    thought which will empower me and enliven me."

If you will practice listening to
  and speaking to Mr. Green Man in this way,
  I promise you that the thoughts he speaks to you
  will begin to lose their power, step by step, each and every day,
  slowly diminishing into your future.

Enjoy!

Try this new idea on for a week.
Listen to and speak to your Mr. Green Man
  in this way and notice how your life begins to change.

Notice the courage that this listening takes.

ॐ

How to always make the right choice

Do you ever feel,
  while shopping for an item in a store,
  that there are *too many* options to choose from?
Whereas, if you go to the store
  and find a selection of three or fewer items,
  you often feel more comfortable in buying.

Isn't this a strange reaction?

We could make choices more easily
  by arbitrarily limiting our range of items to select from.
  Yet we would prefer
    that the outside world do the limiting for us,
  so we can feel more confident
    that we made the "right" choice.

How much does our insistence on making the right choice
  limit our self-expression and participation in life?

Often, when clients are agonizing over making the right choice,
  I will ask them,
    "If you made the right choice, how would you ever *know*
    it was the right choice anyway?"

Did I (Dwight) make the right choice
  to drop out of college after three years?
Did I make the right choice
  to move from Shelby, North Carolina
  to New York City when I was 22?

Did I make the right choice
  to marry in 1983 my wife who I divorced in 1991?
Did I make the right choice in divorcing her?
Did I make the right choice in moving
  from the United States to Asia in November, 1999?

I *believe* I made the right choice in all these circumstances.
But can I prove it? No, I cannot.

Certainly we need to consider the possible costs and benefits
      (as we currently see them)
    for each choice that we make in our life
      (especially the bigger ones).
However, when all is said and done,
    we can never *know* that we made the right choice.
We can only *live as though* we made the right choice.

Do you agonize over choices?
    How does this limit your power and your enjoyment of life?

The next time you are indecisive in a way that doesn't serve you,
    breathe into your fear, and honor yourself
    for choosing the courage to make a choice
    and to declare it "the right choice."

∾

_____
_____
_____
_____
_____
_____
_____
_____
_____
_____

Does everyone inspire you?

I have noticed that,
 as I view the behavior of others
 from the perspective of choosing courage,
 I can be inspired by and/or have compassion for
 almost everyone I meet.

When we begin to appreciate that all choices
 that *either* accept and move through fear
 or avoid fear (in order to feel safer in the moment),
 are opportunities for us to *either* be inspired
 or to feel compassion and understanding,
 then every human being becomes a blessing in our lives.

In looking for the opportunity to feel inspired,
 remember that courage is a *very* personal choice.
  What courage is for you (in terms of a specific action)
   may not be courage for me (and vice versa).
For example, it may not require courage
 for me to ask a clerk in a store for help in finding an item.
 But it may be a choice of courage for my friend to ask for help.
 I can recognize this and feel inspired
  by my friend's courage while I ask myself,
   "Where is the next opportunity *for me*
    to choose courage in my life?"

Remember that if you view your friend's choice of courage
 in relationship to how frightened s/he is,
 then you can appreciate every time that person chooses courage,
 even if s/he seems to play it *very* safe in life.

For the trained eye,
 the inspiration of courage is everywhere and in everyone.

Identify some recent acts of courage
 of at least three people in your life.

Allow yourself to feel inspired by these people.

Now identify at least three choices of courage
 you have made in the last 24 hours,
 and allow yourself to be inspired by those!

๑

_____

_____

_____

_____

_____

_____

_____

_____

_____

People see God every day. They just don't recognize him.
          —Pearl Bailey

I have yet to meet the common man, although I have heard his name mentioned in many circles. The fellow at my elbow in the subway is the most uncommon person imaginable. "Ordinary" is the word much used to describe him, but I find him wholly miraculous and I am sure he finds himself so.

 —E.B. White (1899-1985, American essayist and literary stylist)

When nobody around you seems to measure up, it's time to check your yardstick.   *—Bill Lemley*

Everything is holy! Everybody's holy! Everywhere is holy! Everyday is in eternity! Everyman's an angel!

    —Allen Ginsberg (1926-1997, American poet)

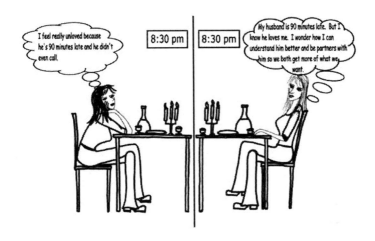

Interpretations:
The power to create your world

Remember the movie, *Pretty Woman*?
"People put you down enough, you start to believe it."
    —Vivian (played by Julia Roberts)
"I think you are a very bright, very special woman."
    —Edward Lewis (played by Richard Gere)
"The bad stuff is easier to believe. Did you ever notice that?"
    —Vivian

Why is the bad stuff easier to believe,
    whether it be about ourselves, about others,
    or about the circumstances of our lives?

Why is it easier to believe that (some) people are evil?
Why is it easier to believe in original sin?
Why is it easier to believe that there is something wrong with us?
Why is it easier to believe that we are not loved?
Why is it easier to believe that we are not special?

Why is it easier to believe that we don't make a difference?
Why is it easier to explain another's actions
 by saying "they don't really care,"
 or "they want to hurt me,"
 or "they are insensitive,"
 or "they are selfish and greedy,"
 or "they are stupid,"
 or "they are lazy,"
 or "they are liars,"
 and so on?
Why is it easier to assess circumstances
 by saying "it's just one of those days,"
 or "it's just my luck,"
 or "there's nothing I can do,"
 or "I don't like it, but what can I do?"
 or "someday, things will be better,"
 or "all the good women are taken,"
 or "the economy is terrible,"
 or "who could enjoy this job?"
 and so on?

It is easier because it *feels* safer.

By buying into
 our often automatic interpretations
 (which we see as facts, not interpretations),
 we lower ourselves to a point where the risk of falling lower
 and suffering further disappointment is minimal.

By buying into our automatic interpretations
 we can avoid the feelings of risk associated
 with *really* understanding others
 as well as *really* understanding ourselves.

Consider the following examples.
    These are just two examples,
    but if you multiply these by the thousands of times
        situations like these occur in your own life
    and the billions of times they occur
        for others around the world,
        imagine the world of difference
        your interpretations can make.

The facts:
    Someone accepts a job for less pay,
        less flexibility and less prestige
    than s/he wanted and felt s/he deserved.

The automatic interpretations:
    This job is beneath me.
    I should be further along in my life by now.
    I'll just have to tolerate this job until I can get a better one.
    I'm embarrassed by what my friends and family
        may think of my doing this job.

New possible interpretations:
    What unexpected gifts might come out of this job?
    What unexpected gifts might I create in this job?
    What breakthroughs might I create for myself
        even when my job circumstances
        do not fit my previous preferences?
    What friends might I make in my new job?
    What new skills might I develop?
    This is an opportunity for me to choose courage
        to do the best job I can and be proud of that,
        while taking the risk that my friends and family
        may think less of me.

The facts:
>A husband comes home from work 90 minutes later
>than he promised to his wife.

His wife's automatic interpretations:
>He doesn't care about me enough to keep his agreements.
>He shows no respect for me.
>He expects me to be here for him, but he's never there for me.
>He's so inconsiderate of me;
>>he keeps his agreements with others, but not with me.

New possible interpretations she could create:
>He cares about me so much
>>in providing financially for me and the kids
>>that he knows when it's important
>>to let a business need override a personal agreement.
>How does my husband experience me
>>that getting home to be with me
>>doesn't seem as appealing as whatever occurred at work?
>>What might I do so that he experiences me differently?
>What benefit might there be in my husband showing up late?
>How I might enroll my husband in being a partner with me
>>so that something like this is unlikely to happen again?

Empowering interpretations
>open up and allow for the *full* range of options and actions
>available in a given set of circumstances.
The art and practice of creating empowering interpretations
>is *not* about boxing yourself (or others) into
>a Pollyanna mindset that prohibits
>powerful and effective action to change the circumstances.

In fact, truly empowering interpretations
will allow a freedom of action
unavailable to us when we are dominated
by our disempowering automatic interpretations.

The next time you find yourself dissatisfied with a situation,
ask yourself,
"How are my automatic interpretations
contributing to my dissatisfaction?"
"What new interpretations can I create to provide myself
with a feeling of empowerment and possibility?"

It is a choice of courage to step into these new interpretations.

༄

_____

_____

_____

_____

_____

_____

Any fact facing us is not as important as our attitude toward it, for
that determines our success or failure.
—*Norman Vincent Peale (1898-1993,*
author of The Power of Positive Thinking)

Experience is not what happens to a man; it is what a man does
with what happens to him.
—*Aldous Huxley (1894-1963, British writer)*

What is the difference between an obstacle and an opportunity?
Our attitude toward it. Every opportunity has a difficulty, and
every difficulty has an opportunity.
—*J. Sidlow Baxter*

Good news:

You may be 100% "at fault"

Imagine that two cars are speeding toward each other
    head-to-head in the same lane,
    the driver of each shouting to the other:
    "Get out of my way!"

The cars crash into each other,
    killing both drivers and all passengers.

Who was at fault?
    Who could have prevented the crash?
    The answer is obvious:
        Either driver could have prevented the crash.
    Both were 100 percent responsible for the crash.

We can look at this behavior and think that it's crazy.
    Only drunken, daredevil, teenage boys
        engage in such foolish behavior, right?
    Wrong!

Look closer and you may find
    similar behavior in your own life.
Look closer and you will notice
    similar behavior in the actions and words of nations.

For example, do you ever say (or know someone who says),
"My job is so stressful. I just can't deal with all the pressure!"?

For you, it looks like the circumstances
    (your boss, your colleagues, etc.)
    are the cause of your stress.

Yet, it is well documented
  that how we view and interpret the circumstances
  of our lives can also be a contributor to our stress.

If your interpretation changed,
  less stress (or even no stress) would be caused.
Or if the circumstances changed, no stress would be caused.
Each and either is up to 100 percent responsible,
  just as in the case of the head-to-head drivers.

Yet, we almost always look outward
  to find the cause of the feelings or circumstances
  that we don't want to have,
  insisting that what's *out there* needs to change.

In doing so, we often miss a gold mine of opportunity
  for discovering how to shift our own responses or behaviors.

As my maternal grandfather would say,
  "For a man with shoes, the earth is paved with leather."

Identify at least three situations in your life
  where the cause of what you don't want
  appears to be external circumstances.

See how you might empower yourself
  by choosing courage to assume that the cause is internal.

❧

_____

_____

_____

_____

_____

_____

_____

Viva la selfishness!

It's very selfish
   to experience the great feelings of deep love.

It's very selfish
   to take good care of your health,
   your energy, your aliveness, and your joy
   in your desire and ability to contribute to others.

It's very selfish
   to want others to feel good around you
   and experience the difference you have made in their lives.

It's very selfish
   to help design a world where each person's selfishness
   easily and naturally contributes to the selfishness of others.

It's very selfish
   to want others to experience selfish pleasure
   in their relationship with you.

Choose courage to be selfish.

❧

_____
_____
_____
_____
_____
_____
_____
_____
_____
_____

Dancing with God

Perhaps life is not really about obeying the rules.

Perhaps life is not really about being a good person.

Perhaps life is an opportunity
    to dance with the universe,
    to allow God and the universe
    to contribute to us and others
    moment by moment, day by day,
    as we engage fully in the experience
    of life and creation,
    letting go of resistance and control where,
    at best, we only have influence.

Come dance with God.
    She is waiting!

℥

And the day came when the risk it took to remain tight inside the
bud was more painful than the risk it took to blossom.
                    —Anaïs Nin (1903-1977,
             French-born American novelist, dancer)

Love God and do what you will.
           —St. Augustine (354-430, philosopher-theologian)

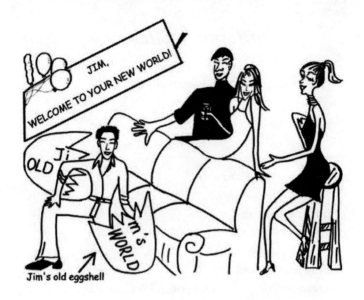

Jim's old eggshell

Your life is over

The life you remember was somebody else's.
It wasn't *yours*.

Your life starts *now*.

The life you *thought* was yours is over.
It's past and gone. The past is past.
In a strange and mysterious way,
    that life somebody else lived
    has prepared you for *this* day—
    the day when *your* life actually begins.

The current circumstances of your life are exactly the same
    as that other person's life s/he just finished living.

Now is the *beginning* of *your life*.

Up until now, the whole purpose
    of this world and everything in it
    has been kept secret from you.
Nevertheless, *everything* has been set up,
    everything has been planned for you
    to be reading this *right now*.

Now is the time to start your life!
Now is the time to wake up!

The secret everyone has kept from you
    is that the whole world, all of nature,
    and all the people in the world
    have been put here as *your* playground
    and as *your* playmates.

The world is your playground!
The world is your opportunity
    for joy and bliss and play and lightheartedness!
The world is your playground
    for drama and intrigue,
    for feeling things to their deepest core.
The world is your playground
    for celebration and accomplishment,
    for creating your life as a work of art.

Welcome to your playground!
Welcome to the fear and excitement!
Choose courage and breathe into the fear
    that is necessary to create the excitement!

It's time to wake up!

♋

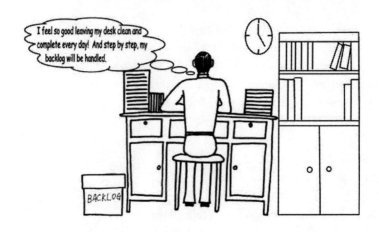

Handle that messy desk once and for all

You can't see the top of your desk.
> Papers are lying around waiting to be filed.
> You can't find the number on a slip of paper
>> for the client you need to call today.
> And so on and so on.
> The backlog is overwhelming and depressing.
> Any intention to turn things around
>> seems doomed to failure in advance.

Here's the simple solution: Divide and Conquer™.

Using one or more large cardboard boxes,
> move all backlog items off your desk, off the floor,
> and from any other areas where you have stored backlog items,
> placing all these items into the cardboard box or boxes.

Now put in place an agreement/promise
    (perhaps with an accountability partner)
    to handle *all new* items before you complete each day.
For example,
    this would include a clean desk at the end of the day
    and all filing handled *before* the end of the day.

The bottom line is simply
    that you may *not* create any *new* backlog.

Now make another agreement/promise
    to spend a minimum number of minutes (e.g., 15)
    each day to work on the backlog items
    that you have put into these boxes.

Once you put this plan into place,
    you will feel an incredible sense
    of freedom, power, and completion
    from the beginning.
Even though it may be a while until all the backlog is addressed,
    you know that, by simply following this very do-able plan,
    you *will* handle all backlog
    and keep yourself current from this point on.

Ask yourself now,
    "If I implemented Divide and Conquer immediately,
        and kept it in place,
        what difference would that make in my life?"
    In a week?
    In a month?
    In a year?
    In a lifetime?

Ask yourself the question,
    "What fears might I have to confront,
        what opportunities for courage might there be

in maintaining and having
a clean and up-to-date workspace?"

Special note: to guarantee that you will keep the promises needed for Divide and Conquer, see the essay Keep ANY Promise You Make to Yourself on page 272.

Take you, step by step, toward your rainbow. Write them down, if you must, but limit your list so that you won't have to drag today's undone matters into tomorrow. Remember that you cannot build your pyramid in twenty-four hours. Be patient. Never allow your day to become so cluttered that you neglect your most important goal—to do the best you can, enjoy this day, and rest satisfied with what you have accomplished.

—*Og Mandino (1923-1996,*
American motivational author, speaker)

The most successful men in the end are those whose success is the result of steady accretion. It is the man who carefully advances step by step, with his mind becoming wider and wider—and progressively better able to grasp any theme or situation—persevering in what he knows to be practical, and concentrating his thought upon it, who is bound to succeed in the greatest degree.

—*Alexander Graham Bell (1847-1922,*
British-born American inventor of the telephone)

As long as we never complete something, we can enjoy the fantasy of how we think it would be if we completed it. We can avoid feeling the risk of how it might actually turn out if we actually completed it.

—*GoldWinde*

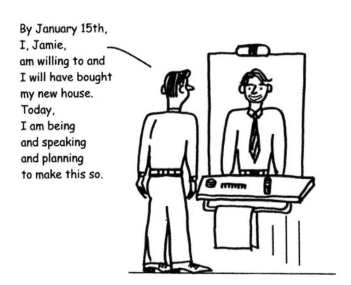

By January 15th,
I, Jamie,
am willing to and
I will have bought
my new house.
Today,
I am being
and speaking
and planning
to make this so.

Create real power now
for any result you want!

Do you have some result
  that you really want to have happen in your future?

Using one simple technique,
  requiring only *one minute* per day
  you can put *real* power behind creating that result.

Let's take a specific example to illustrate how to use this technique.
Imagine that your name is Jamie
  and that you want to buy a new house by January 15, 2005.
  But you're not sure how that can happen.
Then you might write this
  as your "Done Deal™":

"By January 15, 2005,
    I, Jamie,
    am willing to and I will buy my new house.
Today,
    I am being
    and speaking
    and planning
    and acting
    to make this so."

Now here are the full instructions.

For each result you want to create, spend one minute per day
    speaking the Done Deal for your result.
Speak it into your mirror.
Speak it with *nothing* held back,
    so that anyone listening to you (including you, yourself) would say,
    "I can tell this is going to happen
        just by the way you're speaking it."

Go through the Done Deal four times
    (this will take less than one minute).
The first time speak "I" and your name, the way it's written above.
The second time, substituting the word "you" for "I,"
    speak "you" and your name (imagine another person,
        whom you really respect, speaking to you).
    You'll have to change the verb to match the subject
        (e.g., use "are" instead of "am").
The third time speak "he or she" and your name
    (imagine a large group of prestigious people
    talking about the Done Deal that you are creating,
    almost as if it has already happened).
    You'll have to change the verb to match the subject.

The fourth time speak "we" and your name.
    Consider that all parts of you,
    including the part that says, "who are you kidding?"
    and the part that says, "I can do anything,"
    are aligning on the intention that this will happen.
    Again, you'll have to change the verb to match the subject.

For the example with Jamie,
    here's how the whole Done Deal
    would be spoken:

"By January 15, 2005,
    I, Jamie,
    am willing to and I will buy my new house.
Today,
    I am being
    and speaking
    and planning
    and acting
    to make this so."

"By January 15, 2005,
    you, Jamie,
    are willing to and you will buy your new house.
Today,
    you are being
    and speaking
    and planning
    and acting
    to make this so."

"By January 15, 2005,
    he, Jamie,
    is willing to and he will buy his new house.
Today,
    he is being
    and speaking
    and planning
    and acting
    to make this so."

"By January 15, 2005,
    we, Jamie,
    are willing to and we will buy our new house.
Today,
    we are being
    and speaking
    and planning
    and acting
    to make this so."

Take care that speaking the Done Deal
    does not become rote.
Ask yourself after each speaking,
    "Can I tell, just from the way
    that person in the mirror is speaking to me,
    that this is going to happen?"
If the answer is no, then re-speak your Done Deal
    until you are completely congruent
    in your stand and declaration
    that your result will happen.

Choose something you would really like
    to create in your life.
Then write up a Done Deal for it
    and tape it to your bathroom mirror.
Speak it all four ways,
    with nothing held back,
    every day.

Can you tell that to speak your Done Deal
    is a choice of courage?

Honor yourself for the courage you are choosing
    to speak and act on your Done Deal.

∞

_____
_____
_____
_____
_____
_____
_____
_____
_____
_____
_____
_____

And yes I said yes I will Yes.

—James Joyce, Ulysses

It's the repetition of affirmations that leads to belief. And once that belief becomes a deep conviction, things begin to happen.

—Claude M. Bristol (1891-1951,
American author of The Magic of Believing)

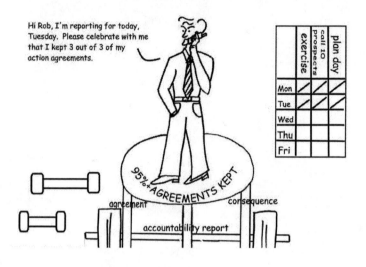

Keep any promise you make to yourself

Here's how you can guarantee
    that you will keep any promise to yourself.

In September of 1986, I was receiving royalties
    from a computer program
    I had designed, developed, and patented.
    (I was a software engineer at that time.)
    The program was called "The Magical Poet."
    It wrote a customized, three-verse limerick
        for (and about) a friend or relative
        based on some information the user provided.
As a result of the royalties,
    I was no longer concerned about my income.
    I took this opportunity to step back and look at my life.

I said to myself,
 "I'm fairly happy and fairly successful,
 but there's one problem that keeps bugging me.
 I don't keep promises to myself very well.
 I promise myself that I will exercise.
  I do it for a few weeks and then I stop.
 I promise that I will call a prospective client each day.
  I might do that for two days and then I stop.
 What a difference it would make in my life
  if I could consistently keep my promises to myself!"
Having studied psychology and motivation for many years,
 I knew that nothing existed that would *guarantee*
 that I would keep my promises to myself.
 But I intuitively felt that I could solve this problem.

After working several months on the idea,
 on December 27, 1986,
 I implemented a technique,
 which later became known as "Consider It Done™."

Being the extremist that I sometimes am,
 I went overboard and made, on average,
 30 promises to myself every day.
 Some of these were small promises,
  like flossing my teeth;
 others were bigger promises,
  like regular exercise.
Over a two-month period,
 I kept over 99 percent of my promises!

I was so delighted and amazed with the results
 that I started telling all my friends about it.
 The most common response was,
 "Dwight, I could use that, too!"

I have since discovered that
    more than 95 percent of the people I talk with
    are willing to admit that consistently fulfilling
    one or more promises to themselves
    would make a significant impact on their lives.

As a result, in April of 1987,
    I changed careers, becoming a life coach,
    and made the "Consider It Done" technique
    part of the service I offered to people.
I have kept statistics on my clients
    who have used "Consider It Done."
    On average, they keep 98.7 percent of the promises
        they make within the "Consider It Done" structure.
I had one salesman increase his income (back in 1991)
    from $2,000 per month to $10,000 per month
    in three months just from "Consider It Done" promises.
I've had countless clients lose the weight they wanted to
    and get themselves into good physical shape.
I've had another client finish writing a book
    he was stalled on.
I've had other clients create structures
    for both accomplishment and leisure in their lives,
    structures that have made a huge difference in their satisfaction.

Even though, at base, "Consider It Done"
    is a powerful support structure,
    it is often a major choice of courage
    to initiate it and continue with it.

Here's how it works.

There are three cornerstones to "Consider It Done."

Cornerstone #1
Choose an action agreement
  that you know you need support in keeping
  (it can be a periodic or a one-time action).

Here are the criteria for choosing this action.

The action must be specific and measurable.
  You must be able to clearly say to yourself after the event:
    "Yes, I did it," or "No, I didn't do it."
  For example, if you say,
    "I will get a good workout
      every Monday, Wednesday, Friday,"
    that is *not* specific and measurable.
  But if you say,
    "I will treadmill at least 4.5 mph
      for a minimum of 20 minutes
      every Monday, Wednesday, Friday,"
    that *is* specific and measurable.

The action must be completely do-able and in your control
  under normal and expected background conditions.
  For example, if you're in sales and you say,
    "I will make a minimum of one new sale each business day,"
    this is probably not do-able;
    you cannot really control
    whether or not you make one sale per day.
  However, if you say,
    "I will place a minimum of five telephone calls
    to prospective clients each business day,"
    that would be within your control
      under normal and expected background conditions.

By consistently controlling what we can control,
    in terms of our actions, then, in the long run,
      we can get the results that we cannot directly control.

The action must be ecologically sound on a personal level.
    This means that you must look at *all* the other
      everyday needs and commitments
      that normally require your time or resources
      and ask yourself,
      "Does adding this action agreement
        to everything else I must do
        and everything else I say I will do make sense?
        Will it all fit on my plate?"
    If it will not fit,
      then you must choose to cancel
      something else, become creative,
      or forget about your new agreement.

Cornerstone #2
Choose a consequence to attach to your action.
You are essentially agreeing that,
    if you do *not* keep the agreement,
    then you will perform the consequence within two days.
The purpose of the consequence
    is to *not* incur the consequence;
    the purpose of the consequence is to guarantee the action.
You want to choose a consequence that is unpleasant enough
    so that, if you're in one of those moods
    in which you might want to ignore your agreement,
    you will look at your consequence and say to yourself,
    "I think I'll just keep my agreement!"

The consequence is *not* a punishment; it is just a consequence.
You have already experienced consequences
    from not keeping this agreement previously,
    much larger consequences than the one you're setting here.
The problem with those natural consequences
    is they haven't been compelling enough
    (in your moment-by-moment awareness)
    to guarantee the action.
With "Consider It Done," we bring the consequences up close,
    we customize them for you, and we make them "for sure."
    In other words,
        we make you an offer you can't refuse and
        we make it compelling.
This way, you perform the action (keep the agreement)
    rather than incur the consequence.
Or, should you incur the consequence, you satisfy it right away.
    It's over with.
    There's no guilt,
    and you get going again immediately with your agreements.
    With "Consider It Done," there is no guilt
    when you don't keep an agreement.

Let me give you some examples of possible consequences.
These are just examples; you can choose your own.

Take a one-minute cold shower.
Burn a $10 bill or flush coins down the toilet.
Eat a teaspoon of dog food.

For some types of agreements,
    it's better to create a pro-rated consequence,
    a consequence which is proportional
    to the quantity of the agreement not kept.

Let's imagine that you make an action agreement
　　to spend one hour per day studying for a test.
　　If you spend the full hour, of course, there is no consequence.
　　However, let's imagine that you spent 45 minutes,
　　　　but not the full hour.
　　If your consequence is to take a one-second cold shower
　　　　for each minute not spent studying,
　　　　then you would have to take
　　　　a 15-second cold shower within two days.
　　If you did not keep *any part* of your agreement,
　　　　you would have to take a cold shower for a full minute!

Special note:
　　Do not make the consequence bigger than it needs to be.
　　This is just a consequence, not a punishment.

You intention is to *not* incur the consequence;
　　it's to support the action.
However, should you incur the consequence,
　　you have to be willing to satisfy it.

Cornerstone #3
Make a daily accountability report to your accountability partner.

You must have a partner to make this process work.
　　Our ability to re-negotiate with ourselves
　　is so well developed that it is important to
　　make our promises not only to ourselves
　　but also to someone else whom we respect
　　and who is willing to hold us accountable
　　for what we say we want in our lives.

Choosing the accountability partner is very important.
　　Use these guidelines and criteria.

(1) Choose someone whom you really respect
    and from whom you want respect.
(2) Do *not* choose a spouse or lover.
  It is generally not a good idea
    to choose a very close friend either.
  With such a person, there is often
    the potential for either collusion
    and/or resentment to develop.
(3) Choose a person you know is willing to be
    very rigorous with you and not let you off the hook.
(4) Choose a person you know is reliable so you are *sure* that,
    should you neglect to make your accountability report,
    s/he will contact you immediately to get your report,
    and collect the non-report consequence (more on this later),
    and get everything going again.
(5) Choose a person who has a voice-mail system
    and/or e-mail system that s/he checks daily,
    so that you can easily report to h/im
    without inconveniencing h/im or yourself.

Here is how your accountability report works.

You can report every day,
    you can report Monday through Friday,
    or you can report on specific days of the week
    that you designate.
    Generally speaking,
      you should make a report for every day
      in which you've made agreements.
    For example, if you only had one agreement
      to exercise every Monday, Wednesday, Friday,
      then it would make sense to report on those days only.

Most people, however,
>   have agreements that cover every day of the week,
>   so it makes it simple and easy to report every day.

The deadline for your report is noon on the day
>   *after* your agreement was scheduled.
>   For example, if your agreements
>   >   are scheduled for Monday,
>   >   >   then you would have until noon on Tuesday
>   >   >   to make your report for those agreements.
>   If you do not report by that time,
>   >   then your accountability partner should get back to you
>   >   before the end of that day
>   >   to get your report for the previous day
>   >   and to confirm the collection of the non-report consequence
>   >   (more about the non-report consequence below).

I strongly recommend that you create the habit
>   of making your report in the evening before you go to bed.
>   Even though you have until noon of the next day to report,
>   >   consider it a safety margin that you don't play with.
As a structure to support yourself in remembering to report,
>   I recommend putting five rubber bands
>   (enough so you will notice them when you brush your teeth)
>   on the handle of your toothbrush.
>   When you are brushing your teeth
>   >   in the evening or the morning
>   >   and you notice those rubber bands,
>   >   if you haven't already made your report,
>   >   *do not* let yourself brush your teeth
>   >   *until* you have made your report!

The content of the report sounds something like this
(whether by voice mail, voice to voice, or e-mail):

"Hi, Pat. This is Jamie.
Please celebrate with me that I fulfilled
all four of my agreements for Monday."

If you did not satisfy all your agreements,
the report sounds something like this:

"Hi, Pat. This is Jamie.
Please celebrate with me that I fulfilled
three out of four of my agreements for Monday.
The one I didn't fulfill completely
was my studying agreement.
I only studied for 45 minutes
of the 60 minutes I agreed to study each day.
The consequence is a 15-second cold shower.
I'll be taking that in the morning
and, when I report tomorrow,
I'll let you know that I satisfied my consequence."

Keep in mind that your consequence
must be satisfied within two days of your unfulfilled agreement,
and report on the status of your consequence daily
until it is satisfied.

Your report might sound like this:
"Hi, Pat. This is Jamie.
Please celebrate with me that I fulfilled
all four of my agreements for Tuesday.
I also took
a 15-second cold shower as a consequence
for not fulfilling one of my agreements on Monday."

Those are the three basic cornerstones of "Consider It Done."
But there are some other points
      that are important in completing the full picture of the process.
The first point is called the "non-report consequence."

As with your other consequences,
      the purpose of the non-report consequence
      is to *not* incur the consequence;
         it's to guarantee the action (of reporting).
The non-report consequence
      results if you do not report as required by the noon deadline.
The non-report consequence should be a dollar amount
      (like $15, for example)
      that is paid/mailed to your accountability partner
      within two business days of its incurrence.
      It should be set high enough so that you, as the action partner,
         will rarely, if ever, incur it.
The reason the non-report consequence
      is paid to your accountability partner
      is to help compensate/motivate h/im
      for the extra time and effort needed
      to call you back and make sure everything
      is okay and back on track.

The second point is called the "ultimate consequence."

The ultimate consequence is a consequence
      for not satisfying a regular consequence
      within the allotted two days.
For example, if you should take a 15-second cold shower
      for an agreement you did not do on Monday,
      and you still haven't taken the cold shower
      by the end of Wednesday,
      then you have incurred the ultimate consequence.

The ultimate consequence is set (in advance)
    at a fairly large dollar amount,
    (usually between $100 and $300),
    that is paid to a charity of your choice,
    above and beyond what you would normally donate.
The check is made out to the charity
    and mailed to your accountability partner
    who mails it to the charity.
Over a thousand people have participated with me
    as their accountability partner,
    and only four people, one time each,
    have ever incurred the ultimate consequence.
Stay far away from this one!

The third point is declaring a vacation or a break.

You have the option of declaring a vacation or a break
    from your agreements and/or your reporting.

After a regular daily report, you would say something like this:
    "I'm leaving on a week's vacation tomorrow.
    I'm suspending my agreements and my reporting
    for the duration of the vacation.
    You can expect my next report a week from now
    for Monday, September 23."

The fourth point is declaring an emergency or opportunity.

When an unanticipated emergency situation
    or unanticipated opportunity situation arises,
    the report might sound like this:

"Hi, Pat. This is Jamie.
    Please celebrate with me that I fulfilled
    three out of four of my agreements for Tuesday.
    I did not keep my exercise agreement
    because I sprained my ankle yesterday.
    I am declaring an emergency on that."

Another example:
    "Hi, Pat. This is Jamie.
        Please celebrate with me that I fulfilled
        three out of four of my agreements for Tuesday.
        I did not keep my study agreement
        because of an opportunity that came up
        with a client who required that extra time."

If, upon listening to a declared emergency or opportunity,
    the accountability partner feels that the action partner
    may be pulling the wool over h/is own eyes,
    then the accountability partner's job
    is to contact the action partner immediately
    and have an honest conversation
    about whether or not the consequence is due.
    Otherwise the accountability partner does not call
        the action partner back
        and the declared emergency or opportunity
        is accepted as such and no consequence incurred.

The fifth point is the policy of making just a *few* basic promises.

You can sabotage your use of "Consider It Done"
    if you require it to handle too many details in your life.
Use "Consider It Done" to support those foundational agreements
    that affect the most important areas of your life.

Examples are:
 regular life reviewing and planning,
 regular exercise,
 eating well,
 good communication with others,
 reading great books,
 focusing on the essential items in your business,
 focusing on the essential items for leisure and renewal.

In addition, when you first start "Consider It Done,"
 begin with one, two, or three agreements.
 Once you're accustomed to fulfilling them consistently,
  you can add more as you like.

The sixth point is to ask yourself the question:
 "Is there any significant possibility
 that I would lie to my accountability partner
 in my 'Consider It Done' reporting?"

If the answer is yes,
 then you need to modify the standard reporting procedure
 so that a customized (for you) truth affirmation
  is spoken before each report.
Here are two disparate examples of truth affirmations.

(1) "I swear upon my relationship with God
 that what I am about to say is completely true and accurate."

(2) "I swear upon the souls of my niece and nephew
 and my relationship with them
 that what I am about to say is completely true and accurate."

If the accountability partner does not hear
    the truth affirmation at the beginning of your report,
    then s/he will contact you immediately
    to hear the report again *with* the affirmation,
    and confirm that you mailed
    the non-report consequence to h/im.

The seventh point is the initiation of a special conversation
    by the action partner and/or by the accountability partner
    in the event that many consequences are incurred,
    especially for one agreement.

Within the context of the "Consider It Done" structure,
    if an action agreement is broken frequently
    and the consequence is thereby incurred often,
    it's important to do a maintenance check.
This breakdown will occur only
    if one or more of the following conditions is present:
    The action agreement does not meet
        the criteria for a valid agreement.
    The consequence is not compelling enough.
    There are too many hidden and/or unacknowledged
        benefits for *not* keeping your agreement.
    You don't have a real desire or commitment
        to the action and/or the result;
        it is only something you feel you *should* do.
    You are not in touch with the benefits
        that you will get from keeping this agreement.

Unless you can address the breakdown,
    I recommend canceling the action agreement in question.

The eighth and last point is ending an agreement
    or terminating "Consider It Done."

Any agreement can be canceled or modified
    with one day's advance notice to the accountability partner.

The entire process can be terminated
    only after a thorough and complete discussion
    with the accountability partner.

When I first designed this process for myself
    and I was ready to try it,
    I was very excited, *but* I was also *scared!*
    In the past, when I had made promises to myself,
    I always knew that I had a back door
    available to me for re-negotiation with myself.
With the "Consider It Done" process,
    I was closing and locking that back door.

For most people, as it was with me,
    it is a major choice of courage
    to step into the "Consider It Done" process.

List at least three agreements that, if kept consistently,
    would make a *big* difference in your life.

Write out the differences you would see and feel in your life
    if you kept these agreements
    consistently over three months, six months, or a year.

Now, call someone appropriate, explain the process to h/im,
    and ask h/im to be your accountability partner.

Honor yourself for the courage to try "Consider It Done."

Let Donald Duck help you stop

Your husband has just done something
    he said he'd never do again.
Your instant, automatic reaction is
    one of hurt, betrayal, and outrage.
You've been down this road before.
You know how it will end
    if you indulge in your feelings to strike back.
At this point, you can vaguely remember your commitment
    to a loving, nurturing relationship with your husband.
But the impulse, the desire, the instinct
    to make him hurt also seems overwhelming.

What can you do?

Try to interrupt your pattern.
Say to your husband,
    "Hold on, honey. Before I scream at you,
    I need to go take a one-minute cold shower."
    Then *take* a one-minute cold shower!
Or you might start singing
    in a high-pitched, Donald Duck voice,
    "Row, row, row your boat gently down the stream . . ."
Or you might say to him,
    "I'm going to get a match and a dollar bill. Don't go away."
    Then get a one-dollar bill and a match
    and burn the dollar bill over the kitchen sink.
Or you might lie down on the floor
    and roll over and over 23 times.
Or you might open a can of Alpo dog food
    that you keep handy for such occasions,
    measure out one level teaspoon, and eat it.

After you have engaged in one or more of these actions
  (or another one that you design for yourself),
  you'll be in a much more resourceful state
  to speak and act in alignment
  with your commitments and deepest desires.

Two other important points:

(1) Have a list of "pattern interruptions" close at hand
  (things you would be willing to do)
  because you may have difficulty thinking of an interruption
  in the throes of anger.
(2) In most cases, let your husband
  (or wife, child, mother, friend, boss,
  employee, or business colleague)
  know in advance that you may be using
  a pattern interruption to assist in your commitment
  to the quality of your relationship with that person.
  You might even ask them to give you a *signal*
  (like looking skyward)
  when you might need to use a pattern interruption,
  because they can see you're about to lose it.

Ask yourself,
  "Is there an important relationship in my life
  in which the use of a pattern interruption
  might be helpful?"
If so, get your pattern interruption prepared
  so that you will be ready to use it the next time
  you find your temper starting to flare with that person.
  Then, let that person know of your commitment
  to the quality of your relationship with h/im
  by informing h/im of your intention
  to use the pattern interruption, should it be needed.

Notice that, in the moment of choosing a pattern interruption
in place of indulging in the automatic reaction,
you are usually choosing the courage of vulnerability.

Give it a try.
It can even be a lot of fun.

&

_____
_____
_____
_____
_____
_____
_____
_____
_____
_____
_____
_____
_____
_____
_____
_____
_____

Let the first impulse pass, wait for the second.
—*Baltasar Gracian (1601-1658,*
Spanish philosopher, writer)

Some persons do first, think afterward, and then repent forever.
—*Thomas Secker*

Words without thoughts never to heaven go.
—*William Shakespeare (1564-1616,*
British poet, dramatist)

What do others think of you?

What power might we have,
    both to give others what they want and need
    and to get what we want and need,
    if we could only read other people's minds.

Some of you may have enjoyed the movie *What Women Want*,
    starring Mel Gibson and Helen Hunt,
    in which Mel is given the freak ability to read women's minds.

Let me introduce you to a technique
    that is the next best thing to reading people's minds.
    I call this technique "How Others See Me" (HOSM).

Whenever I fly by myself,
    I usually request a seat between two other passengers
    who have already been assigned their seats
    (the airline agent is always quite surprised
    by my request, often saying it's a first for h/im).
    But I want to have the maximum opportunity
    for a good conversation on my flight.

The HOSM technique can be used
    with someone you've known for only a few minutes
    or with someone you've known for 20 years or more
    (e.g., your children, your parents, or a high-school classmate).
    In the following example, I speak with
        someone I've known for only a few minutes,
        but the technique is essentially the same,
        regardless of the duration of the relationship.

The challenge of this approach is to act and speak in such a way
that a sufficient feeling of safety
is created for your speaking partner.
You need to make h/im feel safe and comfortable enough
so that s/he will choose the courage
to share h/is candid thoughts and feelings with you.

Let's imagine that I'm sitting beside Bill
and we've been chatting for 20 minutes.

"Bill, I've got a rather unusual favor to ask of you.
Because this favor is out of the ordinary,
I want you to feel comfortable in saying,
'I'd rather not,' if you'd really like to decline.
Can I rely on you to do that should that be the case?"

"Well, let's give it a go. Tell me what you have in mind,"
Bill responds.

"Thank you, Bill.
Recently I've taken on a project
of becoming responsible for how others see me.
It's so easy for me to fantasize that I know
how you (or others) think and feel about me
when, if fact, I have very little knowledge
of what is actually true.
We all have many automatic
thoughts, feelings, opinions, and assessments
about everyone we come in contact with,
very often outside of our conscious awareness.
Even if we know someone only for a few minutes,
we will have some feelings and opinions about this person,
automatic assessments about areas like:
how honest this person is,
how much self-confidence s/he has,
how successful s/he is,

how friendly s/he is,
how trustworthy s/he is,
how charismatic s/he is,
whether or not we would want
    to have a friendship with h/im,
whether or not we would want
    to have a romantic relationship with h/im,
whether or not we would want
    to do business with h/im, and so on.

We may have very little to base our feelings on,
    but we have them anyway, regardless of their accuracy.
The favor that you could do for me
    is to give me your intuitive assessment on a scale of 0 to 10
    regarding various aspects of my personality and character.
When your automatic assessment is very positive,
    it will probably be easy to share it with me.
However, the most valuable feedback
    you can give me would be in those areas
    where your assessment is less than a 9 or 10.
So I would be most grateful for feedback in those specific areas
    where your automatic assessment
    is less than totally favorable, okay?"

"Okay, lead the way," Bill responds.

"Thanks. The first is the trait of 'integrity.'
    On a scale of 0 to 10,
    what is your automatic assessment of my integrity?"

"I'd say a 9 or 10 on that one," Bill replies.

"Okay, thanks.
     The next is the trait of 'good conversationalist.'
     How would you rank me on that one?"

"On that one, I'd give you about a 7."

"Very good. Thanks again.
     I'd be very curious to know, if you can put it into words,
          what about me has contributed to your ranking of me as a 7,
          as contrasted with a 9 or 10?"

"Well, one thing I noticed—
     and this is a little difficult for me to say—
     is that you asked me so many direct questions
     that I felt a bit like you were interrogating me," Bill replies.

"That's very helpful feedback.
     I am sorry my questions caused you some discomfort.
     Is there anything else that could have been different
     in order for you to experience me as a 9 or 10?"

The interview process continues in this manner
     until you have a good feeling for
     and some solid information about
     how Bill sees you from the perspective of his world.

As you interview more and more people using HOSM,
     you will discover some commonalities in how people assess you.
     You will discover changes that you are able and eager to make
          so people see you more as you would like.
     But you will also discover variations
          in the feedback from person to person.
          What people tell you about yourself
          often has a lot to say about them.

HOSM can also be used in a very focused manner.
Imagine that you want to start a new business
and you will need to attract very powerful people
to work with you in building that business.
As you use HOSM with the appropriate people,
you could make the request,
"Please give me a 0 to 10 ranking of how eager
you would be to enter into partnership
with me in this business
(given that you know nothing about the business
except that I am the one starting it)."
Or imagine that you want to attract a romantic partner.
As you are using HOSM with a member of the opposite sex,
you could ask the question,
"Please give me a 0 to 10 ranking
of how irresistible you find me
as a potential romantic partner."
(You'll probably need to reassure h/im
that this is "for information purposes only"
and that it is not a "pick-up" ploy.)

The power of HOSM is limited only by your creativity
and your willingness to choose courage.
To initiate it and follow through
with a HOSM interview is most often a choice of courage.
It is very interesting and exciting!

Choose three people to request
a HOSM session with this week.

Breathe into your fear
and honor yourself for choosing courage.

Really listening is distinct from agreeing or obeying

Most of us, most of the time never really *listen*,
    even though the biggest gift
    that we can often give someone is to *just* listen.

Why?

I believe we find listening difficult for two reasons.

The first reason is that we have confused
    the idea of listening with the idea of
    agreeing with someone or obeying someone.

Really listening *does not* mean that you agree
    with what someone says.

Really listening *does not* mean that you will do anything
    that may be requested.
Listening is distinct from agreeing or obeying.

For example,
    if your spouse says to you,
    "I feel really hurt that
        you didn't cook dinner for me tonight,"
    you can really listen to what s/he says,
    even empathize with what s/he says,
    while responding,
    "I know that you feel really hurt
        that I didn't cook for you tonight."

For these reasons, there is nothing to be concerned about,
    there is nothing to resist in *really* listening.

The second reason is that, on occasion,
    we have insufficient desire or commitment
    to really listen, either because
    we are not experiencing pleasure
    from granting the gift of listening
    to another and/or what the speaker is saying
    is not important, interesting, and/or entertaining to us.

In this circumstance we need to ask ourselves,
    "Am I willing to bring creativity and commitment
        to my listening and my conversation with this person
        so that I can *really* listen to h/im?"
    "Am I willing to choose courage
        to interrupt and say something like,
        'Pardon me. I need your help. I really want to listen to you,
            but I'm having a hard time with it.
            Would you be willing to dialogue
            with me so that I can find a way
            to *really* listen to every word that you're saying?'"

Do you *really* listen
    to your lover/spouse,
    to your mother, to your father, to your children,
    to your boss, to your subordinates, to your clients,
    to your friends?
Do you *really* feel listened to
    by your lover/spouse,
    by your mother, by your father, by your children,
    by your boss, by your subordinates, by your clients,
    by your friends?

Choose courage to *really* listen.

૭

Do you listen to create intimacy?

Do you feel *really* listened to by your romantic partner?
Does your romantic partner feel *really* listened to by you?
(Special note: This essay is about any relationship,
    although a romantic relationship is used as an example.)

With an investment of five to ten minutes per day,
    you and your partner can develop the habit
    of consistently *listening* to each other,
    thereby creating and supporting
    more understanding and intimacy between the two of you.

Here's how it works.

First, make a plan to consistently set aside
    five to ten private and uninterrupted minutes each day
    for the "Listening for Intimacy" process.
Next, alternate days.
    The first day will be "your partner's day."
    The next day will be "your day."
    The day after that will be "your partner's day," and so on.

Two things will happen on "your partner's day."

For this example, imagine that you have set aside ten minutes.
First, during your partner's ten-minute session,
    s/he will share with you something that s/he has had difficulty
        sharing with you in the past.
During these ten minutes,
    your job is to *completely* listen to your partner.
    For purposes of this exercise "completely listening"
        is defined by your partner's response.

Your job is to listen in such a way
    that your partner *feels* completely listened to.

How do you know if your partner feels completely listened to?
    By h/er feedback and coaching.
Your partner's judgment of whether or not
    you are *really* listening to h/er is what matters.
You will give your partner permission to coach you in listening
    such that your partner feels *fully* listened to by you.
You will accept your partner's coaching
    without objection or resistance.
At the same time, your partner will be a great coach,
    encouraging you with gentleness and patience.
S/he will listen to your listening
    to assist you in improving your listening of h/im.

Second, from the beginning of the day,
    your partner will maintain an awareness
    of how well you are listening to h/im.
At the end of the day, your partner
    will give you a 0-10 ranking on how well you listened to h/im.
    A 0 means you were "out to lunch" entirely
    and a 10 means you *really* listened well!
If you get less than an 8 or 9,
    you might want to ask for some specific coaching
    on how you might have listened better during the day.

The next day, when it's your day,
    you switch places with your partner
    and it's your partner's job to *really* listen to you
    (although this doesn't mean
    that you stop listening to your partner!).

Both of you should remember that really listening
    to one another has nothing to do with
    whether or not you agree with
    what the other person is saying.
Listening does not require agreement.

This process can easily be adapted
    to improve the communication and feelings of connection
    between *any* two people, not just romantic partners.

Who might you enroll today
    to participate with you in this "Listening for Intimacy" process?

What differences might it make in your life
    if you were consistent in using this process
    to enhance and maintain the quality of your relationships?

Notice that *really* listening to another
    is often a choice of courage!

Breathe into your fear and honor yourself
    for choosing this courage.

ॐ

The greatest gift you can give another is the purity of your attention.
—*Richard Moss, MD (poet, writer)*

Were we as eloquent as angels we still would please people much
more by listening rather than talking.
—*Charles Caleb Colton (1780-1832,*
British sportsman, writer)

Are you really listening . . . or are you just waiting for your turn to talk?
—*Robert Montgomery (1807-1855, American author)*

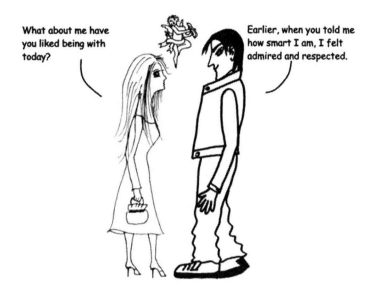

Keep your love shining with just five minutes a day!

Why does our love,
    which often seems so strong at the beginning,
    seem to fade the longer we know another?

One major reason is that we take each other for granted.

Let me suggest a five-to-ten minute exercise
    that you and a partner
    (spouse, lover, friend, colleague, or family member)
    can do at the end of the day
    or at the end of any time that you spend together.
I've received amazing reports on the difference
    this exercise has made for the people who have used it!

It is important that this exercise be approached
    as an "information-gathering" exercise only.
    Whether or not you or your partner
    will be able, and/or willing, to make any changes
    in your behavior with each other
    based upon the information gathered
    is entirely another question.
    The attitude that makes this exercise work is one of
        really wanting to understand the other person
        and how you affect h/im.

Let's say that your partner's name is Jim.

Here's what you would say to him:
    "Jim, what about me have you *liked* being with today?
    Please give me detailed feedback
        on what you've enjoyed or appreciated
        about being with me today."

Really listen to what Jim says.
    Do not assume you know what he will say.
    Keep asking Jim for more feedback
        until he has nothing more to say.
    If you don't fully understand a specific piece of feedback,
        ask for more detail
        so that you can fully understand his feedback.
    If you notice that you are touched by or appreciative
        of anything that Jim says to you,
        express your appreciation to him for what he has said.

After this question has been fully answered,
 ask Jim a second question:
 "Jim, what about me have you *disliked* being with today?
 Please give me detailed feedback
  on anything that you've disliked
  or that has made you uncomfortable
  about being with me today?"

Really listen to what Jim says.
 Do not assume you know what he will say.
 Keep asking Jim for more feedback
  until he has nothing more to say.
 If you don't fully understand a specific piece of feedback,
  ask for more detail
  so that you can fully understand his feedback.
 If it took courage for Jim
  to share openly with you about something,
  express your appreciation for his choice of courage.

If there is anything you might like to change
 about your behavior with Jim in the future,
 consider asking him to support you in making the change
 (by giving you a gentle but an immediate signal)
 should the unwanted behavior occur again in the future.
 Jim is likely to be aware of the behavior he dislikes
 much sooner than you would be.

After you have finished asking Jim these questions
 and fully listening to him, then it's your turn to give feedback.
 Reverse the roles,
  with Jim asking you the same questions
  and with him really listening to you.

Very often it is a choice of courage
    for one or both partners to participate in this process.
    It can be a choice of courage to ask questions.
    It can be a choice of courage to fully and honestly answer them.
    Honor and appreciate yourself and your partner
        each time you participate in this exercise.

If you have never tried this process before
    or if you have not done this process for a while,
    then the choice of courage is often bigger.

Consider the idea that
    if you're not willing to do this process,
    then your relationship is on the rocks
    and it will stay there or even get worse.
    It is probably time to end the relationship.

Whereas, if you and your partner
    are willing to engage in this exercise
    on a daily, or perhaps weekly, basis,
    then the quality of your relationship
    will be consistently maintained and improved.

What do you think?

Choose courage today
    to set up this ongoing exercise with one or more
    of the important partners in your life.

❧

**For more essay(s) on courage and listening,
    see www.GoldWinde.com/Cbook/More/Listening.**

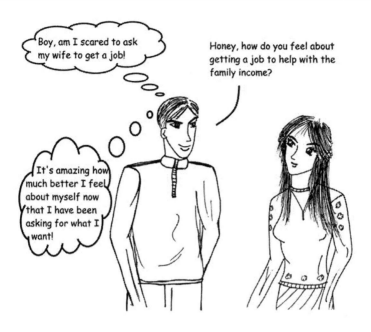

The key to unshakable self-esteem

Self-esteem provides a foundation for creating a life
of both quality and accomplishment.

Self-esteem is the reputation
you have with yourself.
It is the core knowledge
that you are both competent to live
and worthy of living a great life.

Often we think self-esteem
comes from how others view us and relate to us.
Certainly, this is a factor,
especially when we are children.

Sometimes we think that self-esteem
    comes from specific things that we have or do.
    Men often attach their self-esteem to their work.
    Women often attach their self-esteem
        to their partner or their children.
    Often people will base their self-esteem in
        being better than someone else,
        belonging to a certain group, religion, or country,
        having a better education than others,
        belonging to a higher class than others,
        being richer than others,
        being more altruistic than others,
        dressing better than or differently from others,
        and so on and so on.

But the *fundamental* source of true self-esteem
    is the choice of courage.

Every time you choose courage,
    a higher self-esteem is the automatic result.
Every time you default in not choosing courage,
    a lower self-esteem is the automatic result.
Self-esteem is a by-product of choosing courage.
    It is not something you or others can talk yourself into.

Next time you default on choosing courage,
    notice how your reputation with yourself
    deteriorates immediately.

Look for an opportunity to choose courage
    and notice how your reputation with yourself
    improves immediately.

៙

Create more confidence

Clients will often say to me,
    "I want to have more confidence" or
    "I want to be more self-confident."

But what is confidence?
What are people *really* asking for
    when they say they want more confidence?
On occasion, they are simply saying
    they want to have more skill in a given area.
That's easy enough; it just takes practice.

However, what they are usually asking for
    is the ability to act *without* fear.
They want to somehow
    jump over the process of choosing courage entirely
    and go directly to a state of fearlessness.
Confidence, however, cannot be accessed directly.
    It is a by-product of choosing courage consistently.

Allow me to illustrate with an example from my own life.

When I lived in Phoenix, Arizona,
    I would often eat lunch
    at a fast-food Asian restaurant near my home.
Typically, after receiving my order,
    I would look around the restaurant
    at all the people sitting by themselves.
If there were six such people,
    I would then ask myself the question,
    "Which of these six people
    am I most frightened of approaching?"

Then, I would take a deep breath
    and say to myself, "Boy, am I scared!"
Empowered by my choice of courage
    and thus feeling good about myself,
    I would walk up to that person and say,
    "My name is Dwight. I eat here often.
        I thought it would be much more interesting
        to meet somebody new than to sit by myself.
        How would you feel about that?"

During 23 different luncheons, I approached 23 different people.
    Eighteen said I could sit with them
    and five said that I could not.

Did I feel confident when I started doing this?
No, of course not!

Did I feel confident after choosing courage
    to do it 23 different times?
Yes, I did.

Courage is something we create.
Courage is something we choose.
However, we cannot *directly* create or choose confidence.

In what areas of your life would you like to feel more confident?

How might you begin to choose courage today
    so that, over time, you will feel that confidence?

For more essay(s) on courage and confidence,
    see www.GoldWinde.com/Cbook/More/Confidence.

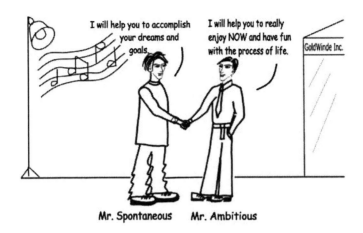

I will help you to accomplish your dreams and goals.

I will help you to really enjoy NOW and have fun with the process of life.

GoldWinde Inc.

Mr. Spontaneous   Mr. Ambitious

Are you friends with ALL of yourself?

I used to have an interesting (but painful) drama
    that plagued my life.

Let's call Dwight #1 "Mr. Ambitious."
Let's call Dwight #2 "Mr. Spontaneous."

Part of the time,
    Mr. Ambitious would be in control of my life.
    He would say,
        "Look at all we could do!
        Look at all we could accomplish!
        Look at all we could become!
        No moment should be wasted!
        Onward, upward, always striving!
        I have promises to keep,
        and miles to go before I sleep."

The rest of the time,
    Mr. Spontaneous would take control of my life.
    He would say,
        "Let's do what we want *now!*
        What difference will it make anyway
        to always accomplish, accomplish, accomplish!?
        Relax. Enjoy. Sleep. Eat.
        Watch TV. Talk with friends.
        Read a good book. Go to a movie. Make love!
        The woods are lovely, dark, and deep."

Mr. Ambitious held the high moral ground.
    He had good PR
        and he knew his position looked very good.
    He knew how to make me feel very guilty
        for the actions of Mr. Spontaneous.

But, when Mr. Spontaneous dug his heels in, no matter the guilt,
    he was the one who had the *power.*
No matter what Mr. Ambitious said,
    Mr. Spontaneous could override him.

For years and years
    (perhaps we could call it "the 40-year war")
    these two sides would wage skirmish after skirmish,
    neither one ever truly winning,
    and both sides losing in many, many ways.

The peace between
    Mr. Ambitious and Mr. Spontaneous came
    only when each side was willing to admit
    the important contributions that the other side
    was trying to make (and was making) in my life.

The peace came
    only after Mr. Ambitious began to support Mr. Spontaneous
        in his desires and concerns
    and Mr. Spontaneous began to support Mr. Ambitious
        in his goals and commitments.

The peace came
    only when they both looked at the bigger picture
    and worked together to create a new lifestyle
    that accommodated both of their desires.

Are you sometimes at war with yourself?
Is there any part of yourself
    that you consider bad
    that you consider lazy
    that you consider irresponsible
    that you consider rebellious
    that you consider weak
    that you consider to be bad or immoral?

Begin to ask yourself,
    "How is this part of me trying to do something important
    for my life?"

How can I begin to honor and pay attention
    to this important intention?

I invite you to make peace with yourself,
    by beginning to honor *all* parts of yourself.

Can you feel the fear associated
    with each side beginning to acknowledge
    the important benefits that
    the other side is trying to provide to you?

Choose the courage to step into this fear (again and again) so that you can create the new peace and joy of a person who is friends with *all* parts of h/imself.

❧

_____

_____

_____

_____

_____

_____

_____

_____

_____

_____

_____

_____

_____

When you say you will or won't do something, do you notice parts of you never got the message?

—*Brad Brown*

I have had more trouble with myself than with any other man I have ever met!

—*Dwight L. Moody (1837-1899, American evangelist)*

As long as a man stands in his own way, everything seems to be in his way.

—*Ralph Waldo Emerson (1803-1882, American writer and philosopher)*

A human being's first responsibility is to shake hands with himself.

—*Henry Winkler (1945-, American actor)*

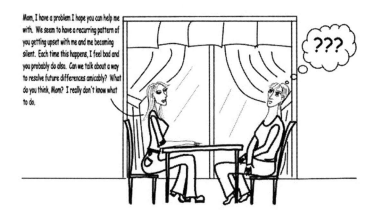

Do you avoid confrontation?

Your spouse just said something that hurt your feelings.
Your boss made a request that seems out of line.
Your employee is not pulling h/is weight.
Your girlfriend is angry with you for a reason
    you don't understand.
Your friend just offended you.

Many of us feel at a loss as to what to do in these situations.
Should we just stuff our feelings inside
    and risk building up our resentment?
Should we try to avoid these people
    or situations in the future?
Should we somehow confront the people involved
    and let them know how we feel?

Each of these options leaves something to be desired.

Let me suggest a new option:
　　the option of partnership.
I'll give you an example from my own experience.

I was staying at my friend's apartment
　　in Shanghai when I first arrived,
　　while I was looking for an apartment to rent.
My friend had another guest drop in
　　from out of town to spend the night.
The guest immediately got on the telephone and started
　　talking with one of his clients.
His vocal volume was off the charts.
　　He spoke as if he were shouting in a large stadium.
I was extremely irritated, as was my friend.
　　However, my friend was unwilling to say anything to him,
　　out of a fear of confronting or offending him.

Once the guest was off the telephone, I said to him,
　　"I have a problem that I hope you can help me with.
　　　　Is it okay to tell you about my problem?"
　　He said, "Okay, sure."
　　"Perhaps I am oversensitive,
　　　　but the volume of your voice when you are on the phone
　　　　automatically makes me feel very uncomfortable.
　　　　I would really like to sleep here for the night and our host
　　　　would like me to sleep here, too.
　　　　But I am afraid that I will need
　　　　to go to a hotel or another friend's place
　　　　if it is necessary for you to speak so loudly
　　　　when you are on the telephone.
　　　　I would appreciate any ideas you might have
　　　　about how we could solve this problem together."

The guest immediately apologized.

He said that many people had told him
about his telephone volume,
but each time he had been unaware
that he was speaking so loudly.

I asked him, should it happen again,
   if I could have permission to give him
   a non-verbal signal of twitching my nose
   so that he could be aware of the need to lower his voice.

He said he would be very grateful.

I then told him that if he really wanted to break this habit,
   he should invite each person he spoke with
   on the telephone to help him by interrupting him,
   should he revert to his "loud mode."
   He thought it was a great idea.

I had no more problems during his visit.
   I didn't have to twitch my nose even one time.

And I felt good about my relationship with him.
   If I had not spoken up in the way that I did,
   even if he did not repeat his behavior during his visit,
   I would have had lingering resentment toward him.

There are two fundamental keys to crafting
   how to speak up in situations like this.

(1) Choose your words and tone of voice
   to invite partnership in solving the problem that is "out there,"
   instead of communicating that you are the problem
   or that s/he is the problem.

(2) Choose your words and tone of voice so that no blame
      is placed on the other person.
    If anything, take the "blame" yourself,
    while inviting partnership in solving the problem.

No matter how well you craft your words,
    speaking in this manner will,
    for almost all of us, be a choice of courage.
    Honor yourself for that courage.

Ask yourself,
    "How could I use this 'partnership approach' in a situation
    where I have been putting up with something
    from someone important in my life?"

    "Am I willing to choose courage to see
    what difference using this new approach might make
    for me and for others?"

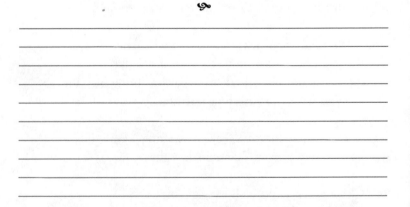

All married couples should learn the art of battle as they should
learn the art of making love. Good battle is objective and honest—
never vicious or cruel. Good battle is healthy and constructive, and
brings to a marriage the principle of equal partnership.
        —*Ann Landers (1918-2002, American advice columnist)*

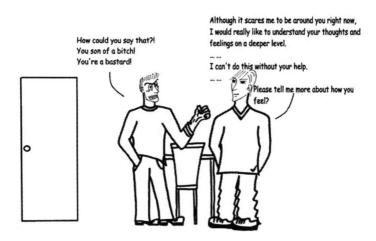

Dissolving blame with partnership

Most of us recognize the damage that we do
    to others, to ourselves, and to our relationships
    when we speak in a way
    that makes others feel threatened or blamed.

Yet, in the moment,
    when we feel threatened or blamed,
    when we feel hurt or angry,
    when we feel irritable or resentful,
    or when we want to feel in control,
    the language of blame
    seems to jump naturally from our lips,
    often with no realization
    that the other person might feel blamed
    by what we are saying and how we are being.

Although words are not everything,
    the most powerful step in shifting a relationship
    from defensiveness and blame to good will and partnership
    is knowing how to speak good will and partnership
    through the words and tone of voice that we choose.

If you are feeling defensive,
    if you are feeling irritable,
    if you are feeling argumentative,
    if you are feeling blamed,
    if you are feeling resentful,
        these are warning signals
        that you must think before speaking
        and craft your response carefully
        with an intent of good will and partnership,
        rather than defensiveness and blame.

It is a proactive art, however,
    to speak with good will and partnership,
    because much of our cultural training
    has focused on defensiveness and blame.

When you are about to speak, ask yourself these questions:
    "Am I choosing words and speaking in a way
        that expresses good will and partnership?"
    "Are the words I'm about to speak
        and the way I intend to speak them
        likely to stimulate a feeling
        of defensiveness or blame in my partner?"

Let's look at some examples
    of what your conversation partner might say
    (that could stimulate defensiveness in you)
    and how you might respond.

Remember that your body language and your voice image
(tonality, timbre, inflection, emphasis, etc.)
must be congruent with and supportive of
the content of your words in order for your speech
to stand a good chance of creating the results you want.

Example #1
"Why did you spend that money on clothes?!"
Your automatic response is one of defensiveness.
Yet, with an intention of good will and partnership,
you might craft your response as:

"You seem upset with me
for buying clothes with the money.
I feel automatically frightened
and automatically defensive
with the thought of your being upset with me
for spending money on clothes.
I would like to understand
more fully what your actual thoughts and feelings are,
and I'd like you to understand mine.
Would you share more deeply and completely with me
exactly what your fears and concerns are, if any,
about my spending the money on clothes?"

Example #2
Your coworker, Jill, seems distant.
You have no idea why she may be upset with you,
if, indeed, she is.
Your automatic defensive tendency
is to withdraw from her and to blame her
for her behavior.
Yet, with an intention of good will and partnership,
you might craft your response as:

"Jill, I need some help and advice with something.
  Do you have a few minutes?
I really value our relationship together in the office.
  But it seems that I may have done or said something
  that has caused you to be upset with me
  and to feel more distant from me.
I could just be imagining things; I sometimes do.
  But I need your help to understand what I might
  have done wrong and how to fix it.
Could you share your thoughts and feelings with me
  about what I am saying?"

Jill may give you some specific feedback
  which you can then respond to in a spirit of partnership.
More likely, she may say,
  "No, nothing is wrong,"
  and you will notice that *her* behavior toward you
  becomes more friendly afterwards.

Example #3
"You never remember my birthday!"
  Your automatic response is one of defensiveness.
  Yet, with an intention of good will and partnership,
    you might craft your response as:

"I sure messed up this time.
  And it wasn't the first time, was it?
I think I can understand
  how hurt and angry you must feel toward me.
And I'm scared.
  I'm scared of you blaming me.
  I'm scared of you withdrawing from me.

I'm not even sure how we can talk about this together
     so that we can both feel closer and more loved
     after we finish talking.
     Sometimes, it seems that our talking just makes things worse.
Can you share your thoughts and feelings
     about our situation and about what I am saying?
     I really need your help on this."

Example #4
"You are such a cruel and insensitive person!
     You #!*#! I hate you!"
     Your automatic response
          is one of fear, hurt, anger, and defensiveness.
     Yet, with an intention of good will and partnership,
          you might craft your response as:

"Although it scares me to be around you right now,
     I would really like to understand
     your thoughts and feelings on a deeper level.
But I have a problem.
     While I want to understand your thoughts and feelings,
          at the same time,
          I am *not* willing to remain in your presence
          if you continue to use abusive words with me.
I can't understand your thoughts and feelings without your help.
     Are you open to telling me more without using abusive words,
     or shall I leave the room for now?
How do you feel? Am I making any sense?"

Notice how, in each example,
     your response is one that assumes and invites partnership
     to solve the problem together, a problem which is "out there,"
     not a problem which is *your* problem or *their* problem.

Even in the last example,
    where a clear boundary was set,
    the boundary was set inside the invitation
    for understanding and partnership.

To act out our defensiveness,
    to blame in response to blame,
    to defend or attach in response to fear
    is often our natural and automatic response.
    Yet it rarely gives us the relationships and results we want.

To embrace our fear
    and use our intention and creativity,
    to craft our response
        with good will, partnership and vulnerability
    is a choice of courage,
    a choice that has a strong probability
        of giving us the relationships and results we want.

Honor yourself for your courage,
    before and afterwards,
    each time you choose to speak in partnership.

∾

_____

_____

_____

_____

_____

_____

_____

_____

_____

_____

Have you let your schooling interfere with your education?

Mark Twain said,
    "I never let my schooling
    interfere with my education."

Most of us, however,
    have not chosen courage
    to do what we need to do
    to ensure that our schooling
    does not interfere
    with our education, our curiosity,
    and our passion for learning.

As young children, we all had a natural passion for learning.
    Where did it go?

The tragedy is that, in the name of education,
    our schooling, from parents,
        from teachers and schools, and from our culture,
    has more often than not just force-fed us "facts,"
    ignoring or devaluing our natural interests and curiosities.
This has been done to us in a manner that often had little to do
    with our own natural curiosities and interests,
    and the experiences of everyday life.

People who enjoy a lifelong romance with learning
    typically choose courage to create their own way,
    outside of, or in addition to, their schooling,
    following their own curiosities
    and natural ways of learning.

How much do you learn every day?
Do you have a passion for learning
    in areas of life that are important to you?
Does your curiosity spur you on
    to keep looking around the next corner?
How might you choose courage and creativity
    to make learning a continuously joyful part of your life?

∽

_____
_____
_____
_____
_____
_____
_____
_____
_____
_____
_____
_____

My idea of education is to unsettle the minds of the young and inflame their intellects.
    —*Robert Maynard Hutchins (1899-1977, American educator)*

Most people are mirrors, reflecting the moods and emotions of the times; few are windows, bringing light to bear on the dark corners where troubles fester. The whole purpose of education is to turn mirrors into windows.
    —*Sydney J. Harris (1917-1986, American journalist, author)*

When you stop learning, stop listening, stop looking and asking questions, always new questions, then it is time to die.
    —*Lillian Smith (1897-1966, American novelist, educator)*

Pride: The killer of life

If children were as resistant to looking foolish
    or making a mistake
    as we adults typically are,
    they would never learn to talk or walk.

Pablo Picasso said,
    "Every child is an artist.
    The problem is how to remain
        an artist once he grows up."

What we often call pride is merely a thin, black veil
    that prevents us from seeing the option of choosing courage.

If, somehow, we could maintain
    the curiosity,
    the unbounded exuberance,
    the indomitable spirit,
    the willingness to make mistakes
        that young children typically have,
    then the veil would fall away
    and our whole life would be open to us!

The key is choosing courage.

Unlike the young child
    who has not yet learned to fear mistakes,
    to fear the disapproval of others,
    to fear even the disapproval of h/imself,
    we adults are bound by these resisted fears.

We have become masters at resisting and avoiding these fears.
We will never go back to being children again.

However, by recognizing our fears,
    by accepting our fears,
    by breathing into the energy of our fears,
    by finding the opportunities for courage in our fears,
    and by honoring ourselves for choosing that courage,
    we can, step by step, move ourselves into that world
        of curiosity,
        unbounded exuberance,
        and indomitable spirit.

Choose an area of your life where you are proud
    (as it is used in this essay).
Become a child again by choosing courage
    and opening up this area
      to excitement, curiosity, and learning.

ℒ

_____

_____

_____

_____

_____

_____

_____

_____

_____

Pride costs more than hunger, thirst and cold.
—Thomas Jefferson (1743-1826,
third president of the United States)

Curiosity will conquer fear even more than bravery will.
—James Stephens (1825-1901, Irish writer)

"Stranger danger." Hogwash!

I am always amazed that many of us assume
    that the people passing us on the street
        (the people who are strangers to us),
    are somehow less safe, less interesting, less friendly,
    than the people we already know
        and consider to be our friends.

Of course, a few people are dangerous;
    but, with just a little caution, they are easily avoided.

Statistics show that *most* interpersonal violence
    is perpetrated by people who are already
    known to us—friends or family, not strangers.

Granted, as a man, I may need to be
    less cautious than a woman;
    however, in all my years of making friends
        with men or women on the street,
    I have yet to be disappointed or to find myself in danger.
More importantly, I have met
    many of my best friends this way.
I would be poorer by far
    if I had been cautious the way so many of us are.

Typically, if you place a group of young children together
    who do not know each other,
    they will immediately become friends.

Somehow, we adults, in our "wisdom,"
    have decided we must be introduced to each other
    or must meet each other in some "safe" venue.
    We cannot trust strangers.

What a shame! What a loss! What a waste!

Publicly, almost everyone is afraid
    to take the first step in saying "hello,"
    concerned that the other person may be a bad person
    or the other person may think
        that you are a bad or foolish person.

What a waste!

How might you begin to choose courage
    to initiate conversations with strangers?

If you saw every stranger as a potential friend,
    how might you act differently?

Honor yourself for the choosing the courage
    to initiate conversations with strangers.

✎

_____

_____

_____

_____

_____

_____

_____

_____

_____

_____

For fun and adventure, try "blind for a day"

Do you ever find yourself wanting a little extra adventure
    but not being sure what to do?

Let me suggest something I have done
    —and thoroughly enjoyed—several times:
I have been blind for a day.

I've done this in New York City,
    in San Francisco,
    in Phoenix, Arizona,
    in Tokyo, Japan,
    and in Shanghai, China.

Let me tell you about the time
    I was blind for a day in San Francisco.

For preparation, I checked the money in my wallet,
    putting in order the $1, $5, $10, $20 bills.
I also had a walking cane
    and some blinders to put over my eyes.

I took the bus to Chinatown.
Standing on the street corner, I put the blinders over my eyes,
    making sure I could not see.
Then I started walking slowly along the sidewalk,
    using the cane as an aid.

Whenever I came to a curb,
    which I could feel with my cane or with my feet,
    I would wait there
    until someone offered to assist me across the street.

I noticed some great smells
    and knew that I was passing a restaurant.
I moved toward the smells
    and was able to feel my way into the restaurant.
The waitress helped me to my seat,
    and I asked her to read
    some items to me from the chicken section of the menu.
After eating slowly and carefully,
    taking special care when I reached for my glass of water,
    I noticed that I enjoyed the food more than I normally would.
Unsure about which bill I had taken
    out of my wallet to pay the check,
    I held up the bill and asked the couple
    at the table sitting next to me
    what the denomination of the bill was.

Once back on the street,
    I decided to walk down to Ghirardelli Square,
    about 12 blocks away.
For the first three crossings,
    I waited for a new person to assist me each time.
On the fourth crossing,
    the man who helped me across insisted on going
    all the way to the square with me.

Once I reached Ghirardelli Square,
    I found a bench to sit on.
Over the next two and a half hours
    I talked with two men about life.
When they asked me about my eyes,
    I made up a story that I had just had
    a radial keratotomy (a type of eye operation)
    and I needed the blinders for only a few days.

In addition to noticing a heightened appreciation
    for the senses of touch, sound, and smell,
        I also noticed another very interesting phenomenon:
I was less judgmental of people when I could not see them!

With the help of some people,
    I was able to get back on the right bus.
Other passengers let me know
    when I should get off the bus.
I ended my adventure by removing my blinders
    once I stepped off the bus.

The world was so fresh and new again!

What new insight about yourself and your life might you discover
    if you were blind for a day?

What courage might you be choosing
    if you were blind for a day?

_____

_____

_____

_____

_____

Adventure is not outside man; it is within.
        —*David Grayson (1870-1946,*
            American journalist and writer)

We live in a wonderful world that is full of beauty, charm and
adventure. There is no end to the adventures that we can have if
only we seek them with our eyes open.
        —*Jawaharlal Nehru (1889-1964,*
            Indian nationalist, statesman)

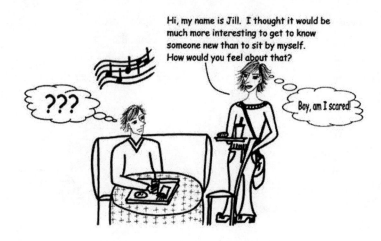

Have fun by turning the tables on fear

Most of the time we resist or avoid fear
    and deal with it (courageously or not)
    only when it is foisted upon us.

But what if we went looking for fear?
    What if we went looking for opportunities for courage?
    What if we tried exercising our courage muscles daily?

If you *really* want to turn the tables on fear,
    if you want to accelerate the process of turning fear into an ally
    (instead of the enemy it seems to be),
    then the "Daily Adventure™" was made for you.

Let me give you an example of a Daily Adventure.
Afterwards, I will tell you how to design Daily Adventures
    that are customized for you and your life.
When I lived in Phoenix, Arizona, my favorite Asian restaurant

was a seven-minute drive from my home.
I would often eat lunch there.

After paying for my "combo chow mein bowl"
    and placing my chopsticks and condiments
        onto my serving tray,
    I would scan all the tables in the restaurant,
    identifying all the people sitting alone.
For this example, let's suppose there were six people sitting alone.

I then asked myself,
    "Which of these six people
        am I most frightened of approaching?"
Then, I would take a deep breath and say to myself,
    "Boy, am I scared!"

Next, I would imagine the five-year-old little Dwight within me
    and say to him,
    "I can see and feel that you're frightened.
    It's okay to feel frightened.
    And I really appreciate and admire you
    for the courage that you're choosing
    in approaching this person."

Then, I would walk up to the person and say,
    "Hi, my name is Dwight. I eat here often.
    I thought it would be much more interesting
    to learn about someone new than to sit by myself.
    How would you feel about that?"
During 23 different luncheons I approached 23 different people.
    Eighteen said I could sit with them and five said that I couldn't.
Regardless of the result, each time,
    I got back in touch with the five-year-old Dwight
    and expressed my appreciation and admiration to him
for thme choice of courage he had just made.

After doing this 23 times, it was still fun,
    but it was no longer a significant choice of courage.
Then I upped the ante. I started approaching tables
    where two or more people were sitting.
    I did this six times.
        Three tables said "yes" and three said "no."
There is always another level of fear to play with!
    Don't worry. You won't run out!

Now let's examine the criteria for designing
    and following through on a Daily Adventure.
1. Choose something that you don't *have* to do.
    Don't choose something that you *should* do.
    This is about having fun with your fear.
2. Choose something that you would like to do
    if it weren't for the fear (e.g., talking with new people).
3. Choose something that stimulates more fear
    than you are accustomed to taking on,
    but not so much fear as to terrify you.
    Inch by inch, life's a cinch; yard by yard, life is hard.
4. Choose something that doesn't involve any real danger.
    Don't be foolhardy.
5. Remember that courage is very individualized.
    What courage is for you is not courage for me and vice versa.
    What courage is for you today
        may not be courage for you tomorrow.
    Don't compare yourself with others (or even with yourself)
        when choosing your Daily Adventure.
6. Once you've tried a given Daily Adventure a number of times,
    you will notice less and less fear associated with your action.
    In order to continue to "exercise your courage muscles,"
        you will need to maintain a level of stimulated fear
        that keeps your muscles in good shape.
    This means you will need to keep changing the adventure.

Here are just a few examples of other possible Daily Adventures.

The possibilities are limited only by
> your level of creativity and willingness to have fun with fear.

1. Say "hello" to every second person you pass on the street.
2. Dress as a beggar and see what you can get.
3. Put some blinders on your eyes and, using a cane,
   pretend to be blind for a period of time
   as you go about the city.
4. Ask a colleague if you can borrow h/is jacket for the day.
5. Start a conversation with a person next to you in line.
6. Call a telephone number randomly
   and see if you can make a new friend.
7. Ask an attractive person for directions that you don't need.

The world is *your* playground.

What Daily Adventure might you take on?
> You could do a similar one every day.
> Or you could invent a new one each day.
> The goal is to have *fun* with *fear!*

Honor yourself for the choice of courage
> to create a Daily Adventure.

**For more essay(s) on courage and adventure,
see www.GoldWinde.com/Cbook/More/Adventure.**

ও

_____
_____
_____
_____
_____
_____
_____
_____
_____

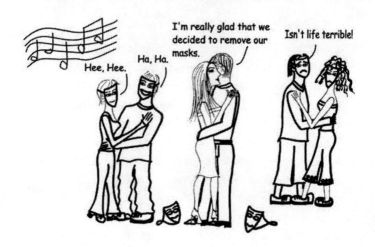

RAFTS: The key to profound intimacy

Do you have a deep connection and intimacy
with your friends,
with your husband or wife,
with your girlfriend, boyfriend, or lover,
with a potential girlfriend, boyfriend, or lover,
with your colleagues,
with your parents or children,
or with other members of your family?

How many friends do you have
with whom you can share everything?
How many friends do you have
with whom you feel safe enough
and close enough
to share yourself vulnerably and fully,
even through your roughest times?

Most of us are starving for safety
    and a feeling of connection with others.
We are starving
    for true friendship,
    for connection,
    and for romance.
But we don't know how to get it
    or we think that there's no one out there
        who can be our true friend.

Now you can have all the intimacy that you want or need.
Let me explain how.

Whenever I meet a new person
    with whom I suspect I might
    enjoy a deeper feeling of connection and intimacy,
    within the first 30 minutes of our conversation,
    I make an invitation such as the following.
"Jill, before I respond to your question
    about why I moved to China,
    in order for me to answer you
    with complete honesty and openness,
    I need to introduce you to a word that I invented, okay?
We've been having a nice conversation for about 20 minutes.
    We've been friendly with each other
        and we've been learning some things about each other.
Even though I have been open with you
    to a certain level, I am also aware
    of some automatic thoughts and feelings
    that I have chosen *not* to share with you.
And I suspect that you've been having
    some automatic thoughts and feelings
    that you haven't shared with me, right?

I have a mask.

> And you have a mask.

We have good reasons for wearing a mask.

> It helps us feel safer, more comfortable, and more secure
>> in the moment.

> If we said everything on our minds,
>> we might feel very afraid of how
>>> the other person would react or feel about us.

Nevertheless, we pay some *big* costs

> in wearing our masks with each other.

I can think of at least two major costs:

> First, it prevents us from truly understanding each other.

> Second, it prevents us from developing deep feelings
>> of connection or friendship.

> Does this make sense?

However, it's not so easy to remove the mask.

So I've invented a special word that—

> if you'll experiment with me in using it—
> will help us remove our masks, step by step,
> in a way that will feel much easier and more fun
> than it otherwise would.

Let me explain the word to you.

The word is 'RAFTS,'

> an acronym that stands for
> 'Reluctant and frightened to share.'

RAFTS sets up a special context for what is said

> immediately after using it.

It puts the other person on notice

> that you are about to share a thought or feeling
> that you might otherwise hide.

It lets your listener know

> that you are frightened
> and that you are choosing courage to share this with h/im.

It lets the other person know that your intention
    is not to hurt or scare h/im
    or in any other way damage your relationship.
Instead, your intention is
    to create deeper understanding and a better relationship.
By speaking the RAFTS word
    you are asking your partner to listen within this context
    as s/he hears what you have to share.
It is asking your listener to hear you in a non-judgmental way
    and with some appreciation for the courage you are choosing.

So, here's how it works, Jill:
Using the RAFTS idea, both you and I
    will begin to notice the automatic thoughts and feelings
    that we are hiding from each other,
    and, when we notice such a thought or feeling,
    we ask ourselves,
    'Would I be willing to choose the courage
    to openly share this thought or feeling with this other person?'
If the answer is 'yes,' then I would say to you,
    'Jill, I have a RAFTS.'
By saying 'I have a RAFTS,'
    I am letting you know that I am frightened
    to share some thought or feeling openly with you.
    I am choosing courage to share it
    with the intention of helping us
    to understand each other better
    and also with the intention of possibly feeling
    more connected with each other.
This helps you to listen to what I have to say
    in a non-judgmental way
    and with some appreciation for my courage.
Do you understand, Jill?
    Would you be willing to experiment in using the RAFTS word?

Thank you.

    Okay, now I am ready to answer your question
    about why I moved to China.

This is a RAFTS for me to share with you, okay?

For various reasons, as I grew up,

    I learned to like women more than men.

    I like men and I have many men friends,

        but, all in all, I prefer women.

For example, if I am at a party

    and a group of women are talking together

    and a group of men are talking together,

    I will always go talk with the women.

    Women, in general, are more interesting to me than men.

And, on top of that,

    I have found that I like Chinese women

    more than any other women in the world!

This is the main reason I moved to China!"

At this point, Jill may or may not do a RAFTS back to me.

If I continue to do RAFTS with her throughout our conversation,

    inviting her to join with me in the process,

    then, most often, a feeling

    of deeper friendship, intimacy and safety

    will occur for both of us.

If you *really* want to accelerate

    the process of connection and understanding,

    then make the following suggestion:

"Jill, why don't we play a game.

    I will ask you a RAFTS question

    (a question in which I feel some nervousness or fear in asking,

    usually a personal question)

    and then you will ask me a RAFTS question.

We'll go back and forth. Okay?

If either one of us doesn't want to answer a given question
    because it is too personal for us,
    then we have the freedom to say,
    'No, I will not answer that.'"

Of course, the RAFTS process, like any other,
    takes some practice.
By asking others to join us in RAFTS
    and by engaging in the actual RAFTS process,
    we are presented with continual opportunities
    for choosing courage.

Introduce at least one person a day
    to the RAFTS process during the next week
    and try it out with them.

Really get into it and see what happens.

Honor yourself for the courage you are choosing.

ℝ

We all wear masks, and the time comes when we cannot remove
them without removing some of our own skin.
    —*Andre Berthiaume (1938-, Roman novelist, essayist)*

We get so much in the habit of wearing a disguise before others
that we eventually appear disguised before ourselves.
    —*Jim Bishop*

Are you a true friend?

I often hear that it's difficult to find a true friend,
    usually implying that I am a true friend.

But what do I offer that others don't?

Do I lend money to my friends?—Typically not.
Do I spend a lot of time with any given friend?—Typically not.
Will I do anything for my friends?—No, I will not.
Do I swear my friendship for life?—No, I do not.
Do I take my friend's side against others?—No, I do not.
Do I always do what my friends want me to do?—No, I do not.
Do I always agree with my friend's opinion?—No, I do not.
Do I sacrifice my needs and desires for theirs?—No, I do not.
Do I say that they are my *best* friend?—No, I do not.

Why then do many people experience me as a true friend,
    sometimes their *only* true friend?

I think it is for two basic reasons.

First,
    by my actions and words, my friends quickly learn
        that I am friends with every part of them,
            including the parts they are not friends with themselves.
They know that they are completely safe with me.
They can say anything to me
        and I will find magnificence in whatever they say.
They know I enjoy them for who they are *now*,
        having no agenda to change them or give them advice.
They know I will support them in whatever they want.

Second,
    I maintain good boundaries with my friends.
    I make sure that my boundaries are set
        so that I am always grateful to my friends,
        never feeling that I am giving more than I am receiving.
    If a particular person cannot accept my boundaries,
        cannot accept my selfishness,
        then we are simply not suited as friends
        and there is no problem.

I provide to others in friendship what I want from them.
    I have so many friends I can be completely open with.
    I have so many friends that I can share any mood with.

If you have trouble finding true friends,
    I suggest that if you start providing to others
    the qualities of true friendship,
    then they will come back to you almost immediately.

Think of someone for whom you might be willing
    to provide true friendship, starting tomorrow.
How might you speak and act so that
    they might experience you as a true friend?

Notice that it is a choice of courage
    to take the actions and speak the words
    to create and maintain such a friendship.

                         ॐ

_____

_____

_____

_____

_____

_____

Are you protecting yourself from love?

Imagine that you were offered an incredible romance:
    a passionate, loving engagement,
    an intimate, once-in-a-lifetime experience,
    with an absolutely fantastic man/woman.
Would you take it?

But what if you knew in advance
    that this romance would inexplicably end
    after six months of passion and bliss,
    after six months of deep learning and growth?
Would you still step into this romance fully?

Or would you protect your heart?

Would you allow yourself
    to reach the heights of intimacy and passion
    if you knew the relationship would end after six months?
How many opportunities for love and self-expression
    do we squander or never take advantage of
    because we are too careful with our heart?
How many possibilities for intimacy and connection do we dismiss
    because we are trying to guarantee our future?
Reflect on how you have kept yourself safe in this way.
Reflect on how you continue to keep yourself safe in this way.

Choose the courage to open your heart,
    embracing and making friends with the fear
    that your most passionate and meaningful relationship
    could also be the shortest.

ॐ

How to destroy the foundations of love

If your relationship
with your lover/spouse ended tomorrow
(for whatever reason),
would you be happy and rejoice
in what you had created and had together?

I don't mean to imply
that you wouldn't experience a feeling of loss;
that feeling of loss could actually be an expression
of how special that person has been for you.

If you are staying in your relationship
only because it might get better,
then your relationship is already shipwrecked
on the shoals of the future.

If you cannot turn to your lover/spouse today
and truthfully say,
"It has been such a privilege and a joy to have you in my life.
Even if, for some reason, our relationship ends tomorrow,
I am so thankful for all I have shared with you.
You have been such a blessing in my life,"
then you are already
in the process of bankrupting your relationship.
(I am not recommending that you *actually* say this;
without the proper context,
it could be taken to mean something different
from the intended meaning here.)

When we find ourselves sticking around
    or putting up with things
    or working on things
    only because our future with this person might be different,
    then we have begun to kill off our experience
    of love and appreciation for this person.

Keep your relationships clean from entanglement.
Do not borrow from the future.
Do not set it up
    so that you feel your relationships *owe* you anything.
Make every interaction with your lover/spouse
    a gift or an immediate trade
    so that you create no debts for the future
    (which are seeds for resentment).
If every transaction is either a gift or a trade,
    where you are clear that you benefit,
    then you will *always* be able to say,
    "What a *blessing* you are in my life!"

Do you have a current relationship in which you cannot easily say,
    "What a blessing you are in my life"?
    If so, how have you borrowed from the future,
        thereby bankrupting your relationship with this person?
    How can you clean this relationship up?

Notice the choice of courage it takes
    to *not* borrow from the future.

❧

_____

_____

_____

_____

_____

_____

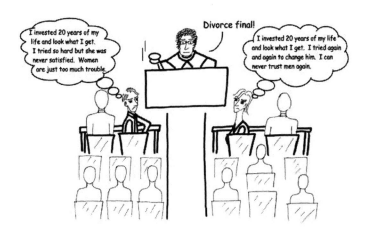

Are you bankrupting your love?

The husband of one of my clients just left her
  and they are getting a divorce.

She feels betrayed,
  after all the effort she made,
  all the sacrifices she suffered,
  all the times she was trying but he wasn't,
  all the times she wanted to leave him
    but held onto hope anyway.

We humans consistently jeopardize
  the quality of our relationships—
  romantic or otherwise,
  by borrowing from the future.

If you cannot honestly say to yourself,
  "If this relationship ended tomorrow, I would be truly grateful
  for the love and friendship I've had with h/im,"
    then your relationship is already
    well on its way to bankruptcy.

How do we get ourselves into this mire of debt
 where we feel that our partner owes us something
 or must change for us
 or our partner feels that we owe h/im something
 or must change for h/im?

Answer: by *not* choosing the courage
 on an hour-by-hour, day-by-day basis
 to make sure that we are satisfied with our boundaries,
 satisfied with our trades (give and take)
 while keeping things complete,
 with no debts built up either way.

You are never doing yourself or your partner
 any favor by having h/im owe you.
And, conversely, s/he is never doing you a favor
 by having you owe h/im.

A relationship only works well when both sides
 insist on arrangements such that
 the selfishness (self-interest) of one dovetails
 with the selfishness of the other.

If, for whatever reason(s),
 such negotiations/arrangements are not made
 so that both sides are consistently satisfied,
  then the opportunity for courage
  is usually available to create a partial or total separation.
To do otherwise is to perpetuate a lose-lose relationship.

Take a look at each of your important relationships.
 Looking at each one separately,
 ask yourself the question,
  "If, by an act of god,
  my relationship with this person ended tomorrow,
  would I be truly grateful for what I had with h/im?"

If the answer is "no,"

then choose the courage to clean up the relationship
or choose the courage to end it.

୨

_____

_____

_____

_____

_____

_____

_____

_____

_____

_____

_____

_____

_____

_____

Disappointment is a sort of bankruptcy—the bankruptcy of a soul that expends too much in hope and expectation.

—*Eric Hoffer (1902-1983, American author and philosopher)*

Today must not borrow from tomorrow.

—*German proverb*

Love never dies a natural death. It dies because we don't know how to replenish its source. It dies of blindness and errors and betrayals. It dies of illness and wounds; it dies of weariness, of withering, of tarnishing.

—*Anaïs Nin (1903-1977,*
French-born American novelist, dancer)

You have NO rights

When problems arise in most relationships,
    whether romantic or otherwise,
    it's because you think you have rights.

You think you have a right
    to be treated fairly by your partner.
You think you have a right
    to be adored, loved, and respected.
You think you have a right
    to enjoy great sex with your partner.
You think you have a right
    for your partner not to have an affair.
You think you have a right
    for your partner to help you out or support you financially.
You think you have a right to get help from your partner
    with the dishes and with the children.

Did you ever wonder why relationships,
    especially romantic relationships,
    are so great in the beginning
    but degrade over time?

One of the major reasons is that,
    at the beginning of a relationship,
    we do not take our partner for granted,
    we do not make assumptions about
    what s/he will or will not do for us;
    we have no rights with h/im.

In the beginning of a relationship,
    when we want something from our partner
    that we're not already getting,
    we have to treat h/im a certain way
    so that s/he gets pleasure in doing it for us.

Yet, after a while,
    we begin to expect things from our partner,
    we begin to think we have rights with our partner.

I once worked with a man
    who had been married for about two years.
    His wife did not want sex as much as he wanted it.
    He was angry and he felt cheated.
    His automatic thoughts were,
    "She is my wife;
        she should want sex with me
        much more often than she does."

I said to him,
    "If there is any possibility
        of you having what you want to have
        with your wife, you will have to let go
        of any rights that you think you have with her.
    When you first met her,
        you did not act as if you had any rights with her.
    If you wanted to make love with her,
        you had to seduce her,
        you had to cherish her,
        you had to enroll her,
        you had to create an atmosphere
        where she wanted to make love as much as you did.
    Feeling like and acting as if you have any rights with her
        will get you exactly the opposite of what you want."

"Now, I don't mean to say
    that you should stay with her indefinitely
    if you don't get what you want with her.
You need to clarify your 'minimum conditions of satisfaction.'
And you might even let her know
    what your 'minimum conditions' are,
    not as a threat, but as a fact
    for her to factor into her commitments and desires."

Letting go of rights is a real choice of courage.
We try to control what we cannot control
    by insisting that we have rights.
And, even if we seem to get what we want sometimes,
    it often comes at a very big cost.

Letting go of rights, letting go of expectations,
    does *not* mean
    not having clear boundaries
    and clear minimum conditions of satisfaction.
In fact, we often hold onto our rights,
    to avoid the fear associated with creating and maintaining
    clear boundaries and minimum conditions of satisfaction.

In which of your personal relationships
    do you think you have rights?
Do these rights really work for you and your relationships?
What courage might you choose to let go of your rights,
    to let go of your expectations,
    and to create what you really want
    with enrollment and good boundaries?

ॐ

How do you know
when to leave your marriage?

Anyone who is successful in playing the stock market
knows one simple rule
about when to sell when the stock is on the downside:

"If I sold this stock at its current price
and I had the money in my hands right now,
would I re-invest that money in the same stock,
knowing what I know now
about its performance and prospects?"

If the answer is "no,"
then the savvy investor gets out and cuts h/is losses.

The investor who hopes the stock will rise
stays in and most often compounds h/is losses.

I believe we would *all* be well served
if we applied this same principle to our marriages.
Certainly, the question of divorce is a more complex decision.
We must calculate the costs of getting out
just as we would factor in the selling commissions
we would have to pay for liquidating
our non-performing stock.
Nevertheless, the same principle applies.

Ask yourself this question,
"Imagine that I am not married to my spouse.
Imagine that I have just met h/im
and I am presented with the option of marrying h/im.

If I knew what I know now:
>   about this person,
>   about how we interact with each other,
>   about how we give each other pleasure and pain,
>   about how we are inspired or discouraged by each other,
>   would I choose to marry this person again?"

If your answer is a definitive "no,"
>   then it's time to get a divorce.

If your answer is "I'm not sure,"
>   then it's time to seek counseling
>   for your relationship.

If children are involved and your answer is "no,"
>   the decision is more complicated,
>   because the benefits and costs to the children
>   must also be considered;
>   but the principle still remains the same,
>   while factoring in those benefits and costs.

Ask yourself the questions,
>   "What are the likely costs and benefits
>   for my children if they continue to live with
>   two parents who get little or no pleasure from each other
>   and often inflict pain on each other?"
>   "By remaining married, what example are we
>   setting for our children about choosing the courage
>   to live a life of genuine love, self-expression, and vitality?"
Then ask yourself the question,
>   "What are the likely costs and benefits for my children
>   if they spend time with parents who are separated
>   (thereby increasing the quality time with each parent),
>   but happier and more satisfied after their divorce?"

Going through a divorce can be rough,
> rough on the parents and rough on the children.
> However, almost *all* of the damage children experience
> > from divorce
> is *not* the result of the divorce itself.
> It is the result of the husband and wife
> > *resisting* the divorce, blaming each other,
> > and feeling guilty for the breakdown of their relationship.
> Separation and divorce can be a time
> > of great celebration and healing,
> > if it is approached powerfully and courageously.

If you are married or in a committed relationship,
> asking yourself these questions
> will probably be a choice of courage.

What are your authentic answers
> when you ask yourself these questions?

For more essay(s) on courage and romance,
> **see www.GoldWinde.com/Cbook/More/Romance**

_____

_____

_____

_____

_____

Better break your word than do worse in keeping it.
> —*Thomas Fuller (1608-1661, British clergyman, author)*

I've been married three times—and each time I married the right person.
> —*Margaret Mead (1901-1978, American anthropologist)*

Are you BEING who you want to be?

Being is distinct from *doing*.
Doing flows easily and naturally out of *being*.
Being does not necessarily flow easily and naturally out of *doing*.

I once worked with a man
    who was a successful manager of a mortgage brokerage house.
Each year, his income was a third of a million dollars or more.
He shared with me an interesting story about himself.
    "Ever since I was small child I always knew
    that I was a $100,000-per-year man.
    Of course, I didn't even know
    what my career was going to be at that time.
    But ever since my early 20s, I've essentially been in the
    $100,000-per-year bracket or better."

Was making $100,000 or more per year hard for him?—No.
It flowed easily and naturally from the person he was *being*.
Yet he took action and risks, and the money was not guaranteed.
And, even when, on occasion,
    he did not make $100,000 or more per year,
    he was still *being* a $100,000-per-year man.

Doing flows easily and naturally from *being*
But if you are *doing* without *being*,
    your *doing* will be hard to do.

We can apply *being* to any area of our life.
Are you *being* irresistible? Are you *being* healthy?
Are you *being* loving? Are you *being* lovable?
Are you *being* adventurous? Are you *being* playful?
Are you *being* lighthearted? Are you *being* passionate?

Being is not necessarily immediately related
    to the current circumstances of your life.
    For example, you can actually have an illness
        while you are *being* healthy.
        Or you can be in debt while you are *being* wealthy.
        Or you can experience hatred while you are *being* loving.
        Or you can notice that someone is saying "no" to you
            while you are *being* irresistible.

Being is the context in which
    the content of your life is perceived and interpreted.

If you are interested in being a certain way,
    these questions will assist you
    in shifting your "ground of being."
I will use "being irresistible" as the example in these questions.
Substitute the "way of being" that you are interested in.

"Am I willing to *be* irresistible?"

"If yes, am I willing to *be* irresistible *now*?"

"How might I act in order to express my *being* irresistible?"

"If I am currently unwilling to *be* irresistible,
    what fear might I embrace
    in order to be willing to *be* irresistible?"

"What do I say that stops me from being willing to *be* irresistible?"

ॐ

How you can have ENOUGH

Do you have enough money?
Do you have enough quality time with your lover or spouse?
Do you get enough sleep?
Are you organized enough?
Do you have enough insurance?
Do you spend enough quality time with your children?

What would be enough leisure in your life?
What would be enough love in your life?
Most of us, in most of our life,
    never clarify "What is enough?"

As a result, it seems that our life is running us,
    instead of us running our life.

If you are not clear about "What is enough,"
    then you will always feel
    the dissatisfaction of never having enough.

How can we answer the question "What is enough?"

Although we can look toward our desires,
    our desires by themselves can never have the final say
    in determining "What is enough?"
Although we must take our desires into account,
    the only way to get true clarity
    about what is enough is by declaration,
    by speaking (out loud, if necessary)
    what is enough for us.

For example, you could declare,
 "Five hours each week of quality time
   with my lover is enough for me,"
 or
 "I can stay organized enough by spending
   20 minutes a day on organization,"
 or
 "Earning at least $4000 a month
   is enough for me."

Of course, once a declaration is made,
 you may need to adjust your actions
 to align with your declaration.

Think of at least one area of your life
 where you have *not* created clarity
 about what is enough.

Honor yourself for the courage
 to decide and declare what is enough.

        ❧

Nothing is enough for the man to whom enough is too little.
   —*Epicurus (circa 341-270 BC, Greek philosopher)*

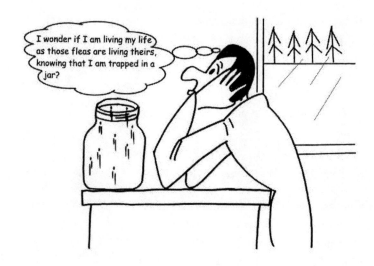

Are you like a flea in a jar?

There is a story about some fleas
>that were put into a glass jar and covered with a lid.

The fleas began jumping very high,
>as fleas are accustomed to do
>when they are fully expressing themselves as fleas.
However, every time they jumped,
>they hit their heads sharply against the lid.
After jumping and hitting their heads many times,
>the fleas restricted their jumping so that
>they jumped just below the height of the lid.

After the fleas had learned to jump within the confines of the jar,
>the lid of the jar was removed.

The fleas continued to jump,
    but only as high as the jar's lid,
    trapping themselves forever
    within the confines of that boring jar.

In what ways might you be like those fleas,
    only jumping so high, only living so much,
    never testing the limits of what you "know"
    to be the boundaries?

What requests are you *not* making
    because you already know the answer?

What actions are you *not* taking
    because you already know what will happen?

Beware of what you know.
It will shut down your life!

Think of some action you might take
    or some request you might make,
    that you've avoided
    because you already "know" the result or answer.

Would you be willing to choose courage
    to test the limits of your "jar"?

❧

_____

_____

_____

_____

_____

_____

_____

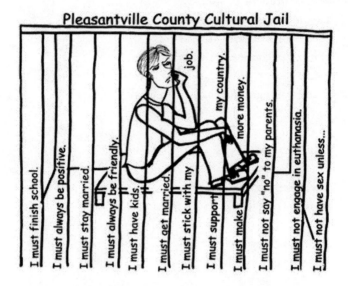

Pleasantville County Cultural Jail

I must finish school.
I must always be positive.
I must stay married.
I must always be friendly.
I must have kids.
I must get married.
I must stick with my job.
I must support my country.
I must make more money.
I must not say "no" to my parents.
I must not engage in euthanasia.
I must not have sex unless...

Has your culture jailed you?

When we look back upon civilizations and cultures of the past
    or when we look at people of other countries
        who share the earth with us,
    we often wonder,
        "How could they possibly believe *that?*"
        or "How could they possibly act *that way?*"

In considering cultures of the past and/or the present,
    try to fathom
    the honorability of suicide in Japan,
    the binding of women's feet in China,
    the crusades and witch hunts of the Western world,
    the sacrificing of humans and animals
        to gods in all parts of the world,
    the condemnation of personal desire
        by most religions and cultures of the world,
    the honorability of killing others for your country,

the willingness of people to obey without question
the wishes or commands of their superiors,
whether those superiors be religious, governmental,
educational, business, or parental,
the consistent vilification of the people
of other regions, religions, and countries,
the intractability and righteousness
of the participants of conflicts and wars,
the certainty by which other people know
that their way
or their religion's way
or their country's way
or their school's way
or their company's way
or their family's way
is the right way.

We may say to ourselves,
"How could other people act or believe this way?"
"I would never do that if I were in their shoes."

Yet, how often do we question our own *current* box
of culture and civilization?
How much of what we do and don't do,
how much of what we say and don't say,
how much of what we believe and don't believe,
is totally driven by and justified by,
usually unseen and unacknowledged
(often implicit) edicts and mandates of
a culture that has us just where it wants us,
while making us think (that's part of the function of culture)
that *we* see things *as they are,*
and *as they should be,*
unlike those "other people"?

Yet, to step outside of culture,
    to stretch the limits of culture
    in a way that tries to consider
    both the benefits and costs of doing so,
    can be the most courageous of all human acts.
Culture's power of enforcement (I am talking about *all* cultures)
    lies in granting approval from others
    and avoiding condemnation and estrangement from others
    (and even from ourselves because we, too, *are* the culture).

Day by day, begin to ask yourself,
    what are the opportunities
    for me to create more benefits and fewer costs,
    both for myself and others,
    by choosing courage
    in the face of the culture and the expectations
        of my society,
        of my country,
        of my school,
        of my company,
        of my family,
        of my friends and colleagues?

Begin to play with these opportunities.

                                   ॐ

_____

_____

_____

_____

_____

_____

_____

_____

_____

_____

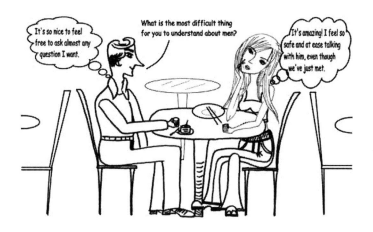

Can you feel the locks and chains of your culture?

We have no idea how tightly
    our cultures bind us and thereby prevent us
    from easily connecting with each other,
    especially when first meeting.

I have discovered a fascinating phenomenon,
    a phenomenon I have never before
    seen mentioned or documented.
Yet it dramatically uncovers
    the alienation we feel with each other
    when our social interactions are
    confined to one's own culture.

Let me give a specific example.
    Although this example is from when I lived in Tokyo,
        it is typical of this previously undocumented phenomenon
        and I've had countless similar experiences here in China.

After selecting my meal at the Meiji University cafeteria,
    I approached an eating table
    where a 20-year-old Japanese student sat.
I asked her if I could join her for English conversation.
    She accepted.

During fifteen minutes of conversation,
    I asked her,
    "What do you like best about yourself?"
    "What do you dislike about yourself?"
    "What is your life dream?"
    "What gives you the most ongoing pleasure in your life?"
    "What is the most difficult thing to understand about men?"

We spoke openly, with energy and liking,
    often looking into each other's eyes.
Then I asked her to notice
    how easy, open, and enjoyable our conversation was.
    She expressed amazement as she agreed with me.
I then asked her to imagine I was a Japanese man
    who had approached her in exactly the same way I had.
    "Would you feel as open and friendly
        with him as you do with me, an American?"
    "No," she replied.

Then I told her that,
    if she were an American woman,
    I would not have felt so open and friendly with her
    as I felt with her as a Japanese woman.
    I would not have felt so safe asking her such personal questions
    and looking directly into her eyes.

In talking with her,
    I was, in some measure, outside my own culture,
    and, yet, I was not inside her culture.
In talking with me,
    she was, in some measure, outside her own culture,
    and yet not inside my culture.
To a degree, we stepped outside of culture.
    This phenomenon is somewhat similar to
    how young children easily connect with other children
    (who were complete strangers beforehand),
    before they learn the unwritten rules
    governing social interactions.

The Japanese student and I both had a freedom (and safety)
    to connect with each other
    that does not exist when we are talking
    with someone from our own culture.

She felt free to be herself with me
    because she did not feel limited by
    the implicit social guidelines of
    approval/disapproval that inhibit her
    within her own culture when speaking
    with a Japanese person/man.

I felt free to be myself with her
    because I did not feel limited by
    the implicit social guidelines that inhibit me
    within my own culture when speaking
    with an American person/woman.

I call this phenomenon the "cross-cultural freedom effect."
It was one of my primary reasons for moving
    to Japan and China.

I can be myself more around people who are not like me
    than I can around people who are more like me!
    Very interesting!

From my own experience and the experience
    of some of my friends,
    this cross-cultural freedom effect
    is more pronounced between two very disparate cultures
        (e.g., a Western culture and an Asian culture)
    than it is between two more similar cultures
        (e.g., U.S. culture and German culture).

Notice the invisible rules
    that inhibit connection between you and another person
    within your own culture.

Experiment with choosing courage
    to talk openly about those rules and their consequences.
    Determine whether you and your partner might be willing
        to experiment with breaking those rules
        in order to create closer connection and understanding.

∽

Borrowing from the future is the root of all evil

If there is any one fundamental habit
　　that gets and keeps us in more trouble than any other,
　　it is the habit of "borrowing from the future."

I see three fundamental ways
　　in which we humans express this habit.

1.　Borrowing *satisfaction* from the future—
　　the most insidious and treacherous form of this habit.

Anytime that we *cannot* honestly say to ourselves,
　　"I'm in love with *this* moment of my life,"
　　then we're likely borrowing from the future.
We're putting up with this moment
　　and justifying it with the hope
　　that some future moment is going to be better.
Of course, if thinking about our future
　　actually creates full satisfaction in this moment,
　　then we're not really borrowing from the future.
However, when we are thinking that life will be great
　　when we graduate from school,
　　　　or change jobs,
　　　　or get married,
　　　　or have a baby,
　　　　or get divorced,
　　　　or retire,
　　　　or discover our life passion,
　　　　etc.,
　　then we are borrowing from our future.

I wrote down a thought that captures
　　the essence of breaking this habit:
"Make love to *this* moment for it's the only one you'll ever have."

2.　Borrowing *time* from the future—
　　the second most damaging form of this habit.

　　We leave the dish in the sink to wash later.
　　We leave the keys on the sofa
　　　　instead of putting them in their place.
　　We leave a piece of paper on our desk
　　　　instead of deciding what to do with it now.
　　We say we'll find time to exercise tomorrow
　　　　instead of doing it today.
　　We'll approach that person we're attracted to later.
　　We'll make that phone call we need to make later.
　　We'll tell our mother how much we love her later.

I have another thought that captures
　　the essence of breaking this habit:
"Just pay the time *now!*"

3.　Borrowing *money* from the future.

Although the damage from this habit is enormous,
　　it does not begin to equal the damage caused by the first two.

Of these three ways of borrowing from the future,
　　however, it is this one that is the most widely recognized
　　and publicly acknowledged as a bad habit.

I do not want to suggest that it is never useful or appropriate
　　to choose to borrow from the future
　　in one or more of these three ways.

If we clearly weigh the benefits and costs in a given circumstance,
    borrowing from the future may indeed
    be the best course of action.
However, for most of us, most of the time,
    we dig our grave with these behaviors
    because they have become our habitual way of living,
    usually without a lot of conscious awareness.

Find and examine at least one example in your own recent past
    for each of these three ways of borrowing from the future.

Notice the fear you feel when you choose the courage
    not to borrow from your future.

❧

_____

_____

_____

_____

_____

Only put off until tomorrow what you are willing to die having
left undone.
    —*Pablo Picasso (1881-1973, Spanish artist)*

The foolish person seeks happiness in the distance; the wise person
grows it under his feet.
    —*James Oppenheim (1882-1932, American poet)*

First I was dying to finish high school and start college. And then
I was dying to finish college and start working. And then I was
dying to marry and have children. And then I was dying for my
children to grow old enough for school so I could return to work.
And then I was dying to retire. And now, I am dying . . . and
suddenly I realize I forgot to live.
    —*unknown*

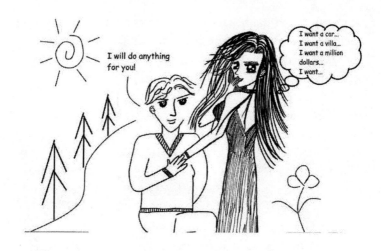

Do you write blank checks?

We all know the idea
    behind writing a blank check.
We just sign our name and somebody else fills in the amount
    that we have just obligated ourselves to pay.
Most of us recognize how foolish it is
    to write blank checks, at least on our bank account.
If we were in the habit
    of writing blank checks against our bank account,
    then either we would have to renege
    on our blank check agreements
    or, with resignation and regret,
    we would have to pay dearly for our foolish promises.

Yet, consider how often you might
        be writing or speaking blank checks
        in other areas of your life,
    creating, in the process,
        upsets and breakdowns and imbalances,
        both for yourself and for others.

How often do you say (either explicitly or implicitly),
    "*Somehow,* some way I'll handle that later," or
    "I'll spend however long it takes to get the job done," or
    "I'll agree to *whatever* request/expectation
        my boss/mother/spouse/lover/friend makes of me"?
Or consider the biggest blank check of our life,
    the one that most of us speak when we get married
    (mistakenly thinking it is good or necessary
    for our spouse and/or our marriage),
    "I'll do *whatever* it takes to make our marriage work," or
    "I'll do *whatever* it takes to make you happy
        and give you what you want,"
    neither specifying any minimum criteria
        for maintaining our promise
    nor under what conditions we would quit the marriage.

Can you see how each one of these is a blank check,
    obligating you, very often,
    to an undetermined and indefinite amount
    of your time and resources?
These are the types of promises,
    these are the types of commitments
    that can bankrupt day-to-day life,
    both for ourselves and for others.

Identify the last time you spoke a blank check?
    What were the results?
Our motivation for speaking blank checks
    is most often to try to feel safer,
    to try to control and guarantee things,
    and/or to look better in the moment.
It can be the choice of courage to say,
    "I will *not* promise when or if it will be done," or
    "I will spend 15 minutes at 4 pm tomorrow
        toward completing this," or

"I will spend two hours per day
    until the job is complete," or
"I will consider *separately* each request/expectation
    from my boss/father/spouse/lover/friend," or
"I will stay married to you *as long as*
        we feel special and loving toward each other
    or I have good reason to believe
        that we can regain those feelings
        within the foreseeable future."

What blank checks have you already spoken (or implied)
    that you need to modify or cancel?

For the future, are you willing to choose courage
    to *not* write or speak blank checks?

ஒ

_____
_____
_____
_____
_____
_____
_____
_____
_____
_____
_____
_____
_____
_____
_____
_____
_____
_____
_____

Poor boundaries will kill off your love

There is so much love and beauty in the world
    that we would appreciate more
    if we would not always expect it
    to make us feel safe and comfortable.
Each one of us is a natural opening
    for love, friendship, and affection.
Yet how many of us are consistently present
    to the feelings of love and goodwill toward,
    not only those around us now, but also
    our former colleagues, friends, lovers, and spouses?

How great it would be
    to still cherish each and every friend you've ever had!
    At one time, you cherished that friend.
How great it would be
    to still admire every boss you've ever worked for!
    At one time, you admired that boss.
How great it would be
    to still be in love with
        every lover you've ever shared intimacy with!
    At one time, you felt very special about h/im.
Most of us
    (unintentionally) kill off our feelings of liking and love
    because we are very unskilled
    at creating and maintaining good boundaries
    and at creating, in a timely manner,
    empowering endings and goodbyes.

Furthermore, the major reason for our lack of skill is that
    we want to feel safe and comfortable in the moment.

It is a choice of courage to assert ourselves
    (in a spirit of partnership)
    to create, change, and/or maintain boundaries
    (so that we don't build up resentment and/or resignation).
It is a choice of courage to assert ourselves
    to create endings and goodbyes
    (with an attitude of partnership)
    so that the needed change in our relationship has occurred
    before resentment or resignation has built up
    and while there are still feelings
    of goodwill, respect, and even love.

For example,
    to end a great romance while it is still good
    can be a supreme choice of courage.
To wait until it's really on the rocks
    and we are beginning to hate the other person
    is when we usually end it,
    holding on until the very last.

Love, and even liking, for most of us,
    quickly devolves into attachment.
When we love, our fear of loss arises immediately,
    and, in our resistance to this fear, we become attached.
We become attached to the belief that the person we love
    will never be upset with us and never disapprove of us.
We become attached to the belief that
    s/he/we will never think of leaving.

We human beings need to become skilled
    at proactively creating good boundaries and great endings,
    instead of waiting until we are pushed against the wall.

I'm not talking about bailing out
    because we are avoiding our fear of the risk of loving or caring.
I'm talking about creating good boundaries
       and powerful goodbyes in support of our love for each other.

For most of us, most of the time,
    especially with our lover/spouse,
    we are very poor at creating
    love-supportive boundaries and timely goodbyes.

Ask yourself,
    "Who in my life right now do I need to say 'goodbye' to
       in one form or another?"
    "Which of my relationships right now
       is suffering from poorly defined boundaries?"
    "What is the opportunity for courage in these circumstances?"

☙

_____

_____

_____

_____

_____

_____

_____

_____

_____

_____

Attachment is the great fabricator of illusions; reality can be attained
only by someone who is detached.
    —*Simone Weil (1910-1943, French philosopher, mystic)*

Love is like quicksilver in the hand. Leave the fingers open and it
stays. Clutch it, and it darts away.
    —*Dorothy Parker (1893-1967, American author)*

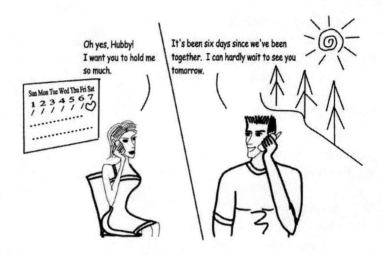

Enrich your relationships with distance

"Absence makes the heart grow fonder."
"Good fences make good neighbors."
"Familiarity breeds contempt."

We've all heard these proverbs.
    But do we apply them appropriately?

When it comes to our relationships
    with our lover, with our spouse,
    with our family, with our friends,
    the common wisdom is that we need more "togetherness."

But often the opposite is true.

More togetherness is not necessarily better.
    Often, it makes things worse.

Certainly, whatever time we do spend together
    should be of the highest quality.
    But quality often goes down as quantity increases.
If you really care about someone,
    perhaps the most loving thing you can do
    is to gently decline h/is request for more time together.

In China, there is a proverb that goes something like this,
    "Marriage is the tomb of love."
I would fine-tune that proverb by saying that
    "the best way to kill off romance is by living together."

A Chinese woman friend of mine has a live-in fiancé.
    She reported to me recently that,
        after coming back from a two-week business trip
        away from home and away from her fiancé, she and he had
        the most incredible and romantic weekend ever.

So why aren't we consistent in maintaining
    a distance (especially a physical distance)
    that will support our "staying hungry for each other,"
    as well as avoiding unnecessary entanglements
    and stepping on each other's toes?
    Because we are resisting the fear
        of the possible loss and/or unsatisfied hunger
        that we might have to endure if we maintain that distance.

What requests might you make
    for additional distance in your relationships
    in order to improve them?
How might you choose courage
    to say "no" to another's request for closeness
    so that you might continue to support
    the best possible relationship with that person?

What actions might you take (unilaterally, if necessary)
to create the distance you need
to really love those in your life
(e.g., moving out of the house)?

_____

_____

_____

_____

_____

_____

Let there be spaces in our togetherness. And let the winds of the
heavens dance between you.
—*Kahlil Gibran (1883-1931, Lebanese poet, philosopher, artist)*

Love is like quicksilver in the hand. Leave the fingers open and it
stays. Clutch it, and it darts away.
—*Dorothy Parker (1893-1967,*
American critic, satirical poet, short-story writer)

Sometimes I wonder if men and women really suit each other.
Perhaps they should live next door and just visit now and then.
—*Katharine Hepburn (1907-2003, American actress, writer)*

Divorce: A resumption of diplomatic relations and rectification of
boundaries.
—*Ambrose Bierce (1842-1914, American author,*
editor, journalist, "The Devil's Dictionary")

Romance and working together don't mix.
The way of being that creates and nurtures romantic intimacy
does not often mix easily with the way of being that creates and
maintains effective working relationships.
—*GoldWinde*

Say "No" if you really love me

Perhaps you've heard the maxim/quote,
    "Good fences make good neighbors."—Robert Frost
The Chinese have a proverb, "Distance creates beauty."

My father was often a very difficult man
    to be around, especially as he got older.
I have no idea how my mother managed
    to stay with him for 41 years before she divorced him.

My father is dead now.
    However, when he was alive,
        I wanted very much that he experience that I loved him.
Yet I knew enough about his behavior
    and about how I responded to his behavior
    to know that, if I spent much time with him,
    it would be quite difficult, if not impossible,
    for all my actions and words to be loving and respectful.

Consequently, I arranged my life (sometimes it took courage)
    to visit with him no more than two days each year.
I knew that I could treat him with love and respect
    if I were with him for no longer than two days.

I also wrote to him (mostly by means of a journal
    that I wrote and shared with others also),
        sending him a letter every two weeks.
I found it easy to express my love and to receive his love
    in the form of letters, back and forth.
If I had demanded of myself that I expose myself to his behavior
    for longer time periods, I would have lost my feelings
    of love for him and he would have known it.

Many of us kill off our relationships
    with our parents, with our children,
    with our spouses, with our lovers,
    with our business associates, and even with our friends
    by living inside the toxic formula,
        "If I really loved/liked this person, then I would . . . ."

Maybe love demands that you *not* live with
    your spouse, your parents, your grown child.

Maybe love demands that you say *no* to a request from
    your friend, your lover, your parent or child.

Love demands that you get clear about the *boundaries*
    that will best serve you in your relationships
    with those you care about.

Togetherness is important.
But *apart-ness* is just as important.

How have you allowed your boundaries to be violated?

How have your relationships been damaged
    because you have not chosen the courage
    to discover and create the appropriate *apart-ness?*

What courage might you choose today to create and maintain
    the boundaries that would enhance
    the quality of your relationships in the long run,
        even though it might create some upset in the short run?

Is your silence killing your friendship?

How can you tell a friend
    that h/is showing up late for your get-togethers
    feels disrespectful to you?
How do you tell a spouse
    that you're feeling less and less safe with h/im
    and withdrawing from the relationship as a result?
How can you tell someone you spend time with
    that h/is breath is unpleasant to you?
How does a woman tell the man whom she really cares about
    that five-minute love-making sessions are not enough for her?

Very often we keep our mouths shut,
    thinking that we'll damage our relationship if we speak up.

But the truth is that, in most cases,
    we will damage the relationship, perhaps beyond repair,
    if we don't speak up.

The truth is that your resignation, resentment, or withdrawal
    will build up.

You'll often blame the other person
    for not being more sensitive, for not being fair,
    for not reading your mind, for not caring about you.

Often your righteousness will reach a point
    where it explodes and your partner's response
    confirms your belief about h/im
    and validates your making h/im wrong
    in the first place.

When you do speak up,
    what you say and how you say it is very important.
    (You might first want to get some coaching on this.)

Nevertheless, no matter how carefully chosen your words are,
    you will still be choosing courage to speak up.

Honor yourself for that courage.

You will be choosing courage
    as an expression of the caring and commitment
    you have for that person and your relationship with h/im.

Think before you speak.

But speak.

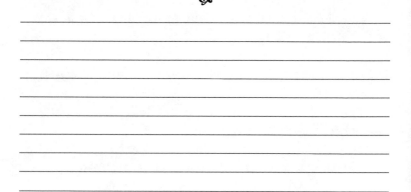

Speak your mind even if your voice shakes.
    —*Maggie Kuhn (1905-1995, American activist, social worker)*

The basic difference between being assertive and being aggressive
is how our words and behavior affect the rights and well being of
others.

    —*Sharon Anthony Bower (American author)*

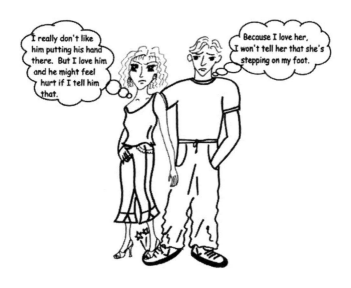

Are you entangled in your relationship?

Choosing the courage to create, clarify, and maintain
boundaries that leave us empowered is the *number one* factor
in having great relationships.
It is especially important in maintaining and enhancing
our relationships once they have started.

Most of us get sucked into the toxic formulas of
"If you really loved me, you would . . ." or
"If I really loved her/him/my child/etc., I would . . ." or
"If I was a good dad/mother/husband/wife/friend, etc.,
I would . . ." or
trying to *prove*
that we love,
that we are a good and/or responsible person,
in an attempt to guarantee that someone
will like us or stick around,

rather than creating and maintaining the clear boundaries
  necessary for a mutually selfish and satisfying
  relationship between two *separate* people.

Most of us have not clarified
  our minimum conditions of satisfaction
  that are necessary for our relationships to work.
As a result, we allow that person to step over our boundaries
  (often while we are also stepping over h/is boundaries),
  because we have not clarified them in the first place.
  Then we resent that person for doing so,
  not realizing our own power and cause in the matter.
As a result,
  our relationships are more often entanglements and dramas,
  rather than relationships that nurture, empower, and excite us.

Establishing clear boundaries
  creates the atmosphere needed for great relationships.
Not establishing clear boundaries
  creates the miasma that slowly poisons our relationships.

To have the quality we want in our relationships,
  we have to be willing to choose the courage
  to potentially lose those relationships,
  and/or be willing to risk
  upsetting those whom we care about.

If we are held hostage by our resistance to the fear
  of disapproval or abandonment,
if we are unwilling to choose the courage, when needed,
  to *not* be a "good guy" or to *not* be a "caring person,"
then we will *never* be able
  to create the rewarding, lasting relationships we want.

Are you clear about when you need to say "yes"?
Are you clear about when you need to say "no"?

If you feel entangled in or victimized by
    your relationships in any way,
    then you are *not* clear about these questions.

Remember, however, that although you are saying "no" firmly,
    you can still say "no" with gentleness, compassion,
    and a clear commitment to the quality
    of your relationship with that person,
    creating and maintaining compassionate boundaries.
Remember the maxim:
    "Be soft on people, but hard on problems."

Ask yourself,
    "Am I choosing courage to say 'yes' when I need to?"
    "Am I choosing courage to say 'no' when I need to?"

∾

_____

_____

_____

_____

_____

_____

_____

_____

_____

> Those who profess to favor freedom and yet depreciate agitation
> are men who want rain without thunder and lightning.
> —*Frederick Douglass (1818-1895,*
> *abolitionist, orator, writer, reformer, diplomat, statesman)*

> We need to find the courage to say NO to the things and people
> that are not serving us if we want to rediscover ourselves and live
> our lives with authenticity.
> —*Barbara DeAngelis (expert on relationships and love, author)*

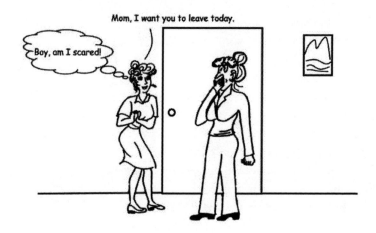

If you're a good guy, it's probably bad

At least in the domain of interpersonal relationships,
   the "good" people consistently empower
   the damaging behavior of the "bad" people,
   encouraging it to persist.

I have a client (35 years old) whose mother
   has consistently dominated and controlled the lives
   of her grown children through
   temper tantrums and threats of disowning them.

And, although her children have, on occasion,
   flared their uncontrolled anger back at her,
   none of them have clarified their boundaries
   and firmly enforced those boundaries with their mother.

Recently, through my coaching,
    my client accepted her mother for a visit,
    making it clear to her mother
    that she was welcome to stay for five days,
    not the ten days her mother had wanted.
    Her mother agreed.
Yet, after five days, her mother showed no signs of leaving.

Taking some deep breaths and saying to herself,
    "Boy, am I scared!" my client sat down with her mother
    and had the following conversation:
"It's been great having you here for the five days
    we agreed upon, Mom.
    Is there anything you need from me
    so that you can leave today?"
"But you need my help with the packers,"
    her mother replied (my client was moving).
"Thank you for your concern for me,
    and I want you to leave today."
"This is no way to treat your mother,"
    her mother replied angrily.
"I know that you feel hurt by my request,
    but I want you to leave today."
"Well, I'm not leaving!
    How can you ask such a thing? I'm your mother!"
"I know my request seems unreasonable to you,
    but I want you to leave today."
"I told you I'm not leaving, you ungrateful bitch!"
"I know that I seem ungrateful to you.
    But if you don't leave, I will call the police.
    I want you to leave today, Mom."
"I'll never speak to you again!
    You're not my daughter anymore."

Her mother left in anger
    without my client having to call the police
    (which she was prepared to do; it was not a bluff).

In the past, my client and her siblings
    had sometimes retaliated in righteous anger
    at their mother's provocation.
    Each time, their mother
        said that she would never speak with them again.
    It was usually less than a month
        before she was back in communication with her children.

Of course, my client had to be willing
    to take the risk that her mother
    might never speak with her again
    (although I think it was a small risk).

All her life, her mother has been allowed
    to get her way by threatening people
    with her anger and righteous indignation.
    She is the grown-up equivalent of the school-ground bully.
Everyone complained about her,
    everyone got sympathy for putting up with her,
    but, up until now,
    no one chose the courage
    to clarify their boundaries with her
    and enforce those boundaries consistently
    in a loving, but firm, manner.
Although, on the surface, it may not seem that way,
    what my client did with her mother
    was the most loving thing she could have done
    for their relationship.

We dishonor our love (or liking) for another
   by allowing that person to consistently violate our boundaries.
Even though we tolerate a loved one
   in the name of love, it's actually
   in the name of feeling safe and more comfortable
      in the moment.
   It was a major choice of courage for my client
      to speak to her mother in the way that she did.
      And her actions really inspired me.

A note about cultural differences.
   For the above example,
      a grown child in the Japanese or Chinese culture
      will typically have to choose a lot more courage
      to clarify and maintain h/is boundaries with h/is parents
      (that is, s/he will have to embrace a lot more fear)
      than a grown child in the American culture.

Take a minute and ask yourself,

   "Is there anyone in my life I am tolerating and allowing
      to consistently step over my boundaries?"

   "What courage would I need to choose
      to clarify my boundaries with h/im
      and consistently maintain those boundaries?"

   "Am I willing to choose this courage?"

   "Is there a way to break the courage into smaller steps
      if I'm not willing to choose it all at once?"

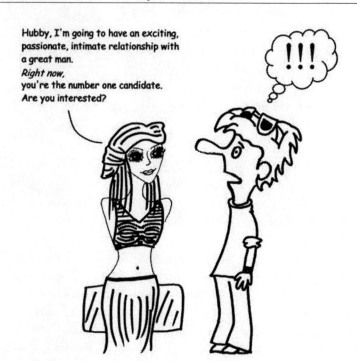

Hubby, I'm going to have an exciting, passionate, intimate relationship with a great man.
Right now, you're the number one candidate. Are you interested?

Are you willing to walk away?

In negotiation tactics, a good negotiator
   is always clear (at least with h/imself)
   what h/is minimum conditions of satisfaction are
   for a satisfactory deal.

A negotiator who is *not* clear
   about h/is minimum conditions of satisfaction
   ends up making many bad deals
   by thinking that s/he "*has to* make the deal."

In other areas of our lives, however,
   most of us never get clear about when we will walk away,
   when our minimum conditions of satisfaction
   are *not* being met in a given area of our life.

It is a choice of courage:
    to embrace our fear,
    to clarify our boundaries,
    to define our minimum conditions of satisfaction,
    and to take consistent, appropriate action.

In your job,
    are you willing to set a standard
    below which you are willing to walk away?
    If you are willing to walk away,
        you have much more power to create the job you want,
        whether it be your current one or a new position.

In your marriage,
    if you were clear that living alone would be better,
    would you be willing to walk away?
    If you are willing to walk away,
        you have much more power
            to create the relationship you want,
        whether it be your current one or a new relationship.

In a friendship,
    if you believed you would be happier without that friend,
    would you be willing to walk away?
    If you are willing to walk away,
        you have much more power to build better friendships,
        whether they include this friend or not.

With a project or a goal,
    if you recognize that the costs outweigh the benefits,
    would you be willing to walk away?
    If you are willing to walk away,
        your projects and goals will be much more satisfying,
        whether or not the current one is finished.

In deciding in which country to live,
    if you believe you would be better off in another country,
    would you be willing to walk away?
    If you are willing to walk away,
        you can live in the country
            that provides the best environment for you,
        whether it's your current country or a new one.

In your life (most probably near its end),
    if you are clear that the pain outweighs the pleasure,
    with no prospect for it getting better,
    would you be willing to walk away?
    If you are willing to walk away,
        then a successful and enjoyable life can be ended
        without the unnecessary and inhumane suffering
            that has no termination, except in your death.

Taking a stand for a magnificent life
    requires that we *not* be willing to settle
    for less than we have the possibility of having.

Where in your life have you not been willing to walk away?

Will you choose the courage to walk away?

                        ⁹∞

_____

_____

_____

_____

_____

_____

_____

_____

_____

_____

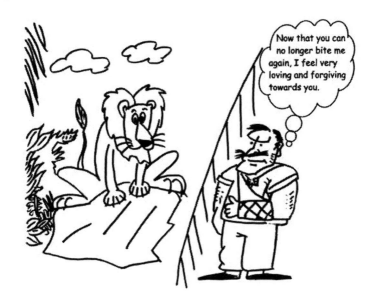

Beware of forgiveness

We often believe that forgiveness
means "putting ourselves again in harm's way."
We think it means exposing ourselves again
to the probability of a similar result.

Nothing is further from the truth.

Forgiveness means *only*
that you let go of blaming or resenting another
for what s/he did or didn't do.
It does not mean that you have not learned
from what happened.

In fact, one of the quickest ways
to assist yourself in forgiving another
is to "remove yourself from harm's way."

For example, a client of mine
managed to forgive his mother for lying to him
(which she does regularly),
by letting go of any expectation or hope
that his mother will tell the truth in the future,
and adjusting his actions accordingly.

For any given incident,
she may or may not tell the truth.
If she tells the truth,
he can experience this as an extra bonus.

He now acknowledges the truth:
he can trust that his mother will probably lie to him again.
He can now forgive his mother
because he is willing to stop lying to himself
that his mother will one day miraculously change her ways.
He can adjust his actions accordingly,
now that he is willing to acknowledge and accept
the risks in doing so,
regardless of how his mother might respond.

In shifting his perspective,
he also eliminates any need to forgive his mother in the future,
because he now knows and accepts that he can trust his mother
to lie to him sometimes.

When we realize that we cannot trust
people to always be the way we would prefer them to be,
when we accept the way
things have been and are likely to be again
(especially in areas where we lack control),
forgiveness and a sense of peace and good will
become an easy and natural part of our living.

Who are you not forgiving?

Choose courage to take whatever actions are needed
    to put yourself "out of harm's way" as much as possible,
    while also accepting the risks involved
    and the possibility that the behavior
    of those you have forgiven could be repeated.

ൣ

Forgiveness does not change the past, but it does enlarge the future.
    —*Paul Boese (author)*

Forgiveness means giving up all hope of a better past.
    —*Landrum Bolling (peacemaker, college president)*

History is a better guide than good intentions.
    —*Jeane Kirkpatrick (American diplomat, syndicated columnist,*
        political scientist, author of "The New Presidential Elite"
        and "The Reagan Phenomenon")

Quitting: The unacknowledged virtue

Perseverance. Don't give up. Never say die.
  Determination. Tenacity. Loyalty.
  Through thick and thin. Persistence.
  At any price. Always do your best.
  Spare no effort. Leave no stone unturned.
  Spare no pains. Go through fire and water.
  Always keep one's word.
  Remember the "Little Engine that Could"!

These are the messages we hear and accept from the earliest age.
  They become a part of our identity.
  And when we see ourselves
      in full or partial violation of these messages,
      we often think badly or are ashamed of ourselves.

Give up. Call it quits. Be a quitter.
  If it's not working, get out.
  If it doesn't fit you, try something else.
  If there's no light at the end of the tunnel,
      maybe it's the wrong tunnel.
  If it doesn't feel easy, it may not be the right way, anyway.
  Cancel your word.
  Knowing when to give up
      is one of the secrets to a successful life.

These are typically the messages that we *don't* hear
  and would consider to be heretical if we did.

Perseverance is great,
  but not all the time and not in every situation.

How many lives would have been saved
    if the Japanese leaders had recognized
    that they were obviously going to lose the war
    and surrendered much earlier than they did?

How many lives would have been saved
    if the leaders of the United States had
    acknowledged what was so clearly an
    un-winnable war in Vietnam
    and pulled out years earlier?

How many loveless, tortured lives,
    for both parents (and sometimes children),
    are unnecessarily endured
    because the spouses are unwilling
    to declare their marriage unworkable?

By always relying on the simplistic formula
    of perseverance, we avoid the challenge
    of thinking for ourselves
    and making difficult and courageous choices
    based upon the context and circumstances
    as well as our deepest desires and commitments.

Wisdom and courage are required to
    ". . . know when to hold them, know when to fold them;
    know when to walk away, know when to run . . .
    knowing what to throw away and knowing what to keep . . ."
Thank you, Kenny Rogers.

Honor yourself for the courage to quit.

                ❧

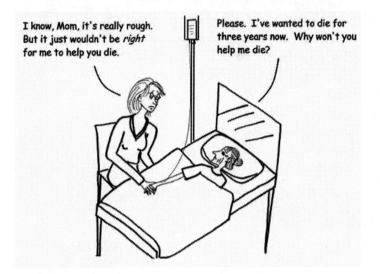

The final ending: The supreme opportunity for courage

My maternal grandmother lived a happy life,
    except for her last eight years.
The last eight years were chronically painful.
She was robbed of her ability
    to do the things she really cherished,
    to walk through her beloved woods
    and read from her many books.
Why should such a beautiful life be tarnished
    by the misery of those last eight years?

So much unnecessary suffering is incurred
    because we resist, rather than embrace,
    the endings that would serve us best.

Consider all the suffering created by our resistance to divorce.
Consider all the suffering created by our resistance to leaving a job.
Consider all the suffering created
    by our resistance to ending unsupportive relationships.

However, the true horror in our modern world
    is the suffering we inflict on ourselves and our loved ones
    by not embracing the *final* ending
    (at least for this earth in this body): death.

When continued suffering of a loved one
    (including yourself) is a foregone conclusion,
    when no one can offer anything other than solace,
    I believe it's time to choose the ultimate act of courage
    to end life with dignity.

Have you faced the question, either for yourself or for a loved one,
    of creating and embracing your death
    (or h/is death) at a time when you can still say,
    "I or s/he have lived a magnificent, fulfilling life,"
    rather than letting nature take its course
    with endless months and years
    of chronic pain and hopelessness?

Honor yourself for choosing the courage
    to face that question now.

ഔ

For more essay(s) on courage and quitting,
    see www.GoldWinde.com/Cbook/More/Quitting.

For further information, read the book *Final Exit: The Practicalities of Self-Deliverance and Assisted Suicide for the Dying,* by Derek Humphry.

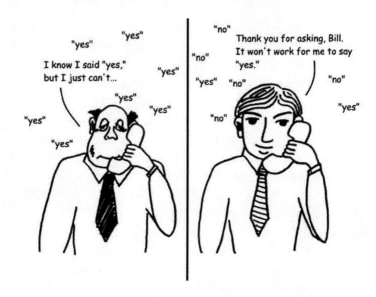

Choose the courage to say "no"

Choosing *no* (and/or saying "no")
is just as important as choosing *yes*.

Very often, we end up feeling
resentful, stressed, overwhelmed,
depressed, ineffective, and guilty
because we neglect to choose *no* with clarity and consistency.

"What am I *not* going to do today?"
"What am I willing to cancel or reschedule so that *this* day can be
fun and productive and guilt-free?"
"In what ways might I choose courage
by choosing *not* to do something?"
"In what ways might I choose courage
by saying 'no' (with gentleness) to another?"

These are questions we must ask ourselves
if we are to create a life of fun, renewal, and accomplishment.

The prevalent idea that we can have it all
    is especially toxic to our lives.

For every *yes* we choose, we must choose *no* a thousand times.
Cramming in one more *yes* just sabotages
    the experience of our lives as works of art
    and destroys or diminishes each *yes* we've already chosen.

How might you choose courage today by saying "no"?

❧

_____

_____

_____

_____

_____

_____

_____

_____

_____

_____

Learn to say no. It will be of more use to you than to be able to read Latin.
    —*Charles Haddon Spurgeon (1834-1892, English preacher)*

Besides the noble art of getting things done, there is the noble art of leaving things undone. The wisdom of life consists in the elimination of non-essentials.
    —*Lin Yutang (1895-1976, Chinese-American writer, translator)*

You have to decide what your highest priorities are and have the courage—pleasantly, smilingly, non-apologetically—to say "no" to other things. And the way you do that is by having a bigger "yes" burning inside. The enemy of the "best" is often the "good."
    —*Stephen Covey (author, lecturer, leadership mentor)*

Why lock yourself in unnecessarily?

My new Chinese friends often ask me,
 "How long will you live in Shanghai?"
My answer is,
 "I will live in Shanghai somewhere
 between 'indefinitely' and 'forever'."
I answer this way to express
 how strongly I feel about the possibility
 of living in Shanghai forever.
However, I see no value
 in committing myself to live here forever
 and much value in leaving the decision open-ended.

Sometimes people ask me,
 "Will you be a life coach forever?"
My answer is,
 "Life coaching is the perfect career for me.
 But if I wake up tomorrow and realize
 that another career provides
 more opportunities for me to experience
 a connection with others,
 interpersonal adventure,
 playfulness, innocence, and romance
 (my five major life inspirations),
 I will change my career tomorrow."

Sometimes it is necessary and powerful
 to lock ourselves in
 to get a specific result.

But often, when we lock ourselves in
    (either implicitly or explicitly),
    our primary motive is
    to try to feel safe and comfortable
    where there is no real safety.
    In such situations, our commitments stifle our lives
        and create much more suffering for us and others
        than is necessary.

Do not confuse what I am suggesting with indecisiveness,
    in which we avoid making a choice
    among two or more necessary alternatives
    because we are unwilling to face the fear
    that accompanies whatever choice we might make.

I am talking about the possibility of making a courageous choice
    not to lock ourselves in,
    not to unnecessarily commit ourselves,
    when the only advantage in commitment is avoiding the fear
        of leaving things open-ended
    and where the ultimate costs
        of locking ourselves in could be enormous.

Ask yourself,
    "Am I currently committing to a project or relationship
        in a way that disempowers me?"

Ask yourself,
    "Do I have a pattern of locking myself in
        because I have been unwilling to choose the courage
        to say, 'No, I will not,'
        either to myself or to others?"

ℬ

You cannot have it all

It has been said that you can have it all.
Total hogwash!

For every "yes" you say, you must say "no" 10,000 times.

For example, by choosing to read this right now,
    you are choosing *not* to do or read an *infinite* number
    of other things you could choose to do or read right now.

When we don't say "no" when we need to say "no,"
    we disempower what we have said "yes" to
    and our capacity to be present to our life,
    to enjoy the processes
    of fully participating in what we have said "yes" to.

Welcome to the opportunity and the *courage* to say "no,"
    both to yourself and to others!

_____

_____

_____

_____

You *have* to choose from among the goods.
          —*K. Bradford Brown (1924-,*
          theologian, family therapist, author,
          co-founder of the Life Training Program)

You can have anything you want, but you can't have everything
you want.
          —*John-Roger and Peter McWilliams*
          in "Do It! Let's Get Off Our Buts"

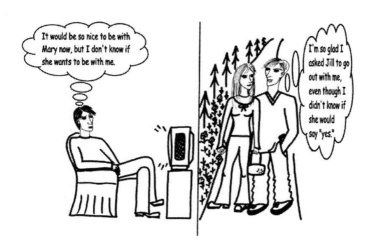

Will you ask for what you want?

With only slight exaggeration, I say to you,
"Everything you want in your life
is available to you through the choice of courage."

Courage can be expressed in many forms.
Two major forms are
saying "no" when you want to say "no"
and making requests when you want something.

How many times have you wanted something
that you did not ask for?
Have you wanted a more fulfilling job
that you did not ask for?
Have you wanted more money for your work
that you did not ask for?
Have you wanted more leisure time
that you did not ask for?

Have you wanted a date with someone that you did not ask for?
Have you wanted attention or love from another
    that you did not ask for?
Have you wanted someone to *really* listen to you
    that you did not ask for?
Have you wanted someone to stop a behavior
    that you did not ask for?
Have you wanted a divorce that you did not ask for?
Have you wanted someone to share your deepest feelings with
    that you did not ask for?
Have you wanted to know what
    someone was thinking or feeling that you did not ask for?
Have you wanted to make love with someone
    that you did not ask for?

How many opportunities have you left unfulfilled
    (for yourself and others) because you did not
    choose courage to ask for what you wanted?
Of course, *how* you ask for something *is* important.
    But, even given a good method of asking,
    you will still have to choose courage to make the request.

Make a list of all the times today
    that you do not ask for what you want.
Then play with the idea of choosing courage
    to ask for what you want (step by step).
You may be amazed with the results of your requests
    and also amazed with how you feel about yourself
       for making these requests!

෨

For more essay(s) on courage and making requests,
see www.GoldWinde.com/Cbook/More/Requests.

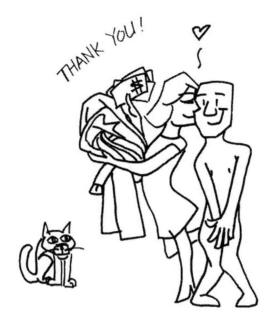

Are you a giver or a trader?

A world of upset and misunderstanding would be eliminated
if we clarified with ourselves and others
what is a trade and what is a gift.

Many interpersonal and business transactions
can be categorized as either trades or gifts,
or a combination of the two.

A problem often arises
because we are addicted to disguising
trades as gifts (not wanting to appear selfish),
not being honest with ourselves or others
that what we represent as a gift is really a trade.

A trade is simple:
I will give you X if you will give me Y.

The following are examples of possible trades.
   I will work for you if you give me $15 per hour.
   I will scratch your back if you will give me a massage.
   I will be friendly to you if you will be friendly to me.
   If you (my husband) will give me financial support and stability
       then I (your wife) will raise our children,
           handle the household items,
           and have sex with you on occasion.

To have clarity with ourselves and our trading partner,
   it is often very helpful to know which of our transactions
   are conditional as trades (and most of them are)
   and which ones are gifts.
Then, we can accept and have peace
   around the conditions of our trades and our gifts.

If we are not able or willing to declare
   that we are getting a good deal in a particular trade,
   then we can re-negotiate the trade or terminate the trade.

The problem arises when we try to disguise trades as gifts
   (not choosing the courage to specify them as trades),
   and thereby default on creating clear boundaries
   about what is expected in return
   and whether or not the other person
   is agreeable to the conditions of the trade.

Consider the source of the following complaints.
   "I am always doing the planning;
       he never initiates anything we do together."
   "I was hurt that you didn't give me anything for my birthday;
       I gave you a great gift on your birthday."
   "Johnny, why do you make a fuss about cleaning your room?
       Don't you appreciate all that we do for you?"

Now let's consider gifts.

The general distinction of a gift (in contrast to a trade)
is that it does not usually require
any necessary action on the part of the receiver
other than getting pleasure/benefit out of the gift
and/or expressing appreciation for the gift.

If we were to be honest with ourselves,
almost all gifts are actually a certain type of trade.

I suggest that you will be very hard pressed to find yourself
consistently giving in any way that does not provide you
with some feedback that you have created
pleasure/benefit for another and/or that you are appreciated
by someone for giving the gift.

Here's an example.

Today, on my way back from grocery shopping,
I noticed a woman's skirt caught in a closed car door,
almost dragging on the street.
I let her know about her dress, which she quickly corrected.

She expressed her appreciation with a smile and a wave.

If I did not typically receive expressions of appreciation
for gifts of this type,
I wouldn't continue giving these types of gifts.

Nor would you.

I am trading the gift
for the appreciation and friendliness I will probably receive.

Even if the recipient of the gift
    never expresses gratitude to us directly
    (as in the case of charitable donations to African children),
    we typically would not continue this type of giving
    if we did not experience
    appreciation and/or pleasure in some capacity
    (perhaps through the acknowledgment
        we get from members of the charitable organization,
        or appreciation and praise expressed by our minister,
        or even appreciation and acknowledgment
        that we give to ourselves).

Let's take one final example:
    the gift of *Courage Now* service to the original subscribers
    (this essay was first distributed
    as part of the free *Courage Now* service).

I received many benefits and pleasures
    in return for my gifts to them.
First of all, I enjoyed the process of thinking and writing about
    fundamental life issues that affect us all,
    knowing that many of the subscribers would read
    what I wrote and apply it to their lives.
In addition, many of them wrote back to me,
    expressing appreciation, and letting me know how my words
    had made a difference for them.

If I had received no feedback on the difference
    my writings were making for them,
    if I had received no pleasure in thinking about how
        what I am saying might enrich their lives,
    if I had received no appreciation
        for creating and distributing *Courage Now*,
        then I would have stopped *Courage Now* immediately.

I was very *selfish* in my gift to them of *Courage Now*.

And, it was important that they let me know immediately
    if they were not getting value from *Courage Now.*
Otherwise, they would not be fulfilling *my* conditions of the gift!

Where have you confused trades *and* gifts in your life?
Have you clarified with yourself
    about what you are getting in return
    for your trades and your gifts?

ॐ

You cannot hold on to anything good. You must be continually
giving—and getting. You cannot hold on to your seed. You must
sow it—and reap anew. You cannot hold on to riches. You must
use them and get other riches in return.
    —*Robert Collier (1885-1950, American writer, publisher)*

Giving is better than receiving because giving starts the receiving
process.
    —*Jim Rohn (American businessman, author, speaker, philosopher)*

The shortest and best way to make your fortune is to let people see
clearly that it is in their interest to promote yours.
    —*Jean de La Bruyere (1645-1696, French moralist)*

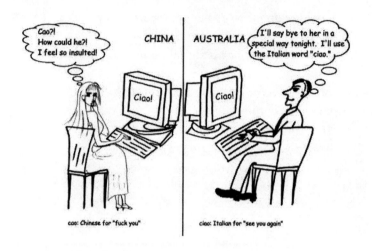

Beware of the unknown assumption!

By "unknown assumption"
    I mean an assumption we are making
        that we are *unaware* is an assumption
        (that may or may not have supporting evidence,
        once we know it is an assumption)
    and which, not knowing it is an assumption,
        we treat like a fact.

When I was ten and my sister was seven,
    we would sometimes have heated arguments
        that were grounded in unknown assumptions.
I remember one argument in particular
    in which I *knew* that cherry ice cream
        was better than vanilla ice cream
    and she *knew* that vanilla ice cream
        was better than cherry ice cream.

As adults we can easily understand
    how this disagreement is grounded
    in at least two unknown assumptions
    (unknown to both my sister and me
        at the time of the argument).
Assumption #1:
    that some objective standard of "better"
        exists concerning the flavors of ice cream.
Assumption #2:
    that one of us would be "damaged"
        if we lost the argument that our flavor was "better."

I recently received an email from a Chinese friend
    that again dramatizes the destructive power
    of unknown assumptions.
"I have a friend who lives in Melbourne.
    He always emails to me to talk about his life and study.
    I also do that. Sometimes we chat in Internet.
    Several days ago, when we finished the chat,
        I said 'good night' to him,
        but I was very shocked that he answered me with 'cao,'
        which is the rudest word in Chinese,
        especially to say that to woman.
    I thought he should not say that
        even if I did something wrong.
    I did not say anything as 'you are impolite' to him;
        I did not hurt him.
    But I was disappointed, and miss the chat in Internet.
    Today I know the word 'ciao' is from Italy
        (I even misread the word also); its meaning is 'see you.'
    I am in deep regret for him.
        So I find if I reply only on my assumption,
            maybe I will make mistake.
        The communication is very important."

It is *so* easy to think our assumptions are facts.
    In fact, it helps us to feel safer
        and more comfortable in the moment;
    it helps us to avoid feeling the fear
        and accepting the risk of not knowing for sure
        what is what and what means what.
However, the cost we pay
    for treating our assumptions as facts is *enormous*.
    Not only does it damage our relationship with others;
    it also damages our relationship with ourselves.

In my friend's case, she was lucky.
    She uncovered the fact that her assumption was *not* a fact.
    She had the opportunity to apologize
        and repair the damage with her friend.
    And, at least for that particular assumption
        (with the word "*ciao*"),
            she is not likely to forget that she cannot assume
            the other person is speaking in the Chinese language.
However, in the case of most assumptions that we take as facts,
    we go through our whole life
    never discovering that our assumptions are assumptions,
    with little or no evidence to support them.
    We harbor feelings
        of hurt, resentment, guilt, resignation, and so on,
        from assumptions we make about others
        and about ourselves.

An *empowering* assumption to make (this is *still* an assumption)
    is that every disagreement, every instance of love lost,
    every instance of upset, every instance of resentment,
    every fight and every war
    lives inside one or more unfounded and toxic assumptions.

An *empowering* assumption to make
    is that every issue and problem
        with others and with ourselves
    is solvable through
    the choices of courage, creativity, curiosity, and context
        (the five Cs; see the essay on page 86).

Create a practice of doubting yourself,
    not a doubt of indecisiveness,
    but a robust and healthy doubt
    of what you *know is true,*
    always being open to and looking for new evidence,
    both for and against your "*truth.*"

Just as an aside, every major advance in science
    has been the result of someone questioning a "fact,"
    revealing it as an assumption,
    with questionable evidence to back it up.

It is a choice of courage
    to doubt and question what you know,
    looking for evidence that might prove you wrong.
    But this choice is the choice
        of power and empowerment.
    This choice is the choice
        that creates new openings for understanding and love.

Pick something you know
    that you might not have solid evidence for.
    Choose the courage to consider your assumption
        from a different perspective.

▪

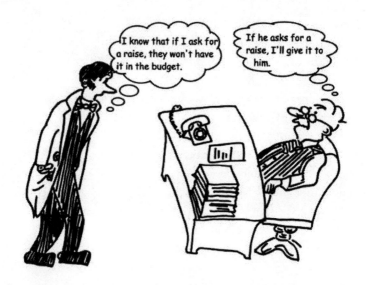

How much do you know that isn't so?

As I talk with my clients and friends,
    I am continually struck by how much they know
        that they have no evidence for knowing.

Here are just a few examples of what they know
    when they often have no evidence to support their knowing.

"I can't get paid for doing what I really like doing."
"If I say that to a man, he will think I am too forward."
"If I ask her out, she will think I am pathetic."
"If I ask for a raise, they won't have it in the budget."
"If I start charging for what I like to do,
    people will think I am selfish."
"If I take a day off for a rest, my office mates will think I'm lazy."
"Everybody knows that it's difficult to get a job now."

"Changing careers will be difficult for me."
"It will damage my kids if I get a divorce."
"I don't have enough courage to say that."
And so on *ad infinitum!*

How many of these beliefs become true
    only because they are believed to be true?
These beliefs (and all their kin) are cages
    constructed of crepe paper,
      ready to be rent asunder by any gust of wind
      that asks if there is any solid evidence to support them.

Maybe you have noticed when someone else
    makes a claim to truth that they probably
    have little to no evidence for.
But how can you discover
    your own superstitions,
    your culture's superstitions,
    your own crepe paper cages
    that crowd you into an ever narrowing world of "security"?

One method is to begin to notice
    when you find yourself giving some reason
    why you *can't* do or say something
    that you would otherwise love to.
Look carefully at each of those reasons
    that you *believe* and ask yourself honestly,
    "What evidence do I have that this is *really* so?"

Question your automatic beliefs.
Question them over and over.
Questioning your beliefs is *not* doubting yourself.

You can grow a deep inner strength
in knowing that you are always eager and willing to question
the evidence and likelihood of your beliefs.

Why is it not more natural and easy to question our own beliefs
(or the beliefs of others that were given to us)?
Because our beliefs provide us with a *feeling* of security,
regardless of their validity.
To live inside the unknown, to live inside a world of likelihoods,
would be a choice of courage,
would be a choice of acknowledging and embracing our fear,
would be feeling an uncertainty and fear
that we don't want to feel.

As a result, many of our beliefs
are direct expressions of our resisted fear.

Find at least one of your beliefs
that you have little to no evidence for
(I'm talking about what we consider to be factbeliefs.
See the essay on page 431 for the distinction of factbelief).

Would you be willing to choose courage
by questioning and dismantling this belief
and stepping into the new action made possible
by this new opening?

ও

Expectation: The source of all upset

The source of all upset is unfulfilled expectations.
If we did not have expectations, we would not become upset.

Expectation, as I use it here, is an attitude that,
if something does or doesn't happen
(depending on the type of expectation), then there must be
something wrong with you,
something wrong with me,
and/or something wrong with the universe.
An expectation is an upset waiting to happen.

Most of us are addicted to expectations.
To let go of our expectations is to let go of a feeling of security
(however false it may be).

I'm *not* talking about
not making commitments,
not having intentions,
not allowing for the possibility that something might happen.
These are all very distinct from having an expectation.

If you simply recognize and embrace
that almost everything in your life has some level of risk,
then you can rejoice and be happy
whenever it comes out the way you intended or wanted!

If we *expect* that things will come out a certain way,
we are setting ourselves up to be upset.
If we *expect*, then we will try to over-control things,
thereby disempowering ourselves even more.

If we accept and embrace the risk that:
    -our child may not do what we request
    -our spouse or lover may not read our mind
    -our friend might lie to us sometime
    -we may be rejected many times for each time we are accepted
    -we may have an accident at any time
    -our computer may not work as desired
    -things may not go as we anticipate and desire
then, if things turn out as unwanted,
    we can find out what happened without becoming upset.
We might experience disappointment, but we won't be upset.

Yet, if they turn out as we intended,
    then we can rejoice in the miracle and blessing
    of this unexpected result!

Paradoxically, when you begin to build your life
    on the understanding that life is risky,
    then you have a much more solid foundation
    than when you *know this* or *expect that*.

When were you upset recently?
    Can you identify the expectation behind that upset?

Choose the courage to let go of expectations,
    again and again.

෨

_____

_____

_____

_____

_____

_____

_____

_____

At what cost is your "safety"?

It's amazing that we can create a world within our minds
and think it is real (although the reality is often quite different)
in order to make ourselves feel safe and comfortable.

"He hasn't returned my call twice now.
He probably isn't really interested in me."
(Therefore, I feel safer and more comfortable by not extending
myself more and possibly feeling very foolish
and risking more rejection.)

"If I ask her to consider this business opportunity,
she'll think I'm being careless and abusing our friendship."
(Therefore, it's not really worth feeling the fear
to open my mouth and invite her to look at it.)

"If I really go for this new job that I want,
they'll think I'm a fool for asking and I'll feel like a failure."
(Therefore, it feels more comfortable
to continue in my unfulfilling current job.)

"If I try to strike up a conversation
with this person sitting beside me on the bus,
she'll think that I want something from her."
(Therefore, I won't make the effort
and I'll avoid any uneasiness.)

"If I ask him out for a date,
he'll think that I'm forward and too available."
(Therefore, I won't make the effort and risk rejection.)

Consider that you know *far less* than you think you know.

And that it's your "knowledge"
    that is severely limiting the possibilities of your life.

Identify something that you
    think you know, yet you really don't.

Choose courage by stepping into this new opening
    of risk and the unknown.

❧

_____
_____
_____
_____
_____
_____
_____
_____
_____
_____
_____
_____

To be uncertain is to be uncomfortable, but to be certain is to be ridiculous.

—*Chinese proverb*

The lust for comfort, that stealthy thing that enters the house as a guest, and then becomes a host, and then a master.

—*Kahlil Gibran (1883-1931, Lebanese poet, novelist)*

Feeling Safe
The more fear you consistently step into by choosing courage, the safer you will begin to feel in life.

—*GoldWinde*

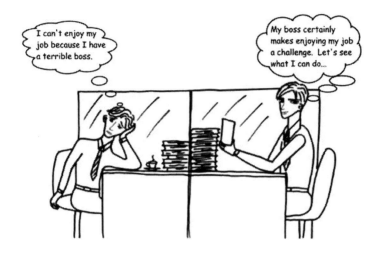

"Because" is a toxic word

"I can't find time for what I really want to do
    because I have to work to make money."

"I can't find the job I want *because* the economy is bad."

"I can't enjoy my current job *because* I have a terrible boss."

"I can't find the partner I want
    because all the good ones are already married."

"I can't really enjoy my life
    because I have to take care of my parents/kids."

"I can't just start something new *because* I'm too old for that."

"I can't say 'no' when I want to
    because someone might become angry."

"I can't ask for what I want
    because they might think I'm too pushy."

"I can't express my true feelings
    because of what they might think of me."

"I can't . . . I can't . . . I can't . . . *because* . . ."

Of course, our reasons for why we can't do something
    might make it more difficult to get what we want.

But these reasons *seldom prevent* us from getting what we want.

With eagerness we grasp onto these reasons
    (which others will usually agree with),
    lying to ourselves and to others,
    because the *real* reason
    we do *not* go for what we want
    is to *avoid the fear* we anticipate feeling
    should we *fully* go for what we want.

What are you *not doing* or what are you *not having*
    "*because* . . ."?

Ask yourself,
    "How can I choose to really go for what I want?"

    "What actions might I take *now*
    to step into choosing that courage?"

✎

Two lies keep your jail door locked

The jail door has two locks. And both locks are lies.
The first lie is that we're powerless to live our lives fully.
The second lie is that "living for others" justifies our resignation.

Both lies protect us from confronting our fear.
Both lies rob us of the opportunity for choosing courage
    and exercising our creativity.

"I can't leave my abusive husband
    because I have no work skills." (I'm powerless.)
"I should stay with him for his sake,
    for the sake of the children,
      in order to set a good example for others,
        and for the sacrament of marriage." (I'm doing it for others.)

"I can't move out of my parents' home
    because I must obey them." (I'm powerless.)
"I should stay with my parents
    because I don't want to upset them." (I'm doing it for others.)

"I can't get the job I love
    because it's not out there." (I'm powerless.)
"I should just accept my situation
    and not expect to have it
      better than others." (I'm doing it for others.)

"I can't find the partner I want
    because all the good ones are already taken." (I'm powerless.)
"It would be unfair to go after just any person I want."
    (I'm doing it for others.)

"I don't have enough free time to enjoy my life
    because I have too many things to do." (I'm powerless.)
"I can't just cancel out or change my commitments.
    That would be unfair to others." (I'm doing it for others.)

In what area of your life do you feel stopped or tied up?

Can you identify the two locks that keep you in this jail?
What opportunities for courage and creativity,
    if taken, might open these locks and set you free?

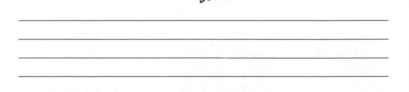

_____

_____

_____

_____

_____

The common good of a collective—a race, a class, a state—was the claim and justification of every tyranny ever established over men. Every major horror of history was committed in the name of an altruistic motive. Has any act of selfishness ever equaled the carnage perpetrated by disciples of altruism? Does the fault lie in men's hypocrisy or in the nature of the principle? The most dreadful butchers were the most sincere. They believed in the perfect society reached through the guillotine and the firing squad. Nobody questioned their right to murder since they were murdering for an altruistic purpose. It was accepted that man must be sacrificed for other men. Actors change, but the course of the tragedy remains the same. A humanitarian who starts with the declarations of love for mankind and ends with a sea of blood. It goes on and will go on so long as men believe that an action is good if it is unselfish. That permits the altruist to act and forces his victims to bear it. The leaders of collectivist movements ask nothing of themselves. But observe the results.

—*Ayn Rand (1905-1982,*
Russian-born American writer, philosopher)

How many package deals are you blindly accepting?

Most of us accept the package deals of life
    because we don't believe it is possible
    to have the benefits of the package
    without the costs associated with the package
    (or without as much of the cost).

Cultural and technological progress
    is often the result of creatively breaking up
    the components of a package deal
    to see if the benefits can still be derived without the costs.

At one time, many people accepted (and today continue to accept)
    the package deal that:
(1)   having sex meant having babies
(2)   having sex outside of marriage meant you were a bad person
(3)   enjoying sex meant a woman was "a whore"
(4)   being a wife meant accepting the domination of a husband
(5)   being a good person meant that you were a Christian
        (or Moslem or . . .)
(6)   getting married meant you could be stuck
        with an unsatisfactory spouse for the rest of your life
(7)   being homosexual meant
        you should probably stay in the closet
(8)   being a patriot meant that you would fight
        for your country on your country's terms
(9)   having a real marriage meant you accepted
        the costs of living together and mixing your money
(10)   working meant doing something
        you wouldn't do if you didn't get paid for it.

These are some obvious package deals that have been broken apart
    to some extent by some people in certain counties and cultures.
However, each of us often unknowingly accepts
    many other less obvious package deals in our day-to-day living.

Look into those areas of your life
    where you have complaints or resignation.
Ask yourself,
    "How might I use my creativity and/or my courage
    to maintain the benefits in this area,
    without the currently associated costs?"
    "Are there any absolute causal connections
    between the benefits and the costs?"

For example, suppose you experience your job
    as unsatisfactory and unfulfilling.
    These are the current costs.
But you also receive money regularly from your job.
    This is the current benefit.

Using your creativity (and the creativity of those around you),
    and a choice of courage,
      you can either create your current job
        as interesting and joyful
      or you can find a new job/career.

Find at least one package deal in your life and try to break it apart.

Honor yourself for the choice of courage to do this.

ও

For more essay(s) on courage and assumptions,
    see www.GoldWinde.com/Cbook/More/Assumptions.

What do you believe about belief?

Can you imagine the transportation breakdowns
    that would be created if, in servicing our automobiles,
we used the same word to describe water and gasoline,
especially if we were not clear
    that there were two distinct liquids
and we were also not clear
    about the criteria for distinguishing water from gasoline.
We might even be tempted to treat water as gasoline
    because it can be acquired much more cheaply.

This, I submit, is the case with the word "belief."
Unknowingly, we use this word to denote
    two very separate, yet interrelated, distinctions.

The *first* meaning of the word "belief" lives inside
    a domain of distinctions called "assertions."
An assertion is a statement of fact
    that one is willing to provide evidence for
    (either directly or indirectly).
Let's call this type of belief a "factbelief."

Here are examples:
"I factbelieve that this floor is wet."
"Scientists factbelieve that water is
    a compound of hydrogen and oxygen."
"I factbelieve that the square root of 144 is 12."
"I factbelieve that my mother is 82 years old."
"I factbelieve that I can buy an airplane ticket
    from Shanghai to Tokyo."
"I factbelieve that I am feeling sad right now."

The *second* meaning of the word "belief" lives inside
    a domain of distinctions called "declarations."
A declaration's power lies solely
    in our listening to it and speaking it
    and in its congruence
    with other pre-existing declarations and factbeliefs.
Although we often can gather evidence
    that a declaration is factually true,
    we could just as easily gather evidence
    for the opposing proposition.
Let's call this type of belief a "fatebelief."

Fatebeliefs live largely undistinguished as such
    (often presenting themselves as factbeliefs)
    inside the subculture of our family,
    inside the culture of our society,
    inside our religions,
    and inside other schools of thought.
Fatebeliefs often masquerade as factbeliefs,
    serving the purpose
    of making us feel safer and more comfortable
    in the moment.
But it is very empowering and helpful
    to distinguish our fatebeliefs from our factbeliefs.

A factbelief
    (which can provide varying degrees
        of certainty based on the available evidence)
    is based on the evidence
    that one is willing to provide or point to
    in support of that factbelief.

A fatebelief, on the other hand,
    (which can provide complete certainty)
    is based on declaration alone
    and the only way to assess the validity of a fatebelief
    is by asking oneself,
    "If I live according to this fatebelief, is it likely to empower me
        in living a fully expressed and joyous life?"
One must also choose fatebeliefs carefully
    so that they are not contradicted by any factbeliefs
    and so that they are congruent with one's other fatebeliefs.
    A fatebelief must stay in the domain of *declaration*
        and not wander into the domain of *assertion*.

Fatebeliefs provide the context of our lives.
Factbeliefs provide the content of our lives.

Together, they determine the quality of our lives.
Mistaken factbeliefs and disempowering fatebeliefs
    can damage our lives.
Accurate factbeliefs and empowering fatebeliefs
    support us in living lives
    of accomplishment and self-expression.

Let me give you an example of one of my fatebeliefs:
"I fatebelieve that everything that occurs in my life is a gift."
Can I prove this? No, I cannot.
Can I disprove this? No, I cannot.
This fatebelief is not open to absolute proof or disproof.
However, the more and more
    that I speak and act according to the idea
    that *everything* in my life is a gift,
    the more and more I find evidence that this is so.

It is also easy to demonstrate that,
    if I live according to the idea
    that everything that happens is a gift,
    then the life that I live, the life that lives me,
    will be a life fully worth living.
Science has become the formalized methodology
    for discovering and propagating certain types of factbeliefs.
Religion and culture (to some extent) have been the vehicles
    for propagating our broader-based fatebeliefs.

Science, for the most part,
    despite some significant breakdowns,
    has been clear about the appropriate criteria
    for establishing valid factbeliefs.
Religion, on the other hand, has often
    (in order to make people feel more secure)
    propagated many fatebeliefs
    that are life-suppressive and divisive.
For example (and there are thousands),
    consider the fatebelief in a devil,
        often propagated by Christianity.
    Can you prove there is a devil? No.
    Can you disprove there is a devil? No.
    It is obviously a fatebelief. It is not a factbelief.
    (Some Christians might say, "You must have faith.")
Certainly one can began to see how belief in a devil
    can make one feel safer.
    A simple way to test this
        (assuming you believe in a devil, even just a little bit),
        is to ask yourself how you might feel
        if it were proven that there was no devil, no hell, etc.?
And there is nothing wrong with wanting to feel safer.

But at what cost?

Anyone who has taken the devil seriously
    and later stepped back to assess the results of this belief,
    will attest to the incredible damage it has caused in h/is life.

Both water and gasoline
    have very important functions in the operation of a car;
    yet they must be kept separate and distinct
    in order to function best.
In a similar way, both factbeliefs and fatebeliefs
    have very important functions in the operation of our life;
    yet they must be kept separate and distinct
    in order to function best.

The most common error is to treat
    a fatebelief as if it were a factbelief.
    We almost always do this
    to help us feel safer and more comfortable.
Fatebeliefs, in some sense, can easily be changed
    just by creating a new declaration.
Factbeliefs, in contrast, are much more
    cut in stone and have an existence
    independent of our speaking them and listening to them.

Let's take a common fatebelief that many of us
    factbelieve about ourselves:
    "I'm not creative."
I may be able to point to my lack of ability to draw;
    I may be able to point to not being selected for the school play;
    I may be able to point to my dead-end job;
    I may be able to give many reasons
        to "prove" that I'm not creative.

But I submit that, if someone
    who believed that s/he were not creative,
    were willing to choose courage
    by taking on the new fatebelief "I am creative,"
    acting as if s/he were creative,
    then s/he would, step by step,
    begin to discover reasons to "prove" h/is creativity.

Write down a list of 25 things
    you believe about yourself.
Question rigorously each of these beliefs, asking yourself,
    "Is this a factbelief or a fatebelief?"
If it is or could be a fatebelief, then ask yourself,
    "Would I wish my best friend
        to have this fatebelief about h/imself?
    If my best friend *really* believed this,
        would it empower and serve h/is life?"

If the answer is "no,"
    what new fatebelief might you create and believe
    to replace this old and disempowering fatebelief?

Do that now.

୨

_____

_____

_____

_____

_____

_____

_____

_____

_____

_____

Are you guilt waiting to happen?

I often notice that a client, without awareness,
    regularly uses the word "should."
    "I should be able to do it in less time."
    "She should have called me first."
    "The company should have a better policy."
    "My husband shouldn't be having an affair."

Sometimes we use the word "should"
    as a substitute for the word "want."
    "I want to do it in less time."
    "I wanted her to call me first."
    "I want the company to have a better policy."
    "I don't want my husband to have an affair."

Sometimes we use the word "should"
    to mean that we predict
    that certain unwanted and unspecified consequences
    will arise if something *doesn't* happen
    (e.g., "I should be able to do it in less time
    or I might lose my job.").

Sometimes we use the word "should"
    to mean that we predict
    that certain desired and unspecified consequences
    will arise if something *does* happen.
    ("The company should have a better policy
    and they would have more satisfied employees
    if they had a better policy.")

Sometimes we use the word "should"
    to mean that we are issuing an unspecified threat
    (e.g., "My husband shouldn't be having an affair
    and, if he doesn't stop, I will leave him.").

Sometimes we use the word "should"
    to mean that almost everyone else would agree with
    out assessment of the acceptability of a certain behavior
    (e.g., "She should have called me first
    and almost everyone would agree with me
    that it was inconsiderate of her not to do so.").

However, we *most often* use the word "should"
    to mean that there is something *wrong* with us (guilt)
    and/or something *wrong* with others (blame)
    and/or something *wrong* with the universe and/or God.

Some of us have become more careful with our language
    and don't use the word "should" very much;
    we use other words and phrases
    that essentially have the same meaning:
    ought to, must, have to, need to, had better,
    it would be good to, it would be bad to,
    it would be right to, it would be wrong to.
Whenever we apply these blame words to ourselves,
    we are often unknowingly and subtly "guilting" ourselves,
    slowly accumulating an atmosphere of guilt
    without ever identifying it as such.

Take on this small project.
    Tomorrow, tally each time you use a "should" word,
    at least in your speaking, if not also in your thinking.

Try to get in touch with the resisted fear
    that the "should" is trying to keep at bay,
    the fear that the "should"
    is trying to keep hidden and unfelt.

Breathe into that fear and ask yourself,
    "Where is the opportunity for courage here?"

༶

_____

_____

_____

_____

_____

_____

_____

_____

_____

_____

_____

_____

_____

When I contemplate the accumulation of guilt and remorse which, like a garbage-can, I carry through life, and which is fed not only by the lightest action but by the most harmless pleasure, I feel Man to be of all living things the most biologically incompetent and ill-organized. Why has he acquired a seventy years life-span only to poison it incurably by the mere being of himself? Why has he thrown Conscience, like a dead rat, to putrefy in the well?
    —*Cyril Connolly (1904-1974, British critic)*

The more sinful and guilty a person tends to feel, the less chance there is that he will be a happy, healthy, or law-abiding citizen. He will become a compulsive wrong-doer.
    —*Dr. Albert Ellis (1913-, American psychotherapist)*

Selfish is a toxic word

Selfish. Selfish. Selfish.
    You are never encouraged to be selfish.
    You have been told not to be selfish.
    It is bad to be selfish.

Typically, people only use the word "selfish"
    in referring to behavior that doesn't fit
    with their own (selfish) desires,
    or doesn't fit with their own standards
    of how one's primary motive in life should be
    to sacrifice one's own desires and needs
    to the desires and needs of others.

The fundamental meaning of selfishness
    is "concern for one's own interests."
Sometimes, it is defined as
    "concern only for one's own interests,"
    implying that one can be concerned for one's own interests
    without being concerned for the interests of others.
But I believe that if you take care of your own interests,
    they will most often dovetail and contribute
    to the interests of others around you.
If you give up your own pleasure and your own interests,
    although you may be praised for it,
    you will rarely make genuine contributions to others
    and you will often damage them and/or
    your relationship with them.

Ask yourself,
>"If I knew that a friend or family member was
>sacrificing h/is own happiness, needs, or desires
>in order to contribute to me,
>would that be a contribution I would want?"

Ask yourself,
>"If I knew that a friend or family member was
>contributing to me
>only out of obligation, guilt, or duty,
>would that really contribute to me?"

The best of all possible worlds
>is a world in which your selfishness
>and my selfishness walk hand-in-hand.

We love to be around people who derive selfish pleasure
>out of being with us and exchanging with us.

Yet most of the tragedies and horrors
>on this earth have been perpetrated
>in the name of unselfishness and altruism.
>Let me give some examples:

Don't think of yourself;
>join the army and kill others for your country.

Don't pursue the type of work that you want;
>your country or parents need you to do other work.

Don't marry the woman you love;
>your parents have chosen someone else for you.

Don't create time for yourself;
>everybody else deserves your time more.

Don't spend money on yourself;
>somebody else needs your money more.

Don't live your passion;
    you'll make others feel left behind.
Don't protect or remove yourself from abuse;
    people might think you don't love them.
Don't flee from this country
    that birthed and taught you
    about the evils of a selfish, greedy, capitalistic country;
    you owe your life to others here and to your society.
Don't be selfish;
    other people's needs are more important than yours.

I particularly like Ambrose Bierce's
    satiric characterization of selfish:
    "Devoid of consideration for the selfishness of others."

How have you shut down your own life
    by giving up your own selfish desires and needs?
And, when you gave up your selfish desires and needs,
    did that sacrifice really serve someone else
    or your relationship with them?

To be truly selfish,
    and thereby serve the long-term needs of yourself and others,
    is often a supreme choice of courage.

ʗ

_____

_____

_____

_____

_____

_____

_____

_____

_____

Trust is a toxic word

Listening to and/or speaking
    the word "trust" may be toxic
    to your life and/or your relationships.

What do you mean when you say,
    "I can trust him," or
    "I cannot trust her," or
    "He betrayed my trust"?

Typically, we look for trust
    (for others to trust us or for us to be able to trust others)
    because we are resisting the fear inherent in life,
    we are resisting the fear inherent in human relationships.

For example, if a new friend shows up late
    for the first three appointments,
    then I know that I am taking a significant risk
    that s/he will show up late the fourth time we meet,
    regardless of what s/he might say
        about h/is promise to be on time.
For me to say to myself and/or others,
    "I trust h/im to show up on time,"
    is an attempt to avoid facing and accepting the probable risk
    that s/he will not show up on time.
I am also avoiding making a clear choice
    of whether *or* not I am willing to continue
    to meet with h/im under these risk conditions.

Typically, people who are betrayed
    are co-conspirators in their own betrayal,
    yet are adamant in denying this fact.

Viva la victimhood!

Trust and mistrust, as they are typically used
    as content-based distinctions (factbeliefs; see page 431),
    are most often toxic words
    pregnant with the seeds of upset and betrayal.

However, trust can be used very powerfully
    as a context-based distinction (a fatebelief; see page 431).
For example, I can say,
    "I *trust* that whatever my friend/spouse/boss does,
        (i.e., whether s/he lies or tells the truth,
        whether s/he keeps h/is word or breaks it,
        whether s/he leaves me or stays with me),
        whatever s/he does will be a gift to me."
This context-based trust is *not* open to proof *or* disproof.
Taken as a stand, this trust is unshakable.
Even if you never understand or see the gift in something,
    you can always live as if it were a gift
    that you haven't yet seen the evidence for.
Living out of this type of trust is an existential choice of courage.

Do you find yourself mistrusted by others?
Do you find yourself not trusting others?
What courage might you choose
    to let go of trying to control with your trust?

Would you be willing to take a stand *now*
    to *trust* that *everything* that occurs in your life is a gift to you?

৯৽

Hope is a toxic word

Warning: listening to and/or speaking
   the word "hope" may be toxic
   to your life and/or to your relationships.

Do you have hope?
I don't hope so.

We are trained to think that hope is positive.
We are trained to think that hope is helpful.
We want to be hopeful.

Yet, at its source,
   hope contains the seeds of betrayal and/or blindness.
At its source,
   hope is a resistance to embracing the risk that life is.
At its source,
   hope is a Pollyanna form of "expectation" (another toxic word).

Let's look at an example.

"I hope I pass the test this time."
   What does this really mean?
   Does it mean,
      "If I don't pass the test, then something is wrong"?
   Does it mean,
      "By hoping maybe it will somehow be given to me"?
   Does it mean,
      "I don't want to face the fear associated
      with the risk of not passing the test,
      so, by hoping, I will try to avoid feeling that fear"?

Does it mean,
  "By hoping I will relieve myself
  of the necessity to really study for this test"?
Does it mean,
  "By saying that I hope,
  I hope others will think I'm a good person"?
Does it mean,
  "By hoping I will avoid the risk
  of taking a stand and creating a firm intention
  that I will pass this test"?

Very often, in hoping, we set ourselves up
  for betrayal and disempowerment,
  should our hopes not come true.

If you examine closely the way you or others use the word "hope,"
  you will see that it is almost always an avoidance,
  an avoidance of feeling some fear, a resistance to fear.

Sometimes hope means something else,
  which can be much more clearly expressed
  without the word hope.

Maybe, in hoping, we are saying,
  "I intend for this to happen
    and I'm in action to make it happen" or
  "I intend for this to happen
    and I will take no more action to make it happen" or
  "I pray to God that this will happen
    and I will accept God's choice as the best" or
  "I am open to the miracle that this will happen
    and whatever happens will be a gift."

These ways of hoping do not contain
   the seeds of betrayal and disempowerment.

Do you live your life in hope?

How much hoping do you do?

What might be the choices of courage
   to let go of hope, stepping instead
   into intention, action, and miracles?

∾

_____
_____
_____
_____
_____
_____
_____
_____
_____
_____

Man is a victim of dope in the incurable form of hope.
   —*Odgen Nash (1902-1971, American humorous poet)*

Hope: Desire and expectation rolled into one.
   —*Ambrose Bierce (1842-1914,*
   American satirist, newspaper columnist, writer,
   The Devil's Dictionary)

Desire is the starting point of all achievement, not a hope, not a
wish, but a keen pulsating desire which transcends everything.
   —*Napoleon Hill (1883-1970,*
   American speaker, motivational writer,
   Think and Grow Rich)

Beware of the assumptions of love

Most of us love to hear the word "love."
And often we love to say the word "love."
"I love you. He loves me. They love us."

It can bring us feelings of warmth, of caring,
    of security, of specialness, of reassurance.

But underneath the veneer of love
    often lie hidden and toxic assumptions
    that can rise up unexpectedly, playing havoc
    with our feelings of affection for each other
    and damaging our relationships.

Assumptions like these:
    "If you love me, you will lend me money."
        (For each of these examples, consider also its mirror image,
            e.g., "If I love you, I will lend you money.")
    "If you love me, you will never have sex with anyone else."
    "If you love me, you will do as I suggest."
    "If you love me, you will not love anyone else."
    "If you love me, you will never leave me no matter what I do."
    "If you love me, you will cook for me."
    "If you love me, you will have sex with me."
    "If you love me, you will have my children."
    "If you love me, you will earn money for me."
    "If you love me, you will pay attention to me whenever I want."
    "If you love me, you will bail me out of jail."
    "If you love me, you will take care of me when I get old."
    "If you love me, you will not move out of the house."
    "If you love me, you will say 'yes' to me."
    "If you love me, you will never lie to me."

"If you love me, you will never divorce me."
"If you love me, your love must be forever
     or it is not true love."
And so on.

When we package our love (and others' love for us)
    with these hidden assumptions,
    we prevent ourselves
    from ever experiencing the joy of unencumbered love.

Why do we do this?
Why do we create these "package deals"?
Answer:
    to avoid the fear we would feel
    if we clarified and asserted both our boundaries
    and/or our minimum conditions of satisfaction
    for a given relationship.
    By creating boundaries, we let go of
        trying to control with our love
        or trying to prove our love for another
        or trying to prove another's love for us.

If you choose courage
    not to lend money to someone,
    it doesn't mean that you don't love that person.
If you choose courage
    to move out of your parents' home,
    it doesn't mean that you don't love your parents.
If you choose courage
    to go against a loved one's wishes (or commands),
    it doesn't mean that you don't love that person.
And so on.

Yet it is necessary and appropriate
   (*especially* for maintaining our experience of love) to have
   clear (and sometimes seemingly unloving) boundaries
   and/or to have minimum conditions of satisfaction
   for each of our relationships.

Examples:
   "For me to be willing to set appointments with you,
      you must generally show up on time."
      (It does not necessarily mean that I don't love you
      if I am no longer willing to set appointments with you.)
   "For me to stay married to you,
      you must generally treat me with respect
      and I can tell you what respectful behavior is for me."
      (It does not necessarily mean I don't love you
      if I am no longer willing to be married to you.)
   "For me to remain living in your house,
      you must allow me to live my own life,
      as long as I don't disturb the household."
      (It does not necessarily mean I don't love you
      if I choose to move out of the house.)
   "For me to lend money to you,
      I require a written agreement
      with your car as collateral."
      (It does not necessarily mean I don't love you
      because these are my conditions for the loan.)
   "If you have sex with another person,
      then I will no longer have sex with you."
      (It does not necessarily mean I don't love you
      because I would not have sex with you
      because you had sex with another.)
   And so on.

Can you begin to see how you can free up
   both your experience of love from others
   and your expression of love to them?

What courage might you choose right now
   to clarify and assert your boundaries
   and your minimum conditions of satisfaction
   so that you can experience your love fully
   and others can more easily love you?

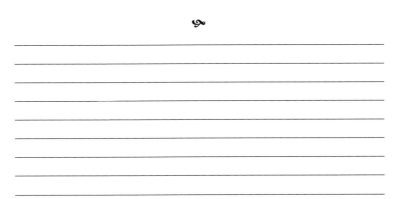

_____

_____

_____

_____

_____

_____

_____

_____

Oh Doris Lessing, my dear—your Anna is wrong about orgasms. They are no proof of love—any more than that other Anna's fall under the wheels of that Russian train was a proof of love. It's all female shenanigans, cultural mishegoss, conditioning, brainwashing, male mythologizing. What does a woman want? She wants what she has been told she ought to want. Anna Wulf wants orgasm, Anna Karenina, death. Orgasm is no proof of anything. Orgasm is proof of orgasm. Someday every woman will have orgasms—like every family has color TV—and we can all get on with the real business of life.

—*Erica Jong (1942-, American author)*

I am speaking now of the highest duty we owe our friends, the noblest, the most sacred—that of keeping their own nobleness, goodness, pure and incorrupt. If we let our friend become cold and selfish and exacting without a remonstrance, we are no true lover, no true friend.

—*Harriet Beecher Stowe (1811-1896,*
American novelist, antislavery campaigner)

Lazy is never lazy

I consider "lazy" to be a toxic word.

Lazy is a make-wrong word,
  which we use either against ourselves and/or against others.
  It only diverts our attention away from the real issue(s).

I believe that being lazy
  is the result of one of the five issues listed below,
  or a combination of these five issues.

Issue #1
You are lazy in reference to a specific action because
  you have no interest in, passion for,
  or commitment to the outcome of that action.
  Your choice to do something is only a "should,"
    usually to avoid disapproval from others.
  "I should study my history book; but I am so lazy about it.
    It just doesn't interest me."

Issue #2
You are lazy because
  you see and/or feel no strong causal connection
  between the actions you are lazy about
  and any results that you're passionate about.
  "My friends say I'm lazy because I won't help them
    on the promotion for the mayor's race.
  I don't see that the promotion
    will make any difference in the results."

Issue #3
You are lazy because
    something else important is not being handled first.
    "I really am interested in getting this done,
        but I feel so lazy right now.
    I am behind on my sleep."

Issue #4
You are lazy because
    the process does not occur as interesting or engaging to you.
    "I want to get in shape.
        But I feel lazy when I think
    of doing the boring treadmill every morning."

Issue #5
You are lazy because
    you are (usually unconsciously)
    trying to do something important for yourself by being lazy.
    "I have no energy for my work anymore.
        I wonder if I'm in the right career."

Do you think of yourself as lazy
    in some important domain of your life?

Calling ourselves (or others) lazy
    is an attempt to control and force
    that which cannot be controlled,
    because it does not address the real issues.
Any seemingly good result that comes from calling ourselves lazy
    comes at a very high cost
    and usually with only temporary benefit.

Choosing to explore the issues underneath laziness
is a choice of courage, a choice of letting go of control.

Identify an area of laziness in your life
and choose courage to examine and address it
with intelligence and compassion.

❧

_____

_____

_____

_____

_____

_____

_____

_____

_____

_____

_____

_____

_____

I'm lazy. But it's the lazy people who invented the wheel and the
bicycle because they didn't like walking or carrying things.
—*Lech Walesa (1943-, Polish political leader)*

Ambition is a poor excuse for not having sense enough to be lazy.
—*Charlie McCarthy (radio comedian)*

People are not lazy. They simply have impotent goals—that is,
goals that do not inspire them.
—*Anthony Robbins (1960-, American author, speaker,
peak performance expert/consultant)*

What is the meaning of life?

What is the meaning of life?
    What's it all for, anyway?

I've noticed a very interesting correlation:
    Whenever I'm thinking about
        or concerned about or anguishing over
        the meaning of life,
        it's always when I am resisting
        some pain, discomfort, or fear.
    Whenever I am happy,
        whenever I am embracing my life
        in all its gloriously diverse expressions,
        especially in moments of pain and fear,
        I have no thoughts or questions about the meaning of life.
        The question, if it occurs to me at all,
            occurs to me as a nonsense question.

Notice that young children
    typically do not question the meaning of life.
    It is not because they are not intellectually developed
        enough to do so.
    It is because they have not yet learned
        to resist their pain and fear.

Questioning the meaning of life (like so many other things)
    is an expression of a resistance to pain and fear.
    It is a resistance to making love to this moment,
        a resistance to embracing the thought that "this is it *now*."

Catch yourself the next time you're preoccupied with
    the question, "What's it all for, anyway?"

Then ask yourself,
"How might I choose courage
to embrace my discomfort, my pain, my fear?"
Notice the difference that makes.

❦

_____
_____
_____
_____
_____
_____
_____
_____
_____
_____
_____
_____

You will never be happy if you continue to search for what happiness consists of. You will never live if you are looking for the meaning of life.

—Albert Camus (1913-1960, French existentialist writer)

When you are deluded and full of doubt, even a thousand books of scripture are not enough. When you have realized understanding, even one word is too much.

—Fen-Yang (947-1024, Zen master and poet)

The wisest keeps something of the vision of a child. Though he may understand a thousand things that a child could not understand, he is always a beginner, close to the original meaning of life.

—John Macy (1877-?, American author)

Breaking a promise may serve your integrity

Keeping your word with yourself and others is important.
Generally, people find that
    I am very reliable in keeping my word with them.
However, most of us confuse the "tools" of integrity
    with the essence of integrity.

When we give our word (to ourselves or to others),
    we always have a higher purpose
    in mind that giving our word is in service to.
When we give our word,
    we always give our word within a certain context
    and within a certain set of circumstances
    and assumed future circumstances.
Our word is there to serve (it is only the "tool") something bigger,
    not to be our lord and master.

I realize there is danger
    in permitting ourselves to change our word,
    in light of new circumstances
    or our shifting view of circumstances.
But there is an equal danger
    in insisting on keeping our word, no matter what.
How many marriages have continued as empty relationships,
    how many careers have continued as spiritless duty,
    how much pain and suffering has been endured
    for the purpose of keeping our word?

When we make keeping our word a god,
    then it becomes very difficult
    to appropriately cancel, change, or renegotiate our word
    when the situation warrants it.

Sometimes we undermine the integrity of keeping our word
    when we don't allow for a new context, new circumstances,
    or a new view or knowledge of our circumstances.

Find a current example in your life
    where keeping your word
    is actually undermining your integrity.

Can you see how it would be a choice of courage for you
    to either cancel, change, or renegotiate
    your word, always taking into consideration
    the benefits and costs of doing so?

**For more essay(s) on courage and shoddy words,
    see www.GoldWinde.com/Cbook/More/ShoddyWords.**

_____

_____

_____

_____

_____

_____

_____

_____

Integrity has no need of rules.
    —*Albert Camus (1913-1960, French existentialist writer)*

Nothing is at last sacred but the integrity of your own mind.
    —*Ralph Waldo Emerson (1803-1882, American poet, essayist)*

Integrity is the essence of everything successful.
                —*Buckminster Fuller (1895-1983,
        American engineer, inventor, designer, architect)*

What are the two types of pain?

Every pain or fear in your life is one of two types:
necessary and unnecessary.

Necessary pain and fear account for less than ten percent
of all the pain and fear we feel.
Unnecessary pain make up more than ninety percent
of all the pain and fear we feel.

Experiences of unnecessary pain and fear
(examples: animosity, anxiety, bitterness, blame, boredom,
complaining, crankiness, cynicism, defensiveness, depression,
feeling betrayed, feeling overwhelmed, guilt, hatred,
indecisiveness, impatience, jealousy, lack of self-confidence,
lack of self-esteem, laziness, perfectionism, procrastination,
resentment, resignation, self-consciousness, self-suppression,
shame, stress, and worry)
are a direct result of resisting and making wrong
the necessary pain and fear.

૭૦

The secret of success is learning how to use pain and pleasure
instead of having pain and pleasure use you. If you do that, you're
in control of your life. If you don't, life controls you.
—*Anthony Robbins (Awaken the Giant Within)*

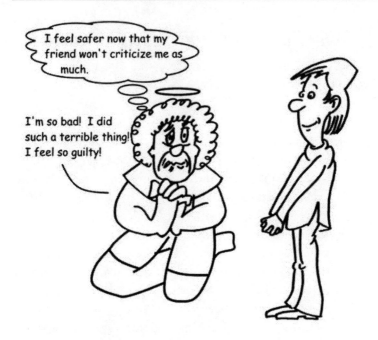

Nineteen benefits of feeling guilty

We get so many benefits from feeling guilty
that it's amazing we don't feel guilty more often.
And all these benefits of feeling guilty
boil down to the benefit of avoiding fear.

Think of something you're feeling guilty about
and see which of these benefits fit for you.

"By feeling guilty, I demonstrate to myself (and others)
that I am a person who has good standards of behavior.
Therefore, by feeling bad about myself (through guilt),
I can avoid the fear that either others or myself
will criticize me for being a fundamentally bad person.
By feeling bad I can be good."

"By feeling guilty I can possibly beat others
   to the punch in blaming me.
   This gives me an added sense of control in my life
      and alleviates some of the fear of others blaming me."

"By feeling guilty maybe I can get others to feel sorry for me,
   thereby lessening the likelihood of their blaming me
   and even getting them to sympathize with me.
   This helps me to feel safer."

"By knowing that I will feel guilty for something
   I am considering doing,
   I know in advance that I will be
      paying the price for it through my guilt.
   Therefore, I can allow myself to go ahead and do it,
      distracting myself from feeling the fear associated
      with the projected consequences of the desired action."

"By feeling guilty I feel like I've paid the penance (price)
   for what I've done and, therefore, I can do it again,
      distracting myself from feeling the fear associated
      with the projected consequences of the desired action."

"When I feel guilty, I feel bad.
   When I feel bad, I give myself permission to try to feel better,
      with things like indulging in food, watching more TV,
         immersing myself more deeply in my work,
         sleeping more, drinking more alcohol, or taking drugs.
      I allow myself to indulge in behaviors
         which give me immediate relief or pleasure
         and I'm able to distract myself
         from feeling the fear associated with the costs
         of indulging in these behaviors.

Therefore, by feeling guilty,
    I am able to dull my fears and sensibilities
    to the costs associated with certain behaviors,
    thereby allowing myself to cash in on
    the immediate, short-term benefits."

"When I feel guilty, I say to myself,
    'I just fell off my horse and got myself all muddy.'
    Then I say to myself,
        'Well, I might as well take advantage of this
        and get myself even muddier;
        it won't really make much difference anyway.
        I'm already bad.'
So then I allow myself to continue with the action(s)
    associated with the guilt and/or allow other actions
    which generate even more guilt.
Therefore, by feeling guilty,
    I am able to distract myself from the fear
        associated with my behaviors,
        allowing myself to cash in on the short-term benefits
        which these behaviors provide."

"By feeling guilty I judge myself
    as an undeserving and unresourceful person
    who has failed at living up to h/is standards.
    Again, as in the above example,
        this deadens my sensitivity to the fear
        associated with the consequences of my actions,
        allowing me to cash in on short-term benefits
        at the expense of my deeper desires and commitments."

"By feeling guilty I get to feel a sense of
    camaraderie and connection with others who also feel guilt.
    I get to avoid my fear of feeling disconnected from them."

"By feeling guilty I distract myself
    from looking at other issues/areas of my life
    that stimulate fear for me."

"By feeling guilty I get to be right about my thought/belief
    that I know the right thing to do.
    By being right about this, I get to feel an added sense of control
        about who I am and what I can do in the universe.
    I get to avoid feeling fear
        through the belief that I am sure about what is right."

"By feeling guilty I withdraw into myself.
    By withdrawing into myself,
        I give myself relief from the demands of others
        (and from the demands I place on myself).
    This gives me a respite from feeling the fears
        associated with these demands."

"By feeling guilty I feel safer
    by having the identification
        of agreement/alignment/connection
    with others and/or my society
        in blaming myself.
    My guilt aligns me with society.
    A child dare not make his parents wrong.
        It would be a scary world indeed
        to think that his parents didn't know what they were doing.
        It's much safer for the child to make h/imself wrong."

"By feeling guilty I can re-stimulate
    those feelings of nurturing/stability
    that I had with my mother and/or father,
    because I often/sometimes felt guilty in their presence.
    This gives me an added sense of safety."

"By feeling guilty I may be stimulated to consider
        possible changes in my actions or attitudes
        which would lead me to feeling safer and more comfortable."

"By feeling guilty about actions that I may take
        which would affect another person,
        who then might say or do something to frighten me,
        I hope to prevent myself from taking that action,
        thereby making myself feel safer."

"By feeling guilty I can intensify the doubt
        of my own choices and judgments,
                thereby relying on
                and/or not rejecting the choices
                that other(s) make for me.
        This gives me an a sense of someone else taking care of me
                because I allow their judgment to supersede mine.
        So again, by feeling guilty, I feel safer."

"By feeling guilty I distance myself from others.
        By distancing myself from others,
                I am less vulnerable to their pain and fear,
                thereby making myself feel safer."

"By blaming myself I can avoid
        the opportunity for choosing courage
        to confront others in creating and maintaining
        the appropriate boundaries with them.
        In this way, I get to feel safer."

Not every benefit applies for every feeling of guilt.
        Discover which ones fit for you
                for any given occurrence of guilt.

Even if you do not see the benefit,
    you can test for the underlying resisted fear
    by taking several deep breaths
    and saying as loudly as you are willing to,
    "Boy, am I scared!" at least five times.

After doing this, notice your guilt again
    and see if it hasn't faded some
    or even disappeared entirely.

The more we can get in touch with the benefits of feeling guilty
    and then step into the opportunities for courage
        presented to us by that resisted fear,
    the more our guilt will diminish,
    the more our actions will adjust appropriately,
    and the closer we'll be to living a life we truly love.

Choose an instance of guilt in your life.
    Keep looking for the benefits you get from feeling this guilt.
    Bless those benefits and then see
        if you're willing to choose courage.

༅

_____

_____

_____

_____

_____

_____

_____

The more sinful and guilty a person tends to feel, the less chance
there is that he will be a happy, healthy, or law-abiding citizen. He
will become a compulsive wrong-doer.
    —*Albert Ellis (1913-, American psychotherapist)*

Let us give thanks for our guilt, etc.

Most of us recognize the power
    of expressing appreciation
    for the things that we like,
    whether in ourselves or in others.

For example,
    by honoring yourself for choosing courage,
    you increase the likelihood that you will exercise courage again.

Other examples:
    By noticing and appreciating
        how good you feel when you exercise,
    you increase your desire and commitment
        to exercise again.

    Or by expressing appreciation
        to a friend for her punctuality,
    you increase the likelihood
        of her being punctual in the future.

However, very few of us recognize
    the power of expressing appreciation
    for the benefits derived from behaviors that we *don't* like.

Typical emotional behaviors that we dislike,
    both in ourselves or in others, are:
        resentment, resignation, depression, guilt,
        fear, whining, righteous anger.

We resist these feelings, these behaviors.

If you will uncover the benefits
  (I've documented 19 benefits of feeling guilty, see page 460)
  that you are getting from one of these feelings,
  and you *really* express appreciation for these benefits,
  then, counter-intuitively, the unwanted feeling
    (in this case, guilt)
  will disappear!

Let's take the feeling of guilt as a particular example.
"Be thankful for feeling guilty?
  You've got to be kidding!"
  I can hear you saying.
Or "There are *no* benefits for feeling guilty,"
  you might protest.
But there are benefits and it is precisely
  by remaining hidden and unappreciated
  that we can cash in on these benefits,
    ensuring that the feelings of guilt will remain in place.
The process is like playing a con game with yourself.

To give you some idea of the possible benefits of feeling guilty,
  I will share three of the 19 here.

1. By feeling guilt, I show to myself (and others)
  that I am a person who has good standards of behavior.
  Therefore, by feeling bad about myself (through guilt),
    I can feel good about myself
    by demonstrating to myself and/or others (through guilt)
    that I am a person of good standards.

2. By feeling guilt, I can beat someone else
    to the punch, blaming myself before *they* blame me.
  This gives me an added sense of control over my life.

3. By knowing that I will feel guilt
        for something I am considering doing,
    I can tell myself that I will be paying the price
        for the action through my guilt.
    Therefore, I can allow myself to go ahead and do it.

I worked with a client in New Mexico several years ago.
He was feeling guilty about the breakup of his marriage
    and how the breakup might affect his two kids
        (even though it was obvious that his kids were better off).
In 20 minutes, he and I were able to identify the benefits
    he was deriving from feeling guilty,
    express gratitude for those benefits,
    and thereby make his guilt disappear!

Select a bad feeling (e.g., guilt, resentment, depression)
    that you are currently experiencing,
    then, with curiosity and patience,
    keep looking for the benefits of having that feeling.
Once you discover a benefit
    (most benefits boil down to wanting to feel safer
    and more comfortable and to avoid fear),
    take as much time as necessary
    to express your appreciation and gratitude for that benefit.

Keep up with this process until you notice that
    the unwanted feeling has disappeared.

Our resistance to the negative is a resistance to fear.
Breathe into and embrace that fear.
Honor yourself for the choice of courage to do this
    —again and again.

૭ৎ

Are you afraid of happiness or success?

Are you afraid of happiness?
Are you afraid of success?
Are you afraid of things being too easy:
>with yourself?
>in your life?
>in your job?
>in your friendships?
>with your romantic partner?

Many of us could benefit from asking the questions,
>"How good am I willing to have it?"
>"How easy am I willing to let it be?"

And often the candid answers are,
>"Not so good" and "Not so easy."

Given all the benefits of happiness and success,
>there is value in discovering the benefits
>of *not* being happy and successful.

Let me suggest a few major ones that may apply.

By remaining unhappy or unsuccessful,
>we remain safe from the possible disappointment
>of becoming happy or successful
>and then losing what we have gained.
>If you don't climb very high, you can't fall very far.

By remaining unsuccessful,
>we avoid the projected costs of maintaining that success.
>Success has its costs as well as its benefits.

If we are unwilling to recognize and accept those costs
 in exchange for the benefits,
  then, of course, we will avoid that success.

If we should become happy,
 if we should become successful,
 if things should come easily to us,
 then maybe we don't deserve it.
 Out of fear that others may resent us,
  envy us, or think badly of us,
  or that "God" will take success or happiness from us,
  we remain in our current state.

Allowing ourselves to be happy,
 allowing ourselves to be successful
 (according to own personal idea of success),
 allowing life to come easily to us
 demands a continual choice of courage.

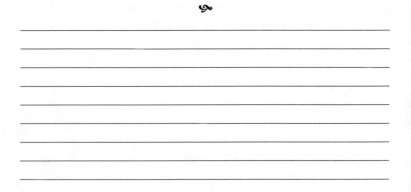

Success is never final and failure never total. It's courage that counts.
     —*Success Unlimited*

Defeat may serve as well as victory to shake the soul and let the glory out.
     —*Edwin Markham (1852-1940, American poet)*

Resignation: Resisted fear at its worst

What is resignation?
Resignation is the everyday man's form of cynicism.

Resignation says that something should be different
    but it's not and there's nothing you can do about it.

Resignation says that
    there's something wrong with you, and/or
    there's something wrong with others, and/or
    there's something wrong with the universe,
    and you're unable and/or unwilling
    to do anything about it.

Sometimes resignation masquerades as a type of acceptance.
    But it is not.
    Resignation resists *what is* by making it wrong.
    Acceptance embraces *what is* with *no* resistance.

Resignation is the most pervasive of all human emotions.
    Why?
    Because of all the great benefits we derive from it.
    The interesting fact about resignation is that
        these benefits must remain hidden and unappreciated
        in order to keep the resignation in place.

Let us examine a particular example.

Let's say that Joe feels resigned
    about the prospects of getting a better job.

If Joe feels resigned,
  this relieves him of the risk of being disappointed
      or looking foolish
  if he unsuccessfully tries to find a better job.
If Joe feels resigned,
  this relieves him of the fears associated
  with the process of finding a better job.
If Joe feels resigned,
  this relieves him of the fear
  that he might not be able to handle the job he wants,
  should he get it.
If, in feeling resigned,
  Joe finds fault with himself,
  this relieves him of facing the fear
  associated with *really* accepting and engaging
  with his current job.
If, in feeling resigned,
  Joe makes others wrong (e.g., his boss),
  this relieves him of facing the fear
  associated with *really* looking
  at his own choices regarding his job
  and his relationship with his boss.
If, in feeling resigned,
  Joe makes the universe wrong,
  this relieves him of facing the fear
  associated with making risky choices in his life.

Resignation has a lot of benefits!
No wonder it commands such a following.

With deep self-examination,
    ask yourself what resignation you might have about:
    your life in general,
    your spouse or lover,
    your lack of a spouse or lover,
    your health and fitness,
    your appearance,
    your job and career,
    your friendships,
    your relationships with family members,
    your relationship with the universe and/or with God.

Look for the "security" that your resignation provides to you.

What are your opportunities for courage here?

❧

_____
_____
_____
_____
_____
_____
_____
_____
_____
_____

If you can't change your fate, change your attitude.
> —*Amy Tan (1952-,*
> *Chinese-American author, The Joy Luck Club)*

Fate, then, is a name for facts not yet passed under the fire of thought; for causes which are unpenetrated.
> —*Ralph Waldo Emerson (1803-1882,*
> *American poet, essayist)*

Can you find the positive in negative?

Especially in the USA,
　　PMA (positive mental attitude) is highly valued and acclaimed.

"Don't be negative."
　　"I shouldn't feel negative."
　　"Always say or think something good."

But I say it's very negative
　　to be negative about the negative.

It is negative to resist the negative.

When we embrace our negativity,
　　when we look for and express gratitude for the benefits
　　that the negative is either providing or trying to provide for us,
　　then we are truly living in a world where everything is a gift,
　　including the negative.

In resisting the negative,
　　notice that you are resisting fear.

To embrace and explore that fear is a choice of courage.

❧

_____

_____

_____

_____

_____

_____

_____

_____

Do you really want to be safe from that?

When you think you're being safe, what are you safe *from*?

If you want to be safe from
finding the job you want,
then don't choose the courage to go for it.

If you want to be safe from
having that man/woman in your life that you're interested in,
then don't choose the courage to ask h/im out.

If you want to be safe from
writing that book you want to write,
then don't choose the courage to start it.

If you want to be safe from
living your life as a magnificent work of art,
then don't choose the courage to go for it.

If you want to be safe from
passionately following your dreams,
then don't choose the courage to say "no" to others.

If you want to be safe from
experiencing deep intimacy and connection with your friends,
then don't choose the courage to speak your heart.

If you want to be safe from
enjoying a life of leisure and adventure,
then don't choose the courage to design your life to make it so.

If you want to be safe from
    living the life you've always dreamed about,
      then don't choose the courage to share yourself openly,
        to make unreasonable requests,
        and to say "no" when you need to.

Are you *really* safe?

∾

_____

_____

_____

_____

_____

_____

_____

_____

_____

_____

_____

It takes a lot of courage to release the familiar and seemingly secure, to embrace the new. But there is more security in the adventurous and exciting, for in movement there is life, and in change there is power.

—*Alan Cohen*

As the ostrich when pursued hides his head, but forgets his body; so the fears of a coward expose him to danger.

—*Akhenaton (BC-1375, Egyptian king, monotheist)*

It is not death that a man should fear, but he should fear never beginning to live.

—*Marcus Aurelius (121-182, Roman emperor, philosopher)*

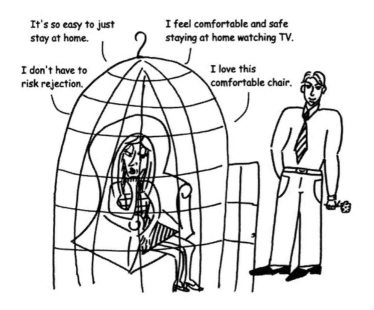

Are you wearing golden handcuffs?

The term "golden handcuffs" typically refers
    to an American executive
    earning a large income
    in a job s/he doesn't really care for
    to support an expensive lifestyle
    to which s/he has become addicted.

For this man (or woman) it seems almost impossible to consider
    getting another job or changing h/is career
    so that s/he might feel more satisfied
    because s/he is handcuffed to h/is situation.
Men and women in this position will often tolerate
    a dissatisfying job for years, if not for the rest of their lives,
    simply because they are unwilling
    to choose courage and use their creativity
    to break out of their golden handcuffs.

Perhaps you too are wearing golden handcuffs.
Consider this example.

Last night, I had dinner with a 25-year-old Chinese woman.
She lives with her parents,
    as is typical in Chinese culture before a woman gets married.
She feels controlled and restricted by her parents,
    especially by her mother.
In various ways, she is forced
    to live her life to suit her parents' wishes
    and to avoid upsetting or scaring them.
However, she has a good job.
    She is bright and confident in her work.
    She has the option of finding her own apartment,
    or perhaps living with a female colleague.

But she is wearing golden handcuffs.

She lives in a much nicer home than she could afford
    if she were living on her own.
Her mother fixes meals for her and pampers her in many ways.
And she knows she would have to face
    the anger and disapproval of her parents
    if she moved out.

After she and I talked, she agreed that she lives in a golden cage,
    where the bars are made of her parents' anger.
    If she tried to move the bars apart to escape from her cage,
    she would stimulate her parents' anger, something that,
    until now, she has not chosen the courage to do.

Again, as always, we are faced with the perennial choice
    between feeling safe and comfortable in the moment
    or living our lives fully.

Golden handcuffs are also often found
   in the context of marriages and even in friendships.

Ask yourself,
   "What golden handcuffs might I be wearing in my life now?"
   "What courage would I have to choose
      if I wanted to break out of these handcuffs?"

❧

_____
_____
_____
_____
_____
_____
_____
_____
_____
_____
_____
_____
_____
_____
_____
_____
_____
_____

Conformity is the jailer of freedom and the enemy of growth.
   —*John F. Kennedy (1917-1963,*
   Thirty-fifth President of the United States)

Be your own palace, or the world is your jail.
   —*John Donne (1572-1632, English metaphysical poet)*

Are you confused?

Confusion is often a symptom of resisted fear.

"I'm confused about my marriage."

Probable translation:
"I want to avoid my fear of examining
    what it might take to make
    our marriage work for me and my spouse.
I also want to avoid my fear
    of looking at what it might take
    to leave my marriage and to create the life I want
    without my spouse.
I also want to avoid my fear of clarifying
    the costs and benefits of
    either staying with my marriage
    or leave my marriage."

"I'm confused about what career I really want in life."

Probable translation:
"I want to avoid my fear
    of uncovering my deepest life inspirations
        (treating life as my playground)
    and intelligently taking on the risks involved
    in selecting/creating a career
    that is a powerful expression of those inspirations.
I want to avoid my fear
    of facing the fact
    that *everything* in life has costs and benefits
    and that *everything* in life has varying degrees of risk."

Now apply similar translations
    to the following expressions of confusion.

"I'm confused about which university to attend."
"I'm confused about what men/women really want."
"I'm confused about the meaning of life."
"I'm confused about which car to buy."

Are there any issues in your life
    that you're confused about?
Ask yourself the question,
    "What fear might I be avoiding that,
        if I were willing to face,
        would likely clear up this confusion?"

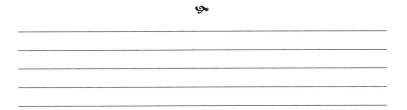

_____

_____

_____

_____

_____

Truth arises more readily from error than from confusion.
          —Francis Bacon (1561-1626,
          British philosopher, essayist, statesman)

Then indecision brings its own delays, And days are lost lamenting over lost days. Are you in earnest? Seize this very minute; What you can do, or dream you can, begin it.
          —Johann Wolfgang Von Goethe (1749-1832,
          German poet, dramatist, novelist)

Indecision is debilitating; it feeds upon itself; it is, one might almost say, habit-forming. Not only that, but it is contagious; it transmits itself to others.

          —H.A. Hopf

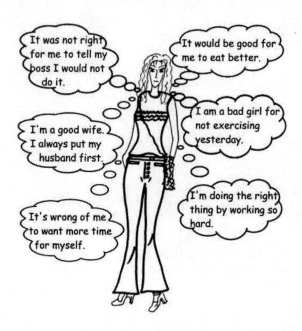

Good and bad are both bad

The basic ideas of good versus bad,
    right versus wrong, fair versus unfair, virtue versus sin,
    have caused humanity more trouble and grief
    than any other single idea in the world.

At best, these ideas are only fit for a child,
    to provide low-context rules for action
    and to ensure that s/he will be approved of
    by those in h/is immediate environment.

The main benefit of allowing these judgmental ideas to control us
    is that we can avoid the fear
    of knowing and taking into account one simple fact:
    Everything has its benefits *and* costs.
    It helps us to avoid facing and accepting
    the fundamental risk that life is.

Only when we *know* that we are good,
    when we *know* that we are right,
    are we able to blind ourselves to
    (or relieve ourselves from looking into)
    the costs of our actions, both to ourselves and to others.

Knowing that we are good (and even that we are bad),
    knowing that we took the right action
        (or even the wrong action),
    knowing that we are "saved" (or even sinners),
    gives us a sense of security that allows us
    to avoid feeling the fear of looking
    at the costs and benefits of our actions.
    It allows us to avoid embracing
        the risks that our actions and non-actions entail,
        including the risks of disapproval from others.

We ignore and/or forget the fact that Hitler
    and all his eager supporters
    knew that they were *right* and *good*
    and that this knowledge enabled them
    to do the horrible things they did.

As a lesser example, we ignore and/or forget the fact
    that the damage that parents do
    to the spirit and happiness of their children
    is most often done by parents who *know*
    the right, good, and proper life that their children should live.

Consider that good and bad have no meaning of their own
    except as they *may*, in *some* contexts,
    describe the benefits and costs of certain actions.

Also consider that benefits and costs
    are ultimately defined by whether or not
    they promote the successful expression of
    joy, pleasure, and rapture in our lives.

Take note that the distinctions of benefit and cost
    must include the parameters
    benefit to whom? and *cost to whom?*
    They must also include short-range
    and long-range considerations.
    They must also include an appreciation
    of the context and environment within which our choices lie:
        we often get attached
        to a particular form or way of doing something,
        forgetting the larger purpose.

For example, we act as if the value of marriage
    is an ultimate value, while forgetting the reasons
    we decided to marry in the first place
    (namely the opportunity to express and feel love
        and to live our lives to the fullest).

Also consider that we often act
    as if having a body with a beating heart is of ultimate value,
    while forgetting that the only reason we really want to be alive
    is to rejoice in our life and rejoice in the opportunities
    for self-expression, pleasure, joy, and contribution to others.

Consider that we often think that a formal education is good,
    without clearly examining the costs and benefits
    as they do or do not serve
    the natural passion, curiosity, and interests
    of the person to be educated.

In doing so, we are not using our creativity and
    choosing courage
to create the structure of that education (formal or not)
that would best serve these basic values.

Is marriage good?
    I can show you contexts where the costs of staying married
    obviously outweigh the benefits.
Is divorce bad?
    Divorce can be a reason for great celebration.
Is keeping your word good?
    Some situations require breaking your word
    in order to maintain integrity.

Tell me anything that you think is
    always good, always bad,
    always right, always wrong,
    always fair, always unfair,
    always approved by God, or always a sin
        and I will demonstrate evidence
        (undiscovered or unacknowledged benefits or costs)
        to the contrary.
    I will show you contexts
        in which the benefits of the bad
        outweigh (often by far) the costs of the bad.
    I will show you contexts in which the costs of the good
        outweigh (often by far) the benefits of the good.

To know what is good, to know what is bad,
    to know what is right, and to know what is wrong
    is incredibly addictive;
    we so yearn for that feeling of security.
Yet this security is the security
    of an ostrich with its head in the sand.

To begin to have what we *really* want (to have a life we love)
    requires an existential choice of courage,
    again and again, day after day,
    to step beyond the dangerously simplistic good-bad world
    and into a more complicated and sometimes messy
    adult world of benefits and costs.

I am amused by a quotation
    from the philosopher Bertrand Russell:
    "The trouble with the world is that the stupid are cocksure
        and the intelligent are full of doubt."

I would take issue with Russell's calling people stupid.
    I don't think people are stupid;
    I think we just want to feel safe and comfortable. (Right now!)
    However, the problem with this feeling of safety
        is that it's often foolishly dangerous to our real life
        and to the lives of those we love.

Experiment with reducing/eliminating the words
    good and bad, right and wrong, fair and unfair,
        from your vocabulary,
    both in your conversation with others
    and in your internal conversations with yourself.

Instead, speak, if you can, in terms of benefits and costs
    (and to whom).

Notice the feeling of insecurity that this stimulates.

Notice the choice of courage that this involves.

৯

Is failure a bugaboo for you?

When we insist on guaranteeing success
    for each and every transaction,
      we often ensure our failure in the larger picture and in life itself.

Failure is an integral part of being alive.
Failure is feedback to guide our actions in life.
Failure is a reminder that life is a glorious risk.
Without the possibility and actuality of failure,
    life would not be life.

If every request you make must be answered with a "yes,"
    if every attempt you make must meet with success,
      then you will be stopped at every corner and every turn.
You will box yourself into smaller and smaller corners,
    trying to avoid anything that confronts the risk that life is.

If, however, we are clear about what we can control
    as contrasted with what we can only influence,
      then, by being willing to stay in action, as we let go of control,
    we can often dramatically increase the influence we have,
    not only with an individual action
    but especially with the results we get in the long run.

For example, a salesperson who insists
    on controlling the outcome with each prospect
    may create a lot of upset
      both for h/imself and for the prospect.
Whereas, the salesperson who gives full effort,
    while letting go of controlling the outcome,
    will often win over the prospect
    and will certainly win over the day.

The most important factor in determining our success in life is our attitude and viewpoint regarding failure and risk.

Welcome to the risk that life is!

Choose the courage to embrace the risk that life is!

ಀ

_____

_____

_____

_____

_____

_____

_____

_____

_____

_____

_____

The fastest way to succeed is to double your failure rate.
—*Thomas J. Watson, Sr. (1874-1966, Founder of IBM)*

Failure is an event, never a person.
—*William D. Brown (1798-1859)*

We pay just as dearly for our triumphs as we do for our defeats. Go ahead and fail. But fail with wit, fail with grace, fail with style. A mediocre failure is as insufferable as a mediocre success. Embrace failure! Seek it out. Learn to love it. That may be the only way any of us will ever be free.

—*Bruce Barton (1886-1967,*
American author, advertising executive)

Rejection projection:
What is really real?

I used to avoid rejection a lot.
I avoided being rejected so much by women
    during my teens and early 20s
    that I didn't have a girlfriend until I was 26.

Avoiding rejection is the *number one* cause,
    not only of loneliness, but also of not getting
    most of the things we want in our life.

"Oh, I couldn't ask for that."
"What if s/he thinks I'm too forward?"
"I don't want to feel the pain if s/he says, 'no'"
"They will think I am too presumptuous."
"I don't want to appear foolish."
"What if s/he thinks I'm desperate?"
"I can't stand it if s/he pays attention to someone else."
"What if they don't want me for the job?"

These are the automatic thoughts that entangle our thinking
    when we consider stepping outside
    the safety of our anti-rejection box.

But what *is* rejection?
If someone says, "No, we will not hire you,"
    does it mean,
    "I don't like you" or
    "I think another applicant will provide me with better value" or
    "I'm going to hire my cousin" or
    "Who would ever hire you!" or
    "I don't want to hire someone with bad breath" or
    (fill in another 1000 possible reasons)?

If someone says, "No, I don't want to go to the movies with you,"
    does it mean
        "I will never go to the movies with you" or
        "I would love to go, but I have a conflict" or
        "I want to go, but I want to play hard to get" or
        "I want to go, but I am too shy to say 'yes'" or
        "I want to go, but not to that movie" or
        "I want to see you, but I don't like movies" or
        (fill in another 1000 possible interpretations)?

Why are we so frightened of rejection,
    especially since we rarely know exactly *what* is being rejected?

In most cases, the fear of rejection is a paper-tiger fear;
    it is an eventuality that has little or no cost
    except for the fear itself.
If you ask someone for a date, there is no real cost in asking,
    even if the answer is "no."
If you ask someone for a job, there is no real cost in asking,
    even if the answer is "no."
But there can be a very big cost
    of *not* asking for a date or
    not asking for a job or
    not asking for whatever it is you want.

Perhaps the biggest (hidden) reason for *not* asking,
    is that we are avoiding the fear of facing the fact
    that we *don't* have control of the situation.
    As long as we don't ask,
        we can live with the illusion
        that we have control in our life
        because everything is predictable
        when we avoid the risk of rejection.

To choose the courage to make requests and risk rejection,
    again and again,
    is to come face to face with the ongoing risk that life is.
We may get what we want and we may not.
But by not requesting, by not risking rejection,
        we feel safer and more comfortable in the illusion
            that our life is under control.

The possibility of rejection is an opportunity for choosing courage.

Take on at least three new opportunities
    of rejection each day for the next seven days.

๑

What I point out to people is that it's silly to be afraid that you're not going to get what you want if you ask. Because you are already not getting what you want. They always laugh about that because they realize it's so true. Without asking you already have failed, you already have nothing. What are you afraid of? You're afraid of getting what you already have! It's ridiculous! Who cares if you don't get it when you ask for it, because, before you ask for it, you don't have it anyway. So there's really nothing to be afraid of.

—*Marcia Martin*

You create your opportunities by asking for them.

—*Patty Hansen (American author)*

You win some, you lose some, and some get rained out, but you gotta suit up for them all.

—*J. Askenberg*

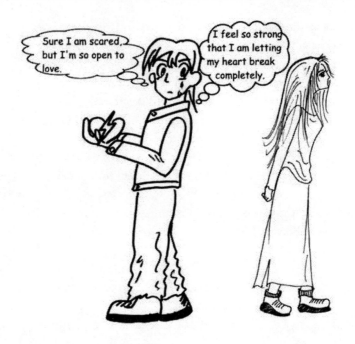

A fully broken heart is an open heart

Are you willing to have a broken heart?
> Are you willing to break another's heart?
> Are you ready for love?

All these questions are the *same* question.

If you're *not* willing to have your heart broken,
> if you're *not* willing to risk breaking the heart of another,
> then you're *not* willing to love fully.

Being willing to fall in love,
> being willing to stay in love,
> (if we keep our eyes open to the risks),
> is the most courageous choice we can ever make.

The experience of romantic love,
  while seeming so lasting when we're in the middle of it,
  is actually quite fragile.
  Even with the best of skills and intentions
  there is never any guarantee of its duration.

In April of 1997, I fell in love with a woman
  more deeply than I had ever fallen before.
  For two months, our romance was the most incredible
  that I'd ever experienced.
One night, we talked on the phone
  from 9:00 PM until 4:00 AM,
  finally ending the conversation
  (even though we wanted to keep talking)
  so that we could get some sleep
  before our date at 11:00 AM!
But after two months, she ended our romantic relationship.

In the following month, I cried more than I had cried
  in all the rest of my life combined.
  I spent many hours on the phone
  with my friends listening to me
  share about my pain and fear
  (fear that I would never find anyone as special as her again).
I continuously encouraged myself
  to breathe into my pain and fear,
  to see and feel it fully
  as an expression of my deep capacity to love.
I wanted to make sure that my heart was *completely* broken.

"A broken heart is an open heart."

After about six weeks,
    I could tell that my process was a success.
    I was more open to love than ever before.
    I was so grateful to my lover for what she had given to me.
    I had a new sense of my self,
        after finding deep strength in my vulnerability.
    Although we were apart,
        I knew I would love her forever.

My women friends here in China often ask me,
    "Do you think true love exists?"
When I ask them what they mean by "true love,"
    they say, "A love that lasts forever."
On occasion, it may happen that a romantic love lasts forever.
    However, it can never be guaranteed or predicted in advance.
    In fact, *trying* to guarantee that love will last
        is the surest way to destroy it.
    There is a Chinese proverb along these very lines:
        "Marriage is the tomb of love."

Imagine that you were given the following choices:

Choice #1:
    Tomorrow you will meet the woman/man of your dreams.
    Being with h/er will bring a sense of peace, joy, and excitement
        deeper than you ever imagined possible.
    You will be deliriously happy.
    Everything will be perfect
        for six months—but only for six months.
    At the end of those six months,
        s/he will leave you, with no explanation.

Choice #2:
    Tomorrow, nothing special will happen.
    Your life will continue for the next six months
        as it has for the past six months.

Which of these two would you choose?

Because love takes us so high, it means there is so far to fall.

To love without guarantees,
    to love with your eyes fully open to the potential risks,
    to love without blame or guilt,
    is a choice of courage, again and again and again.

Will you choose the courage to be open to the gift of love?

ॐ

_____

_____

_____

_____

_____

_____

_____

_____

_____

_____

_____

God is closest to those with broken hearts.

—Jewish proverb

I will indulge my sorrows, and give way to all the pangs and fury of despair.

—Joseph Addison (1672-1719,
British essayist, poet, statesman)

The path of sorrow and that path alone, leads to a land where sorrow is unknown.

—William Cowper (1731-1800, British poet)

Empowerment through vulnerability

Most people associate power with force or
    with the capacity to appear to remain untouched
        by frightening or painful situations.

But there is a different type of power,
    a power that holds a wider context,
    that I call the power of acceptance and vulnerability.

This is the power of letting go of resistance,
    the power of encouraging your heart to break completely
        so that you're more open to love than ever before,
    the power of embracing your fear
        and tapping into its energy to serve your deepest desires,
    the power of allowing your fears and hurts to pass through you,
        knowing that you are bigger than all of them,
    the power to feel fully and deeply the passions of your life,
        knowing that you can choose well within those passions.

Notice the opportunities for vulnerability.
    Breathe into the fear of embracing those opportunities.

Honor your choice of courage to step into those opportunities.

❧

Discover the gold under those rocks

When I was a child,
    my sister (three years younger) and I
    would often trek through the woods behind our house,
    turning over rocks to see what interesting bugs
    might be hidden under them.

Almost all of our resisted fears
    don't occur to us as fears or resisted fears,
    but occur to us in forms we don't recognize
    and are essentially "hiding under rocks."
As long as a resisted fear is hiding under a rock,
    we have no access to shifting or changing it,
    we have no opportunity
    to make a conscious choice about it,
    either through the choice of courage
    or through the choice of coverage
    ("coverage" is a word I have coined
        to mean "choosing to feel safe and comfortable
        in the moment in preference to embracing the fear
        stimulated by choosing courage"; see page 124).

Fundamentally, resisted fear (once identified as such)
    is a gold mine we can tap into;
    it can be the source of expanding aliveness,
        accomplishment, and energy.

Once we suspect or realize that we are frightened
    and we are hiding/resisting a specific fear,
    then we have a clear and straightforward choice.

We can choose courage,
>> taking the appropriate action, if any,
>> breathing into our fear and embracing its energy,
>> and honoring the five-year-old within
>>> for the courage s/he is choosing.
> Or we can choose coverage,
>> expressing compassion for the five-year-old within
>>> for wanting to feel safe and comfortable in the moment.

Let's begin to identify just a few of the many "rocks"
> that resisted fear can "hide beneath."
> Some of these rocks are somewhat transparent;
>> often we can easily see the resisted fear they conceal.
> Other rocks are very opaque
>> and we might never imagine that they hide resisted fear.

Let's look at some of the more transparent rocks first.

Worry

My definition of worry is "an attempt to do away with fear."
> Worry is obviously resistance to fear.

Embarrassment

Embarrassment is resisted fear of how another may be
> seeing us or thinking about us.

Jealousy

Jealousy is resisted fear of loss
> or possible loss of someone we love.

Shyness

Shyness is resisted fear of how others may think or feel about us
> if we were more assertive.

Foolish
Foolishness is resisted fear of how we will look to others
    in a given situation
        because we can't guarantee that everyone
            would heartily approve of our behavior.

Overwhelm
Overwhelm is resisted fear of
    "What will happen if I don't get it all done?"

Now let's consider some resisted fears
    that are less obviously resisted fears,
    hiding under more opaque rocks.

Guilt
The function or benefit of guilt (see page 460 for more benefits)
    is to try to make us feel safer and more secure.
    For example,
        "If I beat myself up first,
        I can beat others to the punch,
        and thereby feel more in control."
    Another example,
        "If I put the blame on myself,
        then I don't have to choose courage
        to maintain my boundaries with another."

Blame
The best way to find the resisted fear in blame is to ask yourself,
    "What fears might I feel
    if I didn't blame this person or these people?"

Resentment
Resentment is often a direct result of not choosing courage
    to create and maintain needed boundaries with others.

Resignation
Resignation is a direct result of not choosing courage to
    either fully embrace and create the situation as a gift
    or to choose courage
        to change the situation in the face of the risk
           that our intention may not be fulfilled.

Stress
Resisted fear is often a factor in accumulated stress.
    When fear is embraced, when courage is chosen,
    then stress is released, not accumulated.

Perfectionism
Perfectionism is resisted fear of what will happen
    or who will disapprove if something is not perfect.

Low self-esteem
Low self-esteem is a direct result of not choosing courage.
    Anyone who consistently chooses courage
        (in all domains of his or her life)
        will have high self-esteem.

Lack of self-confidence
Self-confidence is a secondary result.
    It is not a primary cause.
    Self-confidence automatically occurs
        through the consistent choice of courage
        in a given area or domain.

Self-consciousness
Self-consciousness (second-guessing our own responses)
    occurs out of resisted fear of how others will see us.

Defensiveness
Defensiveness is defending against something that is feared.

Hostility
Hostility is aggression against something that is feared.

Controlling
We usually try to control another through force or blaming
    in order to feel safer and more comfortable.

Withdrawal
We withdraw when we do not feel safe and comfortable.

Indecisiveness
We are afraid of making the "wrong" decision.
    As a result, we are indecisive.

Ingratitude
To get in touch with the resisted fear here, ask yourself,
    "What fear might I feel if I fully expressed
    my gratitude to everyone in my life?"

Laziness
Our laziness is often the result
    of not choosing the courage to go for what we *really* want.

Use this list to find the gold of resisted fear
    underneath the rocks in *your* life.

Whenever you feel any unwanted responses,
    as an experiment,
    take several *deep* breaths and say to yourself,
    ten times over and very loudly (if possible),
    "Boy, am I scared!" to un-resist the fear.
    Notice if there is any shift in the unwanted response
        when you do this experiment.

❧

_____

_____

_____

_____

_____

_____

_____

_____

_____

_____

_____

_____

_____

_____

Things are not always what they seem; the first appearance deceives many; the intelligence of a few perceives what has been carefully hidden.

—*Phaedrus (early Macedonian inventor and writer)*

There comes a time in every rightly constructed boy's life when he has a raging desire to go somewhere and dig for hidden treasure.
—*Mark Twain (1835-1910, American humorist, writer)*

Each problem has hidden in it an opportunity so powerful that it literally dwarfs the problem. The greatest success stories were created by people who recognized a problem and turned it into an opportunity.

—*Joseph Sugarman (American businessman)*

Find strength in your "weakness"

I will often hear my friends in China say that
    what they dislike about themselves is that they are "not strong."
Invariably, when I explore further,
    I find that the strength they are talking about is the strength:
        to not feel fear, to not feel pain, to not cry,
        to not get discouraged, to not feel lazy, to not get tired,
        to not feel depressed.

I find it interesting that I think of myself
    as neither *strong* nor *not strong*.
Yet I have resilience that
    most of my friends and colleagues admire.

I don't try to *not* be afraid;
    I embrace my fear and tap into its energy.
I don't try *not* to feel pain;
    I know that pain is an expression
    of my aliveness and my capacity to love.
I don't try *not* to cry;
    I welcome crying as a beautiful
    and healthy expression of release.
I don't try *not* to get discouraged or lazy;
    I try to discover what's missing in terms of
    uncovering and allowing the natural passions of my life.
I don't try *not* to get tired;
    I pay attention to what my body is trying to tell me
    and make sure I get enough rest.
I don't try *not* to get depressed;
    If I notice some depression,
    I make sure I do some release processes
    that allow me to tap back into my natural passion for life.

Typically, "trying *not* to" (at least in these cases)
    results in more of the same:
        more blocked fear, more buried pain, more unshed tears,
        more discouragement, more laziness, more tiredness,
        and more depression.

To resist these feelings is only to fight with yourself,
    for one part of you to make an enemy of another part.

I am not surprised anymore when,
    upon a new friend's first visit with me,
    she shockingly finds herself
    shedding embarrassed tears in front of me.

Typically, she sees this as weakness.
    I see it as a welcome and much-needed release.

What we often call strength is killing us.
The medicine we have prescribed for ourselves
    is actually a poison,
    compounding the original condition.

Take some time now to ask yourself,
    "How am I actually doing more damage than good
    in *trying to be strong*?"

How might I begin to find my strength in *non-trying*,
    and in *non-resistance*?

Choose courage to allow yourself to be weak.

                  ❧

Worry: An attempt to do away with fear

Worry is an attempt to do away with fear.
Worry is resistance to fear.

When you are worrying,
    you are trying to figure out a way
    to not be frightened, aren't you?

There is nothing wrong with looking
    for a way to reduce our fear.
The problem is our resistance to the fear.
When we resist our fear we reduce our resourcefulness
    and we tend to over-control,
        often getting results that are opposite to our intentions.

The next time you notice that you are worrying,
    pause for a moment.
    Take several deep breaths and relax into the fear,
        allowing it to flow through you.
    Then, as loudly as possible, given the situation you're in,
        shout out with very long breaths,
        "Boy, am I scared!" several times.

Once you've done this,
    notice that the worry
        does not hold you as tightly as it did before.
    Notice the increased feeling
        of self-confidence and resourcefulness.

Fear is not your enemy.
    The energy of fear can be your ally.
    It is resisted fear that is your enemy.

The next time you notice yourself worrying,
    take advantage of the opportunity
    to embrace the energy of your fear,
    bringing its vitality to your desires and commitments.

❧

_____

_____

_____

_____

_____

_____

_____

_____

_____

_____

_____

_____

_____

_____

Worry is interest paid on trouble before it comes due.
        —*William R. Inge (1860-1954, clergyman, scholar, author)*

Worrying does not empty tomorrow of its troubles. It empties today of its strength.

                                        —*unknown*

When I look back on all these worries I remember the story of the old man who said on his deathbed that he had had a lot of trouble in his life, most of which never happened.

                                —*Sir Winston Churchill*

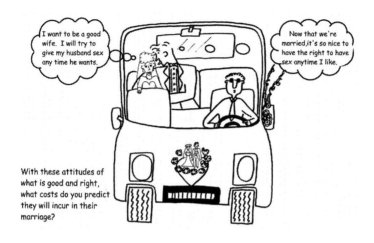

I want to be a good wife. I will try to give my husband sex any time he wants.

Now that we're married, it's so nice to have the right to have sex anytime I like.

With these attitudes of what is good and right, what costs do you predict they will incur in their marriage?

What is your addiction to the "good" costing you?

Can you think of a single movie
    that didn't have a good guy and a bad guy?
    (I know there are a *few*.)

Even such exceptionally enlightened movies
    as *Pleasantville* or *Chocolat*
    have their token bad guys,
    (the mayor in *Pleasantville*, Serge in *Chocolat*).

Have you *ever* read a novel or seen a movie
    in which *both* sides
    (in standard good/bad conflicts,
    for example, the *Axis powers* versus the *Allies* in WWII)
    are portrayed with compassion and understanding.
    If you know of such a book or movie,
        please let me know about it!

Or have you *ever* read a book or seen a movie
>   (aside from horror books and movies which are designed
>   primarily for the fear factor, not the "feeling safe" factor)
>   in which the good guys ultimately lose
>   and the bad guys ultimately win?
>   The book writers and movie makers know instinctively
>   we will not pay money to read or see such fare.

Why?
What function does all this good/bad dramatization serve?
I say that it helps us to *feel* safer (not *be* safer).

If we can believe that if only we are good
>   according to the rules everybody agrees upon,
>   then we will win, we will survive, we will be successful.
>   What a reassurance!

What an incredible cultural fantasy!
A fantasy shared
>   by every culture, sub-culture, and family culture in the world,
>   each with its own official version of the rules regarding
>   what's good and bad, what's right and wrong.

Certainly it is true that many of the rules
>   for being good or doing the right thing
>   have definite and/or probable benefits associated
>   with following these rules.
And, on the other side,
>   it is true that breaking many of the rules
>   and thereby being bad or doing the wrong thing
>   have definite and/or probable costs associated
>   with not following these rules.

The poison that we take,
 the poison that we're addicted to,
 the poison that gives us dose after addictive dose
  of that false sense of security,
 the poison which is part of the culture itself,
 fed to us by almost every book, every movie,
  every sitcom, by our parents and our teachers,
  by our friends, our bosses, our employees,
 is the poison of good and bad,
  the toxicity of right and wrong.

While making us feel inappropriately safe
 because we *know* we are doing the right thing,
 it prevents us from considering
 the costs and benefits of our choices and actions.

While making us feel inappropriately safe
 because we know that by doing the right thing
 others will extol us and not criticize or condemn us,
 and because we will also feel righteous about ourselves,
 it prevents us from considering
  the costs and benefits of our choices and actions.

Since the dawn of language,
 the behavior of seeing life, seeing others, seeing ourselves
 through the lens of good and bad, right and wrong,
 has created and perpetuated more suffering
 in this world than *all* other factors combined.

Knowing what is good, knowing what is right,
 gives us license (and a righteous license, at that)
 to blind ourselves to the costs of good
 and the benefits of the bad.

Why would we pay such an exorbitant price?
>To feel safer and more comfortable in the moment.
>What a deal!

In what areas of your life do you think you are right (or wrong)?
>In what ways do you think you are a good person?
>Or a bad person?
Can you begin to see the continuing choice of courage
>it would take for you
>to begin to guide your choices and actions,
>not on right and wrong, not on good or bad,
>but on costs and benefits
>>for the fullest expression of your life
>>and the lives of those you care about?

❧

_____

_____

_____

_____

_____

_____

_____

_____

_____

_____

_____

_____

Genuine tragedies in the world are not conflicts between right and wrong. They are conflicts between two rights.
>—*Georg Hegel (1770-1831, German idealist philosopher)*

Righteousness is easy in retrospect.
>—*Arthur Schlesinger Jr. (in "Newsweek")*

Are you sure you are right?

People who are unwilling
    to look beyond what they *know to be right*
    contribute blindly
    to more horror and suffering on this earth
    than is ever imagined.

When we know ourselves to be right,
    we feel justified in looking no further
    to discover or examine the consequences
    (the benefits and costs)
    of the stance or actions
    that we initiate, perpetrate, and/or support.

Consider the consequences for . . .

a child *who knows* that he's *right* to obey
    h/is parents, even into adulthood,
    at the expense of creating and living h/is own life.
an adult child who *knows* that euthanasia is *wrong*,
    forcing h/is parents to endure
    years of excruciating pain and hopelessness
    before the final release of death.
a young man who *knows*
    that his country or cause must be *right*
    and patriotically goes off to war to kill others and himself.
a wife who *knows* that divorce is *wrong*
    and loyally submits herself, her husband, and her kids
    to interminable years of upset, resignation, and inauthenticity.

And so on and so on.

We long for the security
    that we feel in the right(eousness)
    of our position, belief, or action!
We long for the security
    that we feel in the right(eousness)
    of the positions, beliefs, and actions of some authority
    (God, church, country, cause, teacher, parents, etc.)!

The psychological purpose
    of right(eousness) is to create
    a (false) feeling of security.

You will be choosing courage consistently
    if you look beyond what you know to be right
    and begin to discover and examine *all* the benefits *and* costs
    of your own (or others') positions, beliefs, and actions.

Where in your life is your righteousness a contributing factor
    to loss of love, to disharmony,
    and even damage to yourself and/or others?

It is a choice of courage to let go of your righteousness
    (i.e., knowing you are right)
    and, instead, take the stance and position
    most likely to enhance your life and others' lives,
    based upon evaluation of the probable costs
    and benefits of your actions.

໑

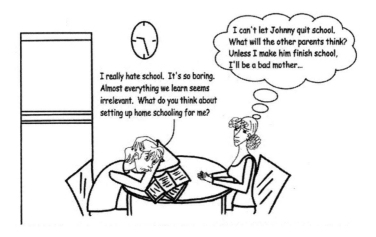

Beware of "Love"

More damage, more "evil" is done in this world
    in the name of love,
        with the appearance of love, with the intention of love
than is ever done by what we consider
to be hateful, unloving, or evil intentions
        (at least 100 times more)!

How many of us lead timid lives,
    not going for what we *really* want
    because we are afraid it will frighten or hurt the ones we love
    (all in the name of and/or with the intention of love)?

How many of us allow
    our resentment and/or hurt to build up
    with a loved one, a colleague or a friend,
    because speaking up would hurt their feelings
    (all in the name of and/or with the intention of love)?

How many of us allow and/or encourage others
    to violate our own boundaries
    (all in the name of and/or with the intention of love)?

How many of us "give" our children too much
    (all in the name of and/or with the intention of love)?

How many of us live our lives through our children,
    imposing *our* expectations and intentions on them
    (all in the name of and/or with the intention of love)?

How many of us tolerate a marriage or relationship
    that is loveless, hostile, vapid, and/or unfulfilling,
    (all in the name of and/or with the intention of love)?

How many of us compel and pressure
    our children into going to school
    where the environment fosters neither creativity nor listening
        for our child's natural passion,
    but conformity and "doing it right"
    (all in the name of and/or with the intention of love)?

How many of us allow and/or compel
    our dying and pain-racked loved ones
    to suffer though a slow and undignified death,
    when we could assist them in ending their suffering earlier
    (all in the name of and/or with the intention of love)?

What are you doing or how are you being
    (either in the name of and/or with the intention of love)
    that, instead of creating loving results
        (especially for the long term),
    is doing exactly the opposite?

It may be a choice of courage for you to act and/or be differently,
so that you have not only the intention of love,
but more loving results.

࿏

_____
_____
_____
_____
_____
_____
_____
_____
_____
_____
_____
_____
_____
_____
_____
_____
_____
_____
_____

History is a better guide than good intentions.

> —*Jeane Kirkpatrick (1926-,*
> *American stateswoman, Academic)*

Hell is paved with good intentions, not with bad ones. All men mean well.

> —*George Bernard Shaw (1856-1950,*
> *Irish-born British dramatist)*

Concentrated power is not rendered harmless by the good intentions of those who create it.

> —*Milton Friedman (1912-, American economist)*

Are you positive about the negative?

Occasionally, I receive feedback that my essays are too negative.

But what does the word "negative" really mean?
When I look deeply into any behavior,
    I can find nothing negative in it.
Some people think that
    guilt, depression, resignation,
        hatred, anger, greed, selfishness, suicide, assisted suicide, etc.
    are negative.
Certainly these feelings and types of behavior
    have costs associated with them,
        often very large ones.
If you are willing to define negative as "having costs,"
    then I agree that I put emphasis
        on examining the costs associated
        with the things we do.
To ignore or blind ourselves to the costs
    associated with our behavior
    will only exacerbate those costs.

However, when I deeply examine the behavior of
    guilt, depression, resignation,
        hatred, anger, greed, selfishness, suicide, assisted suicide, etc.,
    I find that people who behave this way
    derive many benefits from their behavior.

Others would say
    that drugs, broken families, prostitution, pornography,
        school dropouts, gambling, etc.
    are negative.

Certainly these types of behavior have costs associated with them,
    often very large ones.

However, when I deeply examine the behavior of
    drugs, broken families, prostitution, pornography,
        school dropouts, gambling, etc.,
    I find that people who behave this way
    derive many benefits from their behavior.

The major reason we remain unaware of the great benefits
    derived from these types of behavior
    is that we have decided that such behavior is wrong,
    excusing ourselves from the effort of further inquiry.

Still others would say that people who belong to groups
or religions that they themselves don't belong to—
    the New Agers, the Catholics,
        the Protestants, the Muslims, the Buddhists,
        the other "wrong makers,"
        the devil, the atheists, the agnostics,
        the fundamentalists,
        the capitalists, the Nazis, and the Communists—
    are negative.

Certainly the pandemic behavior of making others wrong
    (and of making ourselves and our groups right)
    have costs associated with them, often very large ones.

However, when I deeply examine the behavior of
    making ourselves and others wrong
        (I'm not talking about an issue of accuracy in judgment;
        I'm talking about the condemning of ourselves or others,
        no matter how small that condemning might be),
    I find that the people who behave this way
    often derive many valid benefits from their behavior
        (usually in the domain of feeling more in control
        and trying to avoid fear and pain).

To give up making ourselves wrong and making others wrong
   is, moment by moment, a major choice of courage.
The main benefit of not doing so is feeling
   safer and more comfortable, at least in the moment.
And we all want to feel safe and comfortable, don't we?

Select one aspect of your behavior
   that you consider to be negative.

Examine it carefully and begin to discover
   all the great benefits derived from this behavior.

What new opening do you now see for your life?

Honor yourself for choosing the courage
   to step through this opening.

༄

_____

_____

_____

_____

_____

_____

_____

_____

_____

_____

_____

_____

_____

_____

_____

_____

_____

If you're good, it may be bad

Question what you think is good,
    as well as what you think is bad.

More slaughter and horror has been perpetrated
    in the name of good
    (God, righteousness, loyalty, honor, duty, love, and obedience)
    than in the name of bad (selfishness and greed).

More governments have suppressed or suffocated
    the creativity, enterprise, economy, and spirit of their people
    in the name of charity, security, protecting the innocent,
        and making things fair
    than power-hungry men ever have.

More teachers have suppressed or killed off
    the natural desire for learning and growth in their students
    in the name of education, respect, and doing it the right way
    than perpetrators of ignorance ever have.

More responsible parents have suppressed or throttled
    vitality, curiosity, and joy in their children
    in the name of decency, love, and having responsible kids
    than neglectful parents ever have.

More husbands and wives have strangled
    the intimacy, passion, and connection with each other
    in the name of security, unselfishness, and love
    than being openly selfish ever has.

More friends have suppressed
  the excitement, self-expression, and integrity of their friends
  in the name of conformity and decorum
  than bad influences ever have.

Most of us continue to suppress or kill off
  our own aliveness, energy, and self-expression
  in the name of feeling safe and comfortable,
  being polite, being unselfish, being fair, and being productive
  more than all of our mistakes ever do.

Knowing so clearly what is good and bad
  will give you a very false sense of security.

Welcome to the risk that life is!

Choose an area where you feel like you're being good
  and find an opportunity for choosing courage
  that steps beyond your normal boundaries of safety.

**For more essay(s) on courage and the right-wrong paradigm,
see www.GoldWinde.com/Cbook/More/Right-Wrong.**

To have doubted one's own first principles is the mark of a civilized man.
  —*Oliver Wendell Holmes, Jr. (1841-?,
  American captain, brevet colonel)*

A great deal of intelligence can be invested in ignorance when the
need for illusion is deep.
  —*Saul Bellow*

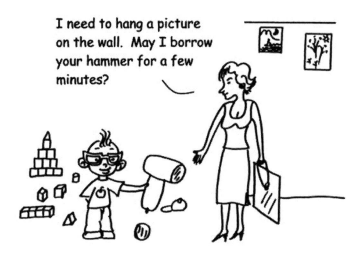

I need to hang a picture on the wall. May I borrow your hammer for a few minutes?

Honor thy children

Do you show honor and respect to your child?

Even if you don't have a biological child,
    I believe you will find much value
      in reading and thinking about this issue.

Parents and other adults frequently complain
    about how children and "the younger generation"
    are disrespectful toward adults.
To the extent that this is true,
    it is a direct result of parents
    not showing respect for their children.
When a child has been treated with respect from an early age,
    he becomes a child (and later a teenager and adult)
    who is respectful of others, particularly his parents.

I have worked with hundreds of parents
    who love their children very much,
    and yet believe their children are disrespectful toward them.
When I ask for specifics about how they treat their children,
    I don't have to hear much
    before I learn about disrespectful behavior
        that the parent is directing toward h/is children.

Loving a child is not enough.
Even though showing love and showing respect are related,
    I believe it is more crucial to a child's development
    to have the experience of being respected,
    than the experience of being loved.
If a parent is consistently showing respect
    to h/is child (in a way that the child experiences as respectful),
    it will be very unlikely that the child
    will not show respect back to the parent.

Some actions, almost always, clearly show respect.
    (1)   Speaking using "please," "thank you," etc.
           and all the other ways of speaking
           that you would accord an adult whom you respected.
    (2)   Knocking on your child's door and waiting for an answer
           before entering h/is room.
    (3)   Being consistent and rigorous in keeping any agreements
           you make with your child.
    (4)   Giving your child as much freedom as possible
           (while maintaining basic safety in those areas
           where you have control)
           to express h/is desires and passions,
           allowing h/im to exercise h/is own ability
           to make decisions,
           and accept and learn from h/is mistakes.

(5) Listening to your child with an intention
to really understand how it is for h/im in h/is world;
reflecting back what s/he said to you
so that s/he can feel that you understand h/im.

(6) Acknowledging your child regularly for the difference
s/he makes in your life,
and for what is great about h/im.

(7) Never trying to control your child's behavior
in circumstances where you have little or no control.
(By attempting to control,
you lose whatever influence you may have
and thereby show disrespect for your child and yourself.)

Some actions, almost always, clearly show disrespect.

(1) Yelling at your child,
or speaking to h/im in a tone of voice
you would not use with an adult whom you respect.

(2) Going through your child's private possessions
without h/is permission.

(3) Talking about your child in front of h/im
as if s/he were not present.

(4) Talking to another person
about your child's undesirable traits in front of h/im.

(5) Not keeping your agreements with your child.

(6) Trying to exercise control in circumstances
where you have only influence.

(7) Using disparaging names or characterizations:
lazy, stupid, insensitive, trouble-maker, rebellious, selfish,
brat, jerk, childish, irresponsible, bad, difficult.

(8) Speaking in a tone of voice that your child
experiences as condescending.

(9) Giving your child a "count down,"
instead of implementing a consequence immediately.

(10)   Administering consequences
       with a "make wrong" attitude toward your child.

(11)   Warning your child
       with condescending (and non-specific) generalizations
       such as "behave yourself," or "be a good girl"
       or "be a good boy."

A more subtle and less obvious form
       of showing disrespect for your child
       is in taking or not taking actions
       that allow your child to mistreat you,
       or to treat you unfairly.
There are many ways in which you might respond
       to disrespectful behavior from your child.
Some ways may be more respectful or powerful than others,
       depending upon you and your relationship with your child,
       and upon the circumstances.
The following are two examples
       that illustrate what I am referring to.

Your twelve-year-old son complains to you
       about how you won't give him money
       to go out with his friends.
His voice gets louder and louder
       and you begin to feel abused by his behavior.
Your tendency is to shout back, argue,
       or try to control him,
       but you know that will only exacerbate
       your current relationship issues with your son.
I suggest these possible responses to his behavior
       that would likely reduce or eliminate your feeling abused
       and stimulate different behavior in your son,
       both immediately and in the future.

(1)   Ask him to tell you *more*
            about how unfair it is for you not to give him money.
        Each time he speaks and you listen
            and you reflect back to him what you heard him say,
            you ask him to share more so you can
            fully understand how it is from his perspective.
        This does not mean you will change your mind
            and give him the money he wants.
        If you embrace his complaining instead of resisting it,
            he will probably run out of steam,
            a space will be cleared,
            and a new opening for a breakthrough
            in your relationship will be created.

(2)   Leave the room immediately without an explanation.
        Do not stay in the presence of his complaining,
            because your presence can often add fuel to the fire.

(3)   Lie down on the floor and roll over and over,
            back and forth, until your son stops complaining.
        Do this in a non-condescending way.
        Your primary intention is
            to shift your own behavior and reaction, not his.

In a second example, your daughter
    does not keep a specific, clear-cut, do-able agreement
    that she made with you.

(1)   If a consequence was attached to the agreement,
            immediately and dispassionately
            impose that consequence.
        To do otherwise is to show disrespect for your daughter
            by suggesting that she is not able to keep agreements
            and/or not able to accept the consequences
            of not keeping her agreements.

(2)   Enroll your daughter in a non-blaming,
non-controling dialogue where you explore together
the benefits and the costs associated with her
not keeping this agreement
and/or other agreements that she makes.
In addition, explore the benefits she received
from *not* keeping her agreement
(every behavior has costs *and* benefits).
and acknowledge those benefits.
Invite your daughter to become a partner with you
in discovering what will work for everybody
(her included, especially)
in the arena of making and keeping agreements.

It is important to distinguish, both for yourself
and for your child, the difference between
an *agreement* and an *imposed condition*.
In an agreement, the child has the option of making
or *not* making the agreement.
The child chooses to make the agreement
because s/he would derive certain benefits
from fulfilling the agreement
to which s/he would not otherwise be entitled.
An agreement is like a trade:
either party can choose to trade or not to trade,
and the only reason for entering into the trade
is that the value to be received
is greater than the value forfeited.
Breaking an agreement is equivalent to
not keeping the conditions of the trade.

Here is an example of an agreement you might offer your son:
"If you will baby sit your little sister tonight
from 7:00 to 10:00, then I will pay you $10.
Would that interest you?"
You son then has the option of accepting
or declining your offer.
It is important for you to be clear
that you will not impose any consequences
if he chooses not to accept your offer.
He is also free to make a counter-offer,
which you may then decline or accept.
As your child develops and matures,
it is increasingly important to provide
h/im with more options to make agreements,
with yourself and others.

In contrast, an *imposed condition*
is *not* an agreement.
You simply state to your child that if s/he takes a certain action
(or does not take a certain action),
you will impose a given consequence.
You do this without h/is consent or agreement;
the only choice your child has
is whether to choose the given behavior
or to choose the consequence.

Here's an example of an imposed condition:
"If you leave your toys in the middle of the living room
and don't put them away in your room
when you're finished playing with them,
I will put your 'Robby Robot' away
where you will be unable to play with him for one week."
Be careful to make the consequence strong enough,
but not stronger than it needs to be.

This is about consequence; it is not about punishment.

As your child develops and matures,
    look for fewer occasions to impose conditions.
However, when you do impose conditions
    and they are not met, be consistent and dispassionate
    in applying the consequences you previously specified.

The manner in which you express yourself
    and the attitude you bring to all of your interactions
    with your child is fundamental
    to h/is experience of your respect for h/im.
Always remember to combine gentleness with firmness.
Act with an intention to nurture and build your relationship.
If you find yourself reacting righteously toward your child
    (if you find yourself being a victim of your child),
    do not disrespect your child by indulging your feelings.
Address those feelings in other ways
    (e.g., see the section "Making Fear Your Friend," page 131).
Dumping them on your child is *not* a valid option.
Your child showing disrespect for you is *never*
    a justification for showing disrespect for your child!
Remember the adage:
    "Be hard on problems but soft on people."

I am deeply grateful to my mother Dorothy,
    whose example always provided me
    with the direct experience of always being treated
    with honor, respect, and profound love,
    as well as an intellectual understanding
    of the distinctions of respect,
        (especially as it applies to parent-child relationships).

Do you have a child (whatever age)?

(Hint: at a minimum, you have your "child within.")

What action might you take today to show respect for your child?

How might it be a choice of courage for you
to show respect either for your biological child
or for the "child within"?

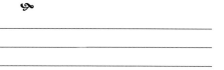

_____

_____

_____

_____

Your children are not your children. They are the sons and daughters of Life's longing for itself. They come through you but not from you. And though they are with you, yet they belong not to you. You may give them your love but not your thoughts. For they have their own thoughts. You may house their bodies but not their souls, for their souls dwell in the house of tomorrow, which you cannot visit, not even in your dreams. You may strive to be like them, but seek not to make them like you. For life goes not backward nor tarries with yesterday. You are the bows from which your children as living arrows are sent forth. The archer sees the mark upon the path of the infinite, and He bends you with His might that His arrows may go swift and far. Let your bending in the archer's hand be for gladness; For even as He loves the arrow that flies, so He loves also the bow that is stable.

—*Kahlil Gibran (1883-1931, Lebanese poet, philosopher, artist)*

Children are not things to be molded, but are people to be unfolded.   —*Jess Lair*

If there is anything we wish to change in the child, we should first examine it and see whether it is not something that could better be changed in ourselves.

—*Carl Gustav Jung (1875-1961, Swiss psychiatrist)*

This is not the only universe

We are normally present to a plus-minus universe.
We act constantly to move away from pain/discomfort (minus)
    and toward pleasure/comfort (plus).
It can be shown that even strange behaviors (e.g., masochism)
    are complex expressions of the plus-minus dynamic.
It is impossible to imagine
    how life could exist and thrive without such a dynamic.

However, for several minutes last Tuesday
    (this essay was written Sunday, May 7, 2000),
        I experienced a *totally* different universe.
If I had not experienced it personally,
    I would have argued vehemently
    that such a universe was impossible.
    I was *completely inside* a *pure-plus universe*.
Moment by moment,
    every sensation, every perception,
    every thought, every feeling
    was glorious, was perfection, was profound,
    was both fully meaningful and totally meaningless,
    was timeless, was change existing in an unchanging world,
    was fully innocent
        in that there was no possibility of anything but ecstasy.

Since then, back in my plus-minus universe,
    I have made a game (admittedly a plus-minus game)
    of noticing that I am in a plus-minus universe,
    perhaps in much the same way that a "thinking" fish,
    who first experiences what it's like *not* to be in water
        might acquire a newfound awareness of the water
            once he returns to it.

I have no complete theoretical model
    in which the plus-minus universe
    and the pure-plus universe can coexist.
I can see, nevertheless, how the plus-minus universe
    can exist inside of the pure-plus universe.
    The reverse, however, would not work.

I can also see that
    while experiencing the pure-plus universe,
    one could play the plus-minus games
    of the plus-minus universe
    with a completeness and fullness
    that's impossible to do
    when living exclusively in the plus-minus universe.

Consider that the ultimate context that supports
    the ongoing choice of courage in your life
    is the same context that allows
    for the unfolding of the pure-plus universe.

❧

_____

_____

_____

_____

_____

_____

_____

_____

> When the mind exists undisturbed in the Way nothing in the
> world can offend, and when a thing can no longer offend, it ceases
> to exist in the old Way . . . . If you wish to move in the One Way do
> not dislike even the world of senses and ideas. Indeed, to accept
> them fully is identical with true Enlightenment.
>
> —*Third Zen Patriarch*

Do you know how to live in the two worlds?

We have "arrived"
 when we are present to two worlds in the same moment.

The first world is the world of playing the game in which
 what isn't is more important than *what is*.
We want to change this. We want to change that.
 We want to arrive there. We want to leave here.
Welcome to the world and the game of change!

The second world is the world
 in which there is nothing to change,
 there is no place to get to, there is nothing to accomplish,
 there is no attachment, there is no expectation,
 there is nothing to do.
Palpably, time stands still; each moment is its own perfection,
 stretching infinitely from the past and into the future.
Welcome to the infinite glory and perfection of it all,
 world without change, cradling within its care
 the world and game of ceaseless change.
Welcome to the perfect world of no-change!

Fathom, if you will,
 the fundamental choice of courage required
 to embrace together the worlds of change and no-change,
 to embrace the world of time
  as well as the no-time world of *now*.

∾

**For more essay(s) on courage and spirituality,
 see www.GoldWinde.com/Cbook/More/Spirituality.**

Essays I could have Written

Almost every day I have the thought, "I want to write an essay on courage about this idea (or that idea)." When dealing with such an all-encompassing subject, the opportunities for further exposition are endless. I have satisfied myself (and, I hope, you also) by sharing with you briefly, below, many of the ideas for the essays that I did not write or had no room to include in this book. Use these ideas to expand your appreciation of how the choice of courage affects your life to the deepest core and from every different angle. Some of these examples will address topics of essays already included in this book. I include them here for both emphasis and completion.

Unlike the previous essays, where my intention was to create a complete and rigorous focus on a given idea, the following will only provide you with seeds for your own possible development of the idea. For those readers who especially like a sense of completion, this section may provide uneasy reading. I invite you to step into the opportunity for courage that may present to you.

These essays ideas are listed in no particular order.

✎ Courage is not blind. It is based upon an open-eyed assessment of costs and benefits, both present and future, for both the actor and those s/he cares about. It is also grounded in one's most fundamental life values and inspirations.

> They called me mad, and I called them mad, and damn them, they outvoted me.
> —*Nathaniel Lee (1653-1692, English dramatist.*
> *on being consigned to a mental institution, circa 17th c.)*

> Take calculated risks. That is quite different from being rash.
> —*Gen. George S. Patton, Jr.*

✎ Trying to always make life safer can often be the most foolhardy risk that we take.

- For some of us, the resisted fear of being blamed or made wrong is the biggest opportunity for choosing courage.
- The misuse and abuse of power is often an expression of resisted fear, for the "victims" as well as the "abuser."
- Sometimes it is a choice of courage to embrace feeling the fear associated with not following the "rule" of choosing courage about something else. One of the ways we try to make ourselves feel safer is by always following some "rule." Seeing the choice of courage as "right" or "wrong" is another example of resistance to fear.
- Perfectionism is often a byproduct of resisted fear.

> The pursuit of perfection often impedes improvement.
> —*George Will (1941-, American columnist)*

> A man would do nothing if he waited until he could do it so well that no one could find fault.
> —*John Henry Cardinal Newman (1801-1890, English catholic cardinal, theologian, catholic apologist)*

> The man who insists upon seeing with perfect clearness before he decides, never decides.
> —*Henri Frederic Amiel (1821-1881, Swiss philosopher, poet)*

- Lack of energy can be a byproduct of resisted fear.
- Stress is often a byproduct of resisted fear.
- Impatience is a result of resisted fear.
- Choose courage to make mistakes.

> The only man who never makes a mistake is the man who never does anything.
> —*Theodore Roosevelt (1858-1919, U.S. president)*

> A child becomes an adult when he realizes he has a right not only to be right but also to be wrong.
> —*Thomas Szasz (1920-, Hungarian psychiatrist)*

- Choose courage to embrace insecurity.
- Over-controlling is resisting fear and trying to create a false feeling of security.
- You have made many trades in your life in which you have selected feeling safe and comfortable in the moment instead of going for what you really wanted. Are you satisfied with the results of these trades?
- The unquestioned dogma of religion is often a resistance to fear.

> People who want to share their religious views with you almost never want you to share yours with them.
> —*Dave Barry (1947-, American humor columnist)*

> God has no religion.
> —*Mahatma Gandhi (1869-1948, Indian spiritual/political leader)*

- A major function of culture is to provide us with blinders and rules so that we can feel safe in the moment. Culture thereby provides us also the most opportunities for choosing courage in the face of this illusion of safety.

> It is curious that physical courage should be so common in the world and moral courage so rare.
> —*Mark Twain (1835-1910, American author, humorist)*

> Every society honors its live conformists and its dead troublemakers.
> —*Mignon McLaughlin (1915-, American journalist, editor, author)*

- Choose courage to consistently nurture a feeling of peacefulness.

> Courage is the price that life extracts for granting peace. The soul that knows it not, knows no release from little things.
> —*Amelia Earhart (1897-1937, American aviator)*

- Choose courage to banish boredom.

🐚 Taking life so seriously is often an expression of resisted fear. Choose courage to lighten up and be playful.

> Time spent laughing is time spent with the gods.
>
> —*Japanese proverb*

🐚 Choose courage to be lusty.

> Sex: the thing that takes up the least amount of time and causes the most amount of trouble.
>
> —*John Barrymore (1882-1942, American Shakespearean actor)*

> I regret to say that we of the F.B.I. are powerless to act in cases of oral-genital intimacy, unless it has in some way obstructed interstate commerce.
>
> —*J. Edgar Hoover (1895-1972, American director of FBI)*

> Nothing is so much to be shunned as sex relations.
>
> —*Saint Augustine (354-430)*

> Of the delights of this world man cares most for sexual intercourse, yet he has left it out of his heaven.
>
> —*Mark Twain (1835-1910, American author, humorist)*

> What most persons consider as virtue, after the age of 40 is simply a loss of energy.
>
> —*Voltaire (1694-1778, French writer)*

🐚 Crisis is an opportunity for courage.

> Out of every crisis comes the chance to be reborn.
>
> —*Nena O'Neill*

🐚 Choose courage to be alone.

Our language has wisely sensed the two sides of being alone. It has created the word "loneliness" to express the pain of being alone. And it has created the word "solitude" to express the glory of being alone.
—*Paul Tillich (1886-1965, German theologian)*

✎ Choose courage to be vigilant for miracles.

To be alive, to be able to see, to walk, to have music, paintings—it's all a miracle. I have adopted the technique of living life from miracle to miracle.
—*Arthur Rubenstein (1887-1982, musician)*

✎ Choose courage to create real security.

It takes a lot of courage to release the familiar and seemingly secure, to embrace the new. But there is more security in the adventurous and exciting, for in movement there is life, and in change there is power.
—*Alan Cohen (author)*

If a nation values anything more than freedom, it will lose its freedom; and the irony of it is that if it is comfort or money that it values more, it will lose that too.
—*W. Somerset Maugham (1874-1965, British novelist, play writer, short-story writer)*

There are risks and costs to action. But they are far less than the long-range risks of comfortable inaction.
—*John F. Kennedy (1917-1963, U.S. president)*

✎ Choose courage to be "unrealistic" or "not practical."

One of the saddest lines in the world is, "Oh come now—be realistic." The best parts of this world were not fashioned by those who were realistic. They were fashioned by those who dared to look hard at their wishes and gave them horses to ride.
—*Richard Nelson Bolles (writer, career consultant)*

🖎 Choose courage to waste. It may serve a bigger purpose by allowing some "waste." This can apply in the area of time, money, food, energy, quality, etc.

> Doing a thing well is often a waste of time.
> —*Robert Byrne (American writer)*

🖎 Choose courage to begin.

> The beginnings and endings of all human undertakings are untidy.
> —*John Galsworthy (1867-1933, author, Nobel laureate)*

🖎 Choose courage to end.

🖎 Choose courage to not use power.

> Power tends to corrupt, and absolute power corrupts absolutely.
> —*Lord John E.E. Dalberg-Acton (1834-1902, historian)*

🖎 Choose courage to decide.

> The indispensable first step to getting the things you want out of life is this: DECIDE WHAT YOU WANT.
> —*Ben Stein (1944-, American columnist, speech writer)*

🖎 Choose courage to leave it undecided.

🖎 Choose courage to reduce fear.

> All problems become smaller if you don't dodge them, but confront them.
> —*Adm. William F. Halsey (1882-1959)*

🖎 Choose courage to grasp now.

> One of the tragic things I know about human nature is that all of us tend to put off living. We are all dreaming of some magical rose garden over the horizon, instead of enjoying the roses that are blooming outside our windows today.
> —*Dale Carnegie (1888-1955, author, public speaker)*

Some men and women have the knack of being so delightfully present that time with them is worthwhile no matter what, whether or not any promises about exclusiveness have been made. There are people in whom freedom is the very essence of their appeal, and those who love them have to make the choice: Is the desire to possess, in and of itself, more worth pursuing than the relationship with that delightful person, and, if so, why? Or is that relationship, whatever it entails, the valuable thing?

—Jane Smiley (American writer)

🖎 Choose courage to risk being unpopular.

If you limit your actions in life to things that nobody can possibly find fault with, you will not do much.

—Lewis Carroll (1832-1898, British poet, writer)

I don't know the key to success, but the key to failure is trying to please everybody.

—Bill Cosby (1937-, American actor, executive producer, author)

🖎 Choose courage to be popular.
🖎 Choose courage to let go of guarantees.

Whether our love last for 3 days, three years, 25 years or until death do us part, let us learn more about opening our hearts to love.

—Susan Jeffers (in "Opening Our Hearts to Men")

🖎 Choose courage to look uncourageous.
🖎 Choose courage to create success.

Whenever you see a successful business, someone once made a courageous decision.

—Peter Drucker

🖎 Choose courage to accept and embrace the costs of your courageous choices.

All blessings are mixed blessings.

> —*John Updike (1932-,*
> *American poet, novelist, short-story writer)*

✍ Choose courage to act on your truth of today while willing for it to be the falsehood of tomorrow.

We have to live today by what truth we can get today and be ready tomorrow to call it falsehood.

> —*William James (1842-1910,*
> *American philosopher-psychologist)*

People learn something every day, and a lot of times it's that what they learned the day before was wrong.

> —*Bill Vaughan (1915-1977,*
> *American journalist, author)*

✍ Choose courage to take leisure.

The time to relax is when you don't have time for it.

> —*Sydney J. Harris (1917-1986, American journalist, author)*

He does not seem to me to be a free man who does not sometimes do nothing.

> —*Cicero (106-43B.C., Roman politician)*

If you treat every situation as a life-and-death matter, you'll die a lot of times.

> —*Dean Smith*

✍ Choose courage to declare what is enough money.
✍ Choose courage to declare what is enough (of quality, of time, of friends, or romance, etc.).
✍ Choose courage to not speak or to stop speaking.

You can suffocate a thought by expressing it with too many words.

> —*Frank A. Clark*

- Choose courage to speak.
- Choose courage to create a partnership between results and process.
- Choose courage to discover and embrace the hidden benefits of your behaviors that you don't like or that you think are "bad."
- Choose courage to discover, to look at, and to embrace the costs of those behaviors that you do like or that you think are "good."
- Discover how the feeling "I'm not good enough" is a protection against a sense of chaos in your childhood. Making your parents "right" and making yourself "wrong" would have definitely made you feel safer in that world where your parents (who were your whole world at that time) had such arbitrary power.
- What are the dangers of taking no risks and choosing no courage?

> If you risk nothing, then you risk everything.
> —*Geena Davis (1957-, American actress)*

> The ultimate result of shielding men from the effects of folly is to fill the world with fools.
> —*Herbert Spencer (1820-1903, British philosopher, sociologist)*

- Choose the courage of ignorance.

> Everybody is ignorant, only on different subjects.
> —*Will Rogers (1879-1935, American humorist, showman)*

> The trouble with most folks isn't so much their ignorance, as knowing so many things that ain't so.
> —*Josh Billings (1815-1885, American humorist, lecturer)*

- Righteousness is an expression of resisted fear.

Perhaps no phenomenon contains so much destructive feeling as "moral indignation," which permits envy or hate to be acted out under the guise of virtue.

—*Erich Fromm (1900-1980,*
German-born social scientist, philosopher)

☙ Choose courage to accept praise.

Sometimes we deny being worthy of praise, hoping to generate an argument we would be pleased to lose.

—*Cullen Hightower (1923-, American salesman, sales trainer)*

☙ Choose courage to really listen when someone is blaming you.
☙ Choose courage to hang up or leave the scene when someone is blaming you.
☙ How is attachment to the result a resisted fear?

Success is never final and failure never total. It's courage that counts.

—*Success Unlimited*

☙ How is attachment to a person a resisted fear?
☙ Choose courage to feel the fear of jealousy.

Him that I love, I wish to be free—even from me.

—*Anne Morrow Lindbergh (1906-2001,*
American writer, aviation pioneer)

No one worth possessing can be quite possessed.

—*Sara Teasdale (1884-1933, American poet)*

☙ Choose the courage to fall in love.
☙ Choose the courage to say "goodbye."
☙ Choose courage to be innocent.

Adults are obsolete children.

—*Dr. Seuss*

Life begins as a quest of the child for the man and ends as a journey by the man to rediscover the child.

—*Laurens van de Post*

> - Choose courage to not "do whatever it takes."
> - Choose courage to set a date or not.
> - Choose courage to act without full preparation.
> - Choose the courage of indecision.

Rather than risk failure, we often accept mediocrity. Human beings, in general, are addicted to premature resolution. We are unable to sustain much tension in our lives unless the ends are very clear to us or the alternatives to not going on are even worse.

—*Richard Moss*

> - Choose courage to do the important over the urgent.

Many important things that contribute to our overall objectives and give richness and meaning to life don't tend to act upon us or press us. Because they're not "urgent," they are the things that we must act upon.

—*Stephen Covey (author, lecturer, leadership mentor)*

> - All resistance to pain/fear is a resistance to now.
> - Choose courage to encourage other people to choose courage.
> - Choose courage to create confidence.
> - The same level of action gets easier as you choose courage again and again.

You gain strength, courage and confidence by every experience in which you really stop to look fear in the face. You are able to say to yourself, "I lived through this horror. I can take the next thing that comes along." You must do the thing you think you cannot do.

—*Eleanor Roosevelt (1884-1962,*
American first lady, columnist, lecturer, humanitarian)

- Choose courage to not ask for permission.

> Poor is the man whose pleasures depend on the permission of another.
> —*Madonna (1958-,*
> *American pop singer, song writer, movie actress)*

- Choose courage to ask for permission.
- When you make something wrong or you resist it, it's difficult for it to turn out well. For example, this is often true with divorce.
- Choose courage to wear a seat belt or a condom.
- Sour grapes is the resistance to the fear of feeling disappointment.
- One's essences (e.g., connection, adventure, playfulness, innocence, romance) are served and supported by specific forms (e.g., living in Shanghai, working as a life coach). The forms are always in service to the essences (or inspirations). To change the form in order to serve the essence better is often an opportunity for choosing courage, since we can easily get attached to a specific form. It is the essence that we are really committed to. If we see that another form would serve the essence better, then to remain in integrity, we must choose the new form.
- Choose courage to act "unfairly" in the service of more benefits and fewer costs.
- What if God is not siding with you against your enemies? What fear might you feel?
- Are your actions trying to justify your past? Choose courage to live from *now* and the open possibilities of your future.
- Choose courage to go your own way and not compare yourself with others.
- Choose courage to disobey the ones you love and who love you.
- Choose courage to live inside of empowering interpretations. To live inside of disempowering interpretations can often feel safer and more comfortable (in the moment).

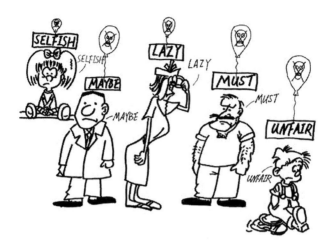

Toxic Words

What do all the following words and phrases have in common: never, because, belief, comfortable, difficult, doing your best, faith, God, hope, important, integrity, maybe, natural, necessary, optimistic, patience, perseverance, responsible, ready, somehow, strong, trust, and why?

In ways that they are often used, they have the potential to damage and/or disempower both the speaker and the listener. This toxic effect is generally neither acknowledged nor intended, but occurs at a subtle level below our conscious awareness.

I could write a chapter, if not an entire book, about each of the toxic words in this section. The purpose of this section is to give you some access, some power in protecting both yourself and the ones you love from your disempowering use of these words.

Unlike in the earlier essays of this book on toxic words, I touch only *very* briefly on each toxic word, seeking to give you some feeling for how it can be used in a way that damages the speaker and/or the listener. I even use some "toxic words" in trying to clarify other toxic words!

To change your life, change your language.

How many toxic words do you use each day?

Words form the core of our experience in the world.
    People love and kill and die for words.
    People suffer and rejoice for words.
    The quality of every moment of our lives
        is shaped by the words that filter and form
        our view of ourselves,
          of others, and of the world.
Yet very few of us realize that
    the manner in which we use language
    is often deeply flawed
    in its ability to provide us with a life we love.

Most of us just accept the everyday language that is given to us
    by our family, by our community, by our books and teachers,
        by our church and religion, by our culture.
We assume that other people
    know the meaning of the words they use,
    and we adopt their usage.
We often do this with little or no consciousness
    of the accuracy of our speaking
    and with minimal awareness the likely effect
    of our words (both on others and on ourselves).

Once we begin to appreciate
    the damage and disempowerment that results
    from the sloppy and imprecise application
    of language to our life,
        we can begin to invent and use
        much more supportive, precise, and empowering language.
Begin to question your language.

I call words that often disempower us "toxic words."
    This does not mean that you will *always*
        create damage when you use them.
    For example, "always" is in my toxic word list.
        However, in the previous sentence
        it is used in a non-toxic way.
    In contrast, if I said,
        "My friend *always* ignores my questions,"
        then that is a toxic use of the word "always."
    I call these words "toxic" so that
        you will have some awareness of the dangers
        that may be involved, both for yourself and for others,
        when you use them.
        The goal is to avoid these dangers
            by choosing different, non-toxic words
            or fully clarifying to the listener
            what you intend by your choice of words.

Words can be toxic for one or more of the following reasons.

1. Lack of context
    Consider the statement,
        "He has no *integrity*. He broke his word with me."
            Integrity is the toxic word.
    The *integrity* of someone can only be assessed within
        a larger context, the context
        of what that person is up to in h/is life.
    Many examples could be given
        in which someone is displaying a *lack of integrity*
        by *not* breaking h/is word,
        because the context (or the understanding of the context)
        changed between the time the person gave h/is word
        and the time h/is word was to be kept.

In general, a word is toxic because of lack of context
    when a benefit or cost is assumed to exist
        (by the speaker and/or listener)
    without reference to or consideration of
        the larger context of values upon which it depends.

2. **Missing qualification**

Consider the statement,
    "He's just not *committed* to me."
        Committed is the toxic word.
In this situation, the exact meaning might be,
    "He's just not committed to marrying me at this time,
        given the benefits and costs he projects
            when he considers what marriage might entail."
The commitment that exists,
    but which is not spoken or acknowledged, might be,
    "He's committed to maintaining
        a romantic and intimate relationship with me
        and he suspects that this will be damaged
        if we get married and live together."
Typically, a specific application of a word is interpreted
    to mean all possible applications of the word.
    The word loses it power of diversity
        and shuts down options and openings.

3. **Make right**

Consider the statement,
    "It's the *right* thing for you to graduate from college."
        Right is the toxic word.
To examine the situation powerfully,
    we might say instead,
    "Given what you really want in your life,
        I have reasons to believe that graduating from college
        would provide more benefits than costs.

How do you feel about sitting down together
and discussing the pros and cons?
I will support whatever choice you believe
has the most benefits and least costs for you."
In general, when a word connotes only benefits
without conveying any consideration for costs,
then it is a "make right" word.

4. **Make wrong**
Consider the statement,
"It's *wrong* for you to get divorced."
Wrong is the toxic word.
To examine the situation powerfully,
we might instead say,
"Given what you really want in your life,
I have reason to believe that, in the long run,
getting a divorce would create more costs than benefits.
How do you feel about sitting down together
and discussing the pros and cons for all involved?
I will support whatever choice you believe
has the most benefits and least costs for you."
In general, when a word connotes only costs
with no sense of possible benefits,
then it is a "make wrong" word.

5. **Hidden meaning**
Consider the statement,
"It is so *selfish* of you to watch only the TV shows you like."
Selfish is the toxic word.
What if you said, instead,
"I automatically feel hurt and disrespected
when you don't consider
my desire to watch the TV shows that I like.

Can we reach a compromise together so
we both feel respected by each other?"
In general, a word becomes toxic
due to a hidden or non-obvious intent or meaning.
If the intent or meaning is made obvious,
the word loses its toxic power.

6. Inaccurate

Consider the statement,
"You are *always* late for our appointments."
Always is the toxic word.
What if you said, instead,
"You have been more than 10 minutes late
for a majority of our appointments together.
I automatically feel hurt and disrespected
when you are late for our appointments.
I am curious about how you were able
to be on time for those times
when you were punctual with me?"
In general, a word may be used inaccurately for emphasis,
yet we rarely acknowledge (to others and/or to ourselves)
that it was used inaccurately.
The inaccuracy usually has the function of creating
a sense of safety by protecting us
from the fear associated with taking a risk.

7. Vague

Consider the statement,
"I am a *weak* person."
Weak is the toxic word.
Does *weak* mean that I don't have a lot of energy
during the average day?
Does *weak* mean I don't keep my word with others?
Does *weak* mean I don't keep my word with myself?

Does *weak* mean I don't make agreements that challenge me?
Does *weak* mean I complain when I feel pain?
Does *weak* mean I feel things very deeply
    and think I am oversensitive?
Does *weak* mean I don't stand up to bullies?
Does *weak* mean I don't put much energy
    into those things which don't interest me?
One might say with clarity,
    "I cry easily when someone is critical of me.
    When this occurs, I am embarrassed
        and I automatically criticize myself for being so sensitive."
In general, words are often vague
    when the speaker's meaning is unclear
    even though the speaker and listener may think,
    without closer examination,
    that what was said was perfectly clear.

A thorough analysis of the subject of toxic words
    could fill a set of encyclopedias.
    Please understand that my comments
        are designed to help you become vigilant about these
        and other similar words and phrases, not to be exhaustive.
These words represent
    only a very small selection of the words that can be toxic.
    And this list does not include a whole slew of "toxic phrases"
    that also are candidates for detoxification.

In addition, consider
    that the toxic impact of the *content* of words
    can pale in comparison with the power of voice delivery,
    the power of our voice image to impart toxicity.

Becoming more aware and rigorous
in choosing to detoxify our language
(as well as detoxifying our voice image)
is almost always a choice of courage
(because it means giving up
the short-term, feeling-safe benefit).
Breathe into the energy of that fear
and honor yourself for choosing this courage.

Here are some of the key words that are often used in a toxic way:

- **Afford**

"I can't *afford* to buy the book."
Does this mean,
"I have no money at all to purchase the book"?
Or does it mean,
"Because my money is limited,
I have balanced the value I would anticipate
from having the book
against the value of other things I could purchase
with the same money,
and I believe there is more value for me
in purchasing the other items instead of the book"?

- **All/always/never/every/everyone**

"*All* attempts at doing this will fail."
It might be more accurate to think and say:
"I have attempted to do this the same way five times
and five times I did not get the result I intended.
I am automatically feeling foolish
for not getting the intended results
and I want to stop feeling foolish
by not attempting this anymore."

"I *always* seem to say the wrong thing."
It might be more accurate to think and say:
    "I notice that once or twice a week
        I say something that stimulates you to be upset with me.
        I also notice that I have a desire
            to exaggerate my sense of guilt about this
        so that you might be more gentle with me."

"You *never* come home on time."
It might be more accurate to say:
    "I notice that I am trying to make you feel wrong
        because I automatically feel hurt and disrespected
        when you come home late."

"*Everyone* believes this is the right thing to do."
It might be more accurate to think and say:
    "My parents told me that everyone
        believes this is the right thing to do
        and I don't want to risk my parents' disapproval
        or the possible disapproval of others
        (even though I don't have much evidence
        of what people really believe about this)."

- **Appropriate/proper/inappropriate/improper**

"It would be *appropriate* to give your grandmother a call."
It might be more accurate to think and say:
    "I want you to give your grandmother a call
        and I will consider you a 'good' person if you call her,"
        or "If you give your grandmother a call,
        she will believe you care about her
        and she will consider you a 'good' grandson."

"Eating with your fingers is really *inappropriate*."
It might be more accurate to think and say:
>"I will be disgusted, embarrassed, and disapproving
>>if you eat with your fingers.
>I am making you wrong for eating with your fingers.
>And I will be grateful if you don't eat with your fingers."

"I really want to be a *proper* woman."
It might be more accurate to think and say:
>"The approval of others is important to me.
>I can maintain that approval
>>by always following the proper rules."

- **Arrogant**

"He's so *arrogant*. He rarely speaks to us."
It might be more accurate to think and say:
>"He has not chosen the courage to speak with us
>>and his mannerisms are a way to help him feel safer."

- **At fault/to blame**

"The man was *at fault* in breaking the law."
It might be more accurate to think and say:
>"I support the particular law that the man broke
>>and I support those who are responsible
>>for enforcing the penalty associated with breaking that law."

"I *blame* my ex-husband for the divorce."
It might be more accurate to think and say:
>"I feel like I was the victim of my ex-husband.
>I feel sorry for myself
>>and I want you and others to feel sorry for me, too.

I want you to take my side against him.
I want him to suffer for the pain he caused me.
I want him to apologize to me for what he did."

- **Because/make/made**

"I felt bad *because* you shouted at me."
"By shouting at me, you made me feel bad."
It might be more accurate to think and say:
    "Given my automatic interpretation
        of what your shouting at me means,
           my unwillingness/inability to re-interpret that meaning,
           our personal history together, my current mood,
           and the context of our current relationship,
           your shouting at me stimulated me to feel bad."

- **Believe/belief**

"Do you *believe* in family values?"
It might be more accurate to ask the following questions:
    What are "family values"
        and what does it mean to believe in them?
        Does it mean that you don't have sex before marriage?
        Does it mean that the husband earns the money
           and the wife raises the kids?
        Does it mean that every person should get married?
        Does it mean staying married when neither party is happy?
    And what does it mean to believe in these values?
        Does it mean that you choose these values for yourself?
        Does it mean that you encourage
           your loved ones to adopt these values?
        Does it mean that you think everybody
           'should' adopt these values?

- **Best/better/good/bad/right/wrong/moral/immoral**

"It would be *best* for you if you got married."

It might be more accurate to ask the following questions:

Got married to *whom* under what context, circumstances, prior agreements, and specific commitments?

Would there be an exit strategy

and clearly defined minimum conditions of satisfaction?

What results do I believe I will achieve in my life

if I choose to get married instead of remaining single?

If I decide that staying unmarried is *best* for me,

will you blame me for that?

Best according to what overall criteria

or standard of measurement?

Best as compared to what else and by what criteria?

What results did I have in mind

when the criteria or standards were designed?

Best according to

what fundamental life inspirations and passions?

Are these my fundamental life inspirations and passions?

What evidence do I have

to support your statement that it would be *best*?

"We should always do what's *right*."

It might be more accurate to think and say:

"I want to feel safe and secure (and righteous)

by always doing what people I respect

(or the church) say(s) is right."

"I know he is a *good* person."

It might be more accurate to think and say:

"By saying that he is a good person,

I can believe that I live in a safer world

and I don't need to keep my eyes open

or choose courage as frequently with him."

"He is a *bad* person."
It might be more accurate to think and say:
    "His reputed behavior scares me.
        He violates certain rules of behavior
        that most of my friends value.
        And I cannot see any valid benefits for his behavior."

- **Braggart**

"He is such a *braggart*, always telling people how great he is."
It might be more accurate to think and say:
    "I feel hurt that he doesn't listen to me
        and doesn't seem interested
        in what I have to say about my life.
    And he doesn't talk about his own life
        in a way that inspires me or interests me.
    I also feel embarrassed when I am in public with him
        because I imagine others
        are critical of him and therefore of me.
        I 'blame' him for this."

- **Busy/lazy**

"You sure keep yourself *busy* with so many things."
It might be more accurate to think and say:
    "I admire and respect you for your active energy
        and the projects you spend your time on."

"You are so *lazy*. You never help with the housework."
It might be more accurate to think and say:
    "I am angry because you don't often help me
        with the housework and I feel disrespected
        and treated unfairly by you as a result of your not helping."

- **Caring/considerate/concerned**

"If you *cared* for me, you would think to introduce me to her."
It might be more accurate to think and say:
> "I automatically feel pleasure when you remember
>> to introduce me to other people.
>
> I automatically felt hurt
>> when you didn't think to introduce me to her.
>
> I want you to reassure me that you want to give me pleasure.
>
> I want to make you feel bad by accusing you
>> of not caring for me,
>
> and I hope my speaking this way will stimulate you
>> to introduce me next time."

"He is really not *concerned* about me.
> He didn't remember my birthday."
It might be more accurate to think and say:
> "I assume that he doesn't care about me
>> because he didn't remember my birthday.
>
> I 'blame' him because I automatically felt hurt
>> when he didn't remember my birthday.
>
> I want to feel sorry for myself
>> and I want you to feel sorry for me.
>
> I want to make him feel bad for hurting me."

- **Comfortable/uncomfortable**

"I don't feel *comfortable* asking for a raise."
It might be more accurate to think and say:
> "I am frightened to ask for a raise
>> and I am unwilling to choose the courage
>> to accept the fear in asking for a raise."

- **Committed/not committed**

"John is never willing to *commit* to me."

It might be more accurate to think and say:

"I am faulting John because he is committed to not marrying me,
    even though he is committed to indefinitely maintaining
    a great romantic relationship with me."

- **Confident**

"I want to feel more *confident*."

It might be more accurate to think and say:

    "I want to be able to act with less fear."

- **Confused**

"I'm *confused* about what I want to do."

It might be more accurate to think and say:

    "Whichever way I think of going
        stimulates more fear for me than I am willing to feel."

- **Coward/wimp**

"He is such a *wimp* when it comes to his wife."

It might be more accurate to think and say:

    "His wife's behavior stimulates a fear in him which
        he is unwilling to risk escalating
        by taking more assertive action with her.

- **Deserve/worthy/unworthy**

"I don't feel like I *deserve* to get all this attention."

It might be more accurate to think and say:

    "I feel guilty for getting all this attention.
    I am frightened to get all this attention.
    I am frightened that it won't last.
    I am also frightened that others will disapprove of me
        for getting all this attention."

"I don't think I am *worthy* of his love."
It might be more accurate to think and say:
"I am frightened of seeking his love and not getting it.
I am unwilling to take the risk
of seeking his love and not getting it.
Therefore, I will feel safer for now
by thinking and feeling that I am not worthy of his love."

- **Difficult/hard/struggle/tough**

"Looking for a job is *hard*."
It might be more accurate to think and say:
"I am resisting the fear associated with taking
the actions necessary to get a job.
I am not using my creativity to make looking for a job fun."

"Life is a *struggle*."
It might be more accurate to think and say:
"Whenever and wherever there are opportunities
for choosing courage in my life,
I usually choose to feel safe in the moment."

- **Doing one's best/giving 100 percent**

"You should always do your *best*."
It might be more accurate to think and say:
"I think I will look good (to myself and others)
if I say 'you should always do your best.'
I also feel that I can control things better if I have that attitude.
However, I cannot really tell you
how I or anyone else would ever know
if we had done our best."

• **Duty/obligation**

"It is a young man's *duty* to fight for his country."
It might be more accurate to think and say:
"I will use my influence and my vote
to make sure that, by threat of incarceration,
all able-bodied young men
are required to serve in the armed forces,
even against their conscience,
while being paid less than the free market
would allow them to be paid otherwise."

"We have an *obligation* to stay married."
It might be more accurate to think and say:
"It frightens me to know
that my spouse has the option to choose divorce
for no other reason than
preserving h/is own happiness."

• **Ego/egoist/self-centered**

"His *ego* is bigger than this house."
It might be more accurate to think and say:
"I don't feel connected with him when he talks.
I 'blame' him because he doesn't give me
and others the attention and focus
that I want and I think others want.
I am unwilling to choose the courage
to speak with him about this.
I prefer to 'blame' him."

• **Excuse**

"She's just making *excuses*."

It might be more accurate to think and say:

"I 'blame' her for not taking the action and for giving reasons
   that she thinks justify not taking the action.
   I don't think her reasons
      are the real reasons she did not take the action
      and I am uninterested in discovering the real reasons.
   I am unwilling to sympathize with her reasons."

• **Failure/success**

"I'm a *failure* in my marriage."

It might be more accurate to think and say:

   "I blame myself because my marriage turned out
      differently than I intended and promised.
      By blaming myself, I avoid looking at the fear
         I have to face to either create my marriage
         the way I want it to be or to get out of my marriage.
      I am not acknowledging any good parts
         of my relationship with my spouse.
      I am not acknowledging everything
         I have learned in this marriage.
      I am resisting the pain of loss in my marriage."

• **Fair/unfair/just/unjust**

"It's *not fair* that my wife has a lover."

It might be more accurate to think and say:

   "I blame my wife for having a lover.
   I feel automatically hurt, angry, and disrespected
      that my wife has a lover.
   Her affair stimulates my fear that I'm not important to her
      and my fear of what might happen to our marriage.

Her affair also stimulates my fear of what I think of myself.
I want to force my wife to give up her lover
    and apologize to me."

"It's very *unfair* of you to take a vacation by yourself."
It might be more accurate to think and say:
    "Because of the way I automatically interpret it,
        I feel hurt that you are going on a vacation by yourself.
    Because I am your wife,
        and because I have done so many things for you,
        I believe you owe it to me to take me with you."

- **Faith**

"We have *faith* that the Bible/Koran/etc. is the word of God."
It might be more accurate to think and say:
    "If we believe that the Bible/Koran/etc. is the word of God,
        then we will feel reassured that following His word
        will provide us with the safety and rewards
        only available from a being as powerful as God.
    We can also avoid the fear we might feel
        if we explored outside the boundaries of His word."

- **Fear (instead of resisted fear)**

"I was stopped by my *fear*."
It might be more accurate to think and say:
    "I am using my energy to resist my fear.
    I really don't want to feel my fear.
    I want to feel safe in the moment instead.
    Therefore, to feel safe in the moment,
        I chose not to take the action
        and I lied to myself that I made that choice
        of feeling safe over taking the action
        by saying that 'I was stopped by my fear'."

- **Force/no choice**

"My teacher *forced* me to re-take the exam."

It might be more accurate to think and say:

"My teacher told me she would fail me
     if I did not re-take the exam.
I chose to re-take the exam to avoid failing the class."

"I had *no choice* but to sell the house."

It might be more accurate to think and say:

"Of all the options I considered,
     selling the house seemed to be the least painful one."

- **Forgiving/not forgiving**

"I should *forgive* him."

It might be more accurate to think and say:

"I am blaming myself for continuing to blame him.
Forgiving him seems to include
     putting myself in harm's way again
     and I am frightened and unwilling to do that."

"Every time I *forgive* him, he just does it again."

It might be more accurate to think and say:

"I think he will change his behavior if I forgive him
     and then I can avoid choosing courage
     to create necessary boundaries with him."

- **Giver/taker**

"She's a *giver*, not a *taker*."

It might be more powerful to ask the following questions:

Does she take pleasure in giving?
Does she take care of herself by giving?
When she gives to others, does that empower them
     or does it encourage a disempowering dependence?

Is she a 'better' person because she is a giver?

Does she give to others by receiving their gratitude
and letting it touch her?

Is taking care of one's own needs and desires 'wrong'?

If everybody was a giver and there were no takers,
who would the givers give to?

- **Goal/deadline**

"We must do what it takes to reach our *goal*."

It might be more powerful to ask the following questions:

Is the process of reaching the goal worthwhile
in and of itself?

Is the benefit/cost ratio of reaching the goal favorable?

What is the bigger purpose that the goal serves?

Have circumstances changed so that the goal
holds a different value than when it was originally set?

What will be the costs if we don't reach the goal?

What are the alternative ways to achieve similar results
without the associated costs?

- **God/Allah/Satan/the devil**

"*God* wants us to please Her by following Her laws."

It might be more powerful to ask the following questions:

How do we know that God has desires?

What evidence (not faith) do we have
that She might *not* have desires?

How do we know that pleasure is an issue for Her?

How do we know *Her* laws?

What evidence might we discover
that the laws are not Her laws?

For what higher purposes
did God propose these laws for us
(other than to please Her)?

In what contexts would following a given law
    provide more benefits than costs?
In what contexts would following a given law
    provide more costs than benefits?
If the full expression of my life is my highest value,
    does following this law (within a stipulated context)
    provide me with more benefits than costs?
Wouldn't She want me to have more benefits than costs?

"She is influenced by the *devil*."
These questions are usually ignored or dismissed:
    What evidence do I have that the devil exists?
        What benefit do I derive by believing in a devil?
        How does it help me feel safer?
    What benefits is she trying to gain for herself
        by taking actions I disapprove of?
    What evidence could I provide in order
        to support my statement
        that she is influenced by the devil?

- **God's will/fate/destiny**

"I think it's just my *destiny* to never find someone
    who really loves me."
It might be more accurate to think and say:
    "I am very resigned about not having found
        someone to really love me.
    I am unwilling to choose courage and risk rejection
        any more than I already have.
    I am unwilling to look at what I might be doing or not doing
        that prevents me from getting what I want.
    I want to give up and just call it 'destiny'."

- **Good enough/not good enough**

"Maybe I am *not good enough* to do the job?"

It might be more accurate to think and say:

"I am frightened that others might think
   that I didn't do a good job.
I am unwilling to feel that fear by taking on the job."

- **Greed**

"I don't like *greedy* people."

It might be more accurate to think and say:

"When someone else asks for what s/he wants,
   I don't want to face my fear by saying 'no' to h/im.
And when others don't say 'no' to this person
   I feel sorry for them and want to rescue them.
This person is asking for more than s/he needs.
   S/he is getting more than others and that is 'unfair'."

- **Have a right to/don't have a right to**

"I *have a right* to sex with my wife."

It might be more accurate to think and say:

"I don't want to feel the fear
   associated with my wife saying 'no' to me.
I don't want to feel powerless when my wife says 'no' to me.
I don't want to feel the frustration I will feel
   if I can't have sex with my wife when I want.
I don't want to feel cheated in my marriage.
I will try to control the circumstances by 'blaming' her
   if she doesn't want to have sex with me."

"I *don't have a right* to have more than one boyfriend."

It might be more accurate to think and say:

"I am resisting my fear that others will blame me
    if I have more than one boyfriend.
    I am resisting my fear that,
        if I have more than one boyfriend,
        my boyfriends will get angry at me or leave me.
    I am resisting my fear that my friends will be jealous of me
        if I have more than one boyfriend.
    I am resisting my fear that people will think
        I am a slut if I have more than one boyfriend."

- **Have to/must/must not**

"I *must* get this all done today."
It might be more accurate to think and say:
"I want to avoid the consequences
    that I anticipate if I don't get all this done today.
    I don't want to choose the creativity and courage
        necessary to lessen or eliminate those projected consequences
        if I am not able to get everything done today."

"I *must not* think of him."
It might be more accurate to think and say:
    "I want to avoid
        what I will feel and/or do if I think of him."

- **Have courage (instead of choose courage)**

"I didn't *have the courage* to say it."
It might be more accurate to think and say:
    "I chose to feel safe in the moment and believed that you
        would think badly of me for *choosing* to feel safe.
    Therefore, I will imply
        that I did not have the choice
        by saying, 'I did not have courage'."

- **Honest/dishonest**

"I hate it when someone is dishonest with me."
It might be more accurate to think and say:
    "I think dishonesty is 'bad.'
    I feel frightened and out of control
        if I find out someone has lied to me
        or might have a pattern of lying.
    If someone lies to me,
        I am the victim and s/he is the 'bad' guy.
    I have no interest or curiosity
        in discovering how that person was trying
        to take care of h/imself by lying
        and what I may have done to stimulate h/im
        to feel so unsafe that s/he wanted to lie to me."

- **Hope/hopeless**

"I *hope* that my boss will give me a raise."
It might be more accurate to think and say:
    "I intend to get a raise
        but I am unwilling to choose the courage
        to improve my work and/or ask for a raise
        in order to encourage my boss to give me a raise.
    By 'hoping,' I will avoid the fear that I will probably not
        get a raise given my current behavior."

"We must always have *hope*
    that things will improve for our sick son."
It might be more accurate to think and say:
    "To accept the possibility/probability that things
        will not improve for our sick son
        is more fear than I am willing to face."

"Our situation is *hopeless.*"
It might be more accurate to think and say:
"I don't want to face the fear of risk associated
with maintaining a commitment
to either improve our situation
or to choose another course of action.
By saying it is hopeless, I can relax and accept my 'fate'."

It also might be more accurate to think and say:
"I am unwilling to fully accept things as they are.
Our situation 'shouldn't' be the way it is.
I feel safer by calling it 'hopeless'."

- **Important/unimportant**

"Getting a good education is *important.*"
It might be more powerful to ask the following questions:
Important for whom?
Important in order to get what results?
Are these results desired by the person
who will receive the good education?
What evidence supports the claim
that a good education will achieve these results?
What constitutes a good education?
How does this differ from a poor education?
Are there better or easier ways to get the results
without the costs associated with getting a good education?

- **Independent/dependent**

"It's important to be *independent.*"
It might be more powerful to ask the following questions:
Independent from what and from whom?
Independent in what circumstances?
What is the evidence of "being independent"?

For specific instances of independence,
>   what are the short—and long-term benefits and costs?
What fears might be associated
>   with "depending upon another?"

- **Integrity/keeping your word**

"I think it would compromise your *integrity* if you quit school."
It might be more accurate to think and say:
>   "You said you were going to finish school.
>   You are breaking your word if you quit.
>   Integrity is about keeping your word
>>   and fulfilling your obligations to others.
>   It has nothing to do with
>>   listening to other important parts of yourself
>>   that may be encouraging you to quit school."

- **Jealous**

"You make me feel *jealous* when you talk with other men."
It might be more accurate to think and say:
>   "When you talk with certain other men,
>>   it automatically stimulates my fear of losing you.
>   I want to prevent you from stimulating my fear of losing you."

- **Justify/justification**

"There is no *justification* for your behavior."
It might be more powerful to ask the following questions:
>   What are the criteria upon which justification is based?
>   Do all parties involved agree upon these criteria?
>   Do these criteria take into account
>>   the potential short—and long-term benefits
>>   and costs for everyone affected by the behavior?
>   Is the speaker interested in discovering the benefits
>>   that the actor may have derived from h/is behavior?

- **Lazy/hard working**

"You are very *lazy* when it comes to doing the dishes."
It might be more accurate to think and say:
> "You derive no personal value from doing the dishes
>> and, by calling you lazy,
>> I want to make you feel bad enough
>> so that you'll do the dishes."

"John is such a *hard worker*."
It might be more accurate to think and say:
> "John places his work above many other things in his life
>> and I like that I can rely on him for that."

- **Listen to (meaning "obey")**

"My husband doesn't listen to me
> when I ask for more time with him."
It might be more accurate to think and say:
> "My husband doesn't grant my request
>> when I ask him to spend more time with me."

- **Love/unconditional love/true love**

"If you *loved* me, you would buy gifts for me."
It might be more accurate to think and say:
> "I feel loved when you buy gifts for me.
> I automatically interpret your buying gifts for me
>> as evidence that you love me.
> I automatically interpret your not buying gifts for me
>> as evidence that you don't love me."

"If I *loved* my 23-year-old son,
> I would pay for his traffic tickets."

It might be more accurate to think and say:
  "I don't want my son or other people
    to think or say that I don't love him
    if I don't pay for his traffic tickets."

"I am waiting for *true love*."
It might be more accurate to think and say:
  "I am waiting for that person who will love me forever
    and I will somehow know that our love will never die.
  I am unwilling to face the fear
    of knowing that I cannot guarantee and cannot know
    if I will love anyone forever
      or that s/he will love me forever."

- **Loyal/disloyal**

"She was *disloyal* to her husband when she had an affair."
It might be more accurate to think and say:
  "She had an agreement with her husband
    not to have sex with other men.
  She broke that agreement
    (without letting him know or without his approval).
  I disapprove of her breaking that agreement."

- **Manipulate/manipulation**

"The media just *manipulate* people."
It might be more accurate to think and say:
  "People are influenced by the media in ways
    they are not aware of and which do damage to them.
  I also want to influence people by telling them that they
    are being manipulated;
  I think this influence will be good for them."

- **Maybe/perhaps**

"*Maybe* I will be able to make the telephone call."
It might be more accurate to think and say:

> "I know I can make the call
> > and I probably won't choose to make the call.
> > But I want to shield myself
> > from the possible disapproval that I might receive
> > if I told you I will probably choose not to make the call."

- **Money**

"They just want to make *money*,"
It might be more accurate to think and say:

> "I am frightened of feeling cheated if I buy their product.
> Without further examining the possible value
> > I might receive from their product,
> > I feel safer by implying that they want to make money
> > without providing any real value in exchange."

- **Natural/unnatural**

"If it's *not natural*, I won't put it in my mouth."
It might be more accurate to think and say:

> "I am unwilling to consider the possible benefits and costs
> > that may be associated with ingesting something
> > that is unnatural or artificial."

"Oral sex seems so unnatural."
It might be more accurate to think and say:

> "I am unaccustomed to thinking and feeling
> > that I could enjoy oral sex."

- **Necessary/not necessary/need**

"It's *not necessary* for you to buy that CD."

It might be more accurate to think and say:

"Given my desires and value structures,
I would choose to keep the money
instead of buying the CD.

I feel anxious watching you spend your money
on that CD and I want to influence your actions
by telling you it is 'not necessary'."

"I *need* to be able to work faster."

It might be more accurate to think and say:

"If I am not able to work faster,
there will be consequences I am frightened of facing."

- **Not enough time**

"I don't have *enough time* to do what I want to do."

It might be more accurate to think and say:

"Given all the other choices that I make,
to do what I want to do
or to avoid things I don't want to happen,
I currently see no options
to include more things that I want to do."

- **Optimism/pessimism**

"He's so *optimistic*."

It might be more powerful to ask the following questions:

Is he aware of the risks involved in taking
any particular action that he is optimistic about?

Is he denying or suppressing
his automatic feelings of hurt or fear?

Can he feel empathy for those who are in touch with
their feelings of hurt or fear?

"She's so *pessimistic*."
It might be more powerful to ask the following questions:
> How is she trying to feel safe by projecting the worst?
> What courage might she choose
>> to embrace her fear instead of resisting it?

- **Overcome**

"We must *overcome* anything that gets in our way."
It might be more accurate to think and say:
> "We will use resistance and force
>> to subdue anything that obstructs our path.
> We will not consider the possibility
>> of forming a partnership with that which appears to resist us.
> We will not examine closely the costs likely to be incurred
>> by using resistance and force."

- **Overwhelmed**

"I am so *overwhelmed*."
It might be more accurate to think and say:
> "I currently don't see a way
>> to finish everything that I said I would finish.
> And I am resisting the automatic fear
>> associated with leaving some things unfinished."

- **Patient/impatient**

"He wasn't *patient* enough to finish college."
It might be more accurate to think and say:
> "He didn't see the value, or wasn't in touch with the value,
>> of finishing college.
> The costs of finishing college seemed larger to him
>> than the benefits.
> He was not enjoying the process of going to college."

- **Permission**

"May I have *permission* to touch your hand?"

It might be more accurate to think and say:

"If I touch your hand without asking your permission,

I risk your possible disapproval or rejection.

To avoid that fear, I will ask your permission first."

- **Perseverance**

"She keeps trying no matter what. I admire her *perseverance*."

It might be more powerful to ask the following questions:

Has she carefully assessed the costs and benefits

of all the options before her, including the option to quit?

Does she keep trying even when it's obvious

that the costs outweigh the benefits?

Is she resisting a fear that she would have to face

if she decided to cancel her original commitment?

- **Polite/impolite/rude**

"She was so *rude* and *impolite*.

She told me she didn't want to see me again."

It might be more accurate to think and say:

"I automatically felt hurt and humiliated

when she said she didn't want to see me again.

I want to hurt her feelings; I want to control her.

I want to get sympathy from others

by calling her rude and impolite."

- **Politics**

"They are just playing *politics*."

It might be more accurate to think and say:

"In making their decisions,

they are responding to costs and benefits

other than the ones that I think are legitimate."

- **Practical/impractical**

"I'm a *practical* woman when it comes to marriage."
It might be more accurate to think and say:
    "I believe that wealth and the ability to make a good living
        are the most important factors in choosing a husband."

"To major in acting is very *impractical*."
It might be more accurate to think and say:
    "Actors often have to choose a lot of courage and creativity
        to find work that pays well. And still it's a risk."

- **Pressure**

"My parents *pressured* me into taking piano lessons."
It might be more accurate to think and say:
    "I chose to avoid my parents' potential anger
        by agreeing to take piano lessons."

- **Procrastinate**

"It's so terrible that I *procrastinate* on things."
It might be more accurate to think and say:
    "I feel safer and avoid discomfort in the moment
        by delaying things.
    Now I feel safer in the moment
        by beating myself up about doing that."

- **Promiscuous**

"It really says something about her character
    that she is so *promiscuous*."
It might be more accurate to think and say:
    "I feel very uncomfortable with a woman
        expressing her sexuality with many men,
        especially in the open way that she does.
    Something about her behavior scares me.

So I feel safer if I insult her
by saying she has bad character and that she is promiscuous."

•   **Racism/prejudice**
"He's a *racist*."
It might be more accurate to think and say:
"Some of his words and/or actions
about certain people seem to be influenced
by ethnic differences.
I disapprove of certain types of words and/or actions
based upon such differences
and I want others to join me in my disapproval."

•   **Ready/not ready/don't feel ready**
"I'm *not ready* to look for a new job just yet."
It might be more accurate to think and say:
"I am frightened to look for a job now.
I'm hoping that I will have less fear later.
I am waiting for that moment to arrive."

"I *don't feel ready* to start my own business."
It might be more accurate to think and say:
"I don't want to feel the fear I would anticipate feeling
if I started my own business.
I am unwilling to take that risk."

•   **Rejection**
"I can't stand *rejection*."
It might be more accurate to think and say:
"When someone says 'no' to me,
I automatically interpret it to mean something 'bad'
about me and I am unwilling to feel the fear and pain
associated with this automatic interpretation."

- **Respectful/disrespectful**

"When you disobey me, it is so *disrespectful*."
It might be more accurate to think and say:
> "I automatically feel disrespected when you don't do as I ask."

- **Responsible/irresponsible**

"Johnny, be *responsible* and do your homework."
It might be more accurate to think and say:
> "Johnny, I will be pleased if you obey my order
> to do your homework."

- **Right choice/wrong choice**

"I don't know which is the *right choice*."
It might be more accurate to think and say:
> "Every option that I consider seems risky and scary to me.
> I want to feel safe and secure.
> I imagine there is a choice that will make me feel this way,
>> but I do not know what it is."

- **Selfish/unselfish**

"It was so *selfish* of him to do what he wanted."
It might be more accurate to think and say:
> "He didn't seem to consider
>> the selfish interests of the other people
>> around him when he did what he did."

- **Sensitive/insensitive**

"He's so *insensitive* to my feelings.
> It proves he doesn't care about me."
It might be more accurate to think and say:
> "I felt automatically hurt
>> when he did not notice I was sad.
> I want to protect myself from my own hurt by 'blaming' him."

- **Sexist**

"I felt very offended by his *sexist* remark."

It might be more accurate to think and say:

"I automatically interpreted his remark
as disrespectful to women
because he often generalizes about women
in a way that seems to limit their self-expression.
I also dislike his focus on women
as the objects of men's sexual desires."

- **Should/shouldn't/ought/supposed to**

"You *shouldn't* get involved with that."

It might be more accurate to think and say:

"Given your deepest desires and commitments,
I believe the costs outweigh the benefits
for you to get involved with that."

"I *should* be a better person."

It might be more accurate to think and say:

"If I choose courage more often, I will feel better about myself.
Therefore, I will choose courage more often."

"I *shouldn't* feel the way that I do."

It might be more accurate to think and say:

"I am frightened that others will disapprove of the way I feel.
By disapproving of my feelings first,
I will beat them to the punch
and thereby feel more in control;
I will feel safer and more secure."

• **Sin**

"It's a *sin* if you commit adultery."

It might be more accurate to think and say:

"I will condemn you if you commit adultery.

I accept as a fatebelief that the Bible is the word of God.

The Bible says that committing adultery is a sin.

Therefore, God will also condemn you if you do that.

And neither She nor I will allow any contextual exceptions

or considerations of the costs and benefits

involved in any particular act or acts of adultery."

• **Someday/sometime/somehow**

"We should get together *sometime*."

It might be more accurate to think and say:

"I have some desire to get together with you.

I also want you to think well of me

for suggesting that we get together,

even though I am not likely to take

any further action to make it happen.

I am unwilling to feel my fear of setting a time right now."

"*Somehow* I will find the time to do this later."

It might be more accurate to think and say:

"I have an intention to make time for this.

However, I am not willing to take time now

to schedule the time for handling this.

I am also unwilling to put any other structure

in place right now that will increase my chances

of finding time for it later.

Knowing myself, it is very likely

that I will forget about this intention

until and unless I am reminded

that I didn't find the time for it."

- **Strong/weak**

"I'm a *strong* person.
   I can push myself to always keep going."
It might be more accurate to think and say:
   "I find myself less sensitive to some of my own feelings
      than others are of their own feelings
      and/or I have the ability to ignore or suppress
      feelings that others do not or will not
      so that I can keep myself in action when others will stop."

It might also be more accurate to think and say:
   "I have the skill to stay in touch
      with the value of what I am doing more than others do."

"I'm *weak*. I seem to keep changing my mind
   and I can't stick with things that are important."
It might be more accurate to think and say:
   "The parts of me that are trying to do good things for me
      haven't figured out a way to get along together
      so that all parts of me can win."

It might also be more accurate to think and say:
   "I haven't yet developed the skills and habits
      to stay in touch with the value
      of what I consider to be important."

- **Stubborn**

"She'll never budge from her position,
   no matter what. She's *stubborn*."
It might be more accurate to think and say:
   "I have not been able to help her see
      how a different position could benefit her more.
   Maintaining her position helps her feel safe."

- **Stupid**

"That's a very *stupid* thing that you did."

It might be more accurate to think and say:

"I think you made a big mistake
that, to me, seems easy to avoid.
I don't know the factors
that contributed to the mistake,
but I want you to feel bad about yourself
for making the mistake so that you won't make it again."

- **Tolerate/tolerant**

"You must be *tolerant* of your husband's behavior."

It might be more accurate to think and say:

"It is inconsiderate of you to insist upon
minimum conditions of satisfaction
in your relationship with your husband.
Being married means that you cannot establish
boundaries with your husband."

- **Trust/betrayal**

"I just don't feel like I can *trust* my husband anymore."

It might be more accurate to think and say:

"I trust that my husband will act in the future
as he has acted in the past.
And I'm unwilling to face my fear
if I admit that I trust him to continue
his behaviors that I don't like."

- **Try**

"I'll *try* to give him a call."

It might be more accurate to think and say:

"I know that it is within my control to give him a call,
but I want to avoid the fear
of saying I will definitely call him and following through with it.
I also don't want to face my fear
of telling you that I will not call him."

- **Waste/wasteful**

"Don't *waste* your time watching TV, Johnny!"

It might be more accurate to think and say:

 "I disapprove of you watching TV.

 I think the value of doing something else (e.g., studying)
  is greater than the value of pleasure (or whatever else)
  you get from watching TV.

 I want to stop you from watching TV
  by making you feel bad about watching TV
  and by frightening you with my disapproval.

 I am a better judge of what is valuable for you than you are."

"It's *wasteful* of you to throw those clothes away."

It might be more accurate to think and say:

"Without considering the value of your time
 in comparison to the value of your money,
 without considering the value of
 the freed up space in your closet and in your mind,
 I believe the cost of throwing those clothes away
  is more than the benefit you would derive
  if you kept the clothes or took the time
  to give them to someone who needed them."

- **Why/why not**

"Why did you miss class today?"

It might be more accurate to think and say:

 "I am critical of you for missing class
  and I want you to apologize
  and assure me that you will not miss class again."

"Why do you want to hold my hand?"

Does it mean,

 "What feeling do you anticipate having if you held my hand?"
 "What response do you want from me in holding my hand?"
 "What do you want to express by holding my hand?"
 "What sexual motivations do you have in holding my hand?"

"What evolutionary forces explain why you want to
     hold my hand?"
"What immediate environmental factors contribute to
     your desire to hold my hand?"
"What actions do you want to stimulate by holding my hand?"
"Why do you want to hold my hand instead of her hand?"
"Why do you want to hold my hand now?"
"Why didn't you want to hold my hand yesterday?"
"Do you promise to want to hold my hand tomorrow?"
and so on.

∽

_____

_____

_____

_____

_____

_____

_____

_____

_____

_____

_____

Words can sometimes, in moments of grace, attain the quality of
deeds.

—*Elie Wiesel (1928-, author, activist)*

A different language is a different vision of life.
—*Federico Fellini (1920-, Italian film-maker)*

Learn a new language and get a new soul.

—*Czech proverb*

A year in my life

I have never wanted to be anyone else. My life is the best life I know of. I am certain others may be happier, others may be richer, others may have reached enlightenment, others may be healthier, others may have had more advantages than I, but no one has a more fascinating and adventurous life (at least for me) than I do! And many of my friends seem to agree with me on this point.

Over the course of every two to three weeks, I write an eight-page, 6,500-word journal of my life experiences and thoughts. I share it with over 60 of my friends and family members in China, Japan, Europe, Australia, and the U.S. In this section, using my journals as the source material, I open up my personal life to you. I take you from a few months before my move from California to Tokyo (when I was visiting Tokyo and made the decision to move there) and bring you up through the time when I decided to move from Tokyo to Shanghai. My friend and colleague, writer par excellence Trish Coffey, has extracted and rewritten the essential 25% of my journal entries from this time period. Because both my life and this book are about the choice of courage, we have selected mostly those portions of the journals that share about my own journey along the path of courage. Some other parts of the journals are included because we felt they were otherwise especially interesting or because they are important to the continuity of the story line.

Two technical notes: (1) When the full time and date are given, as in "10:02 p.m., Thursday, April 29, 1999," it indicates the time that I was sitting down to write in my journal. Whereas, when the time appears without a date, as in "6:03 p.m.," it indicates the time of the event I am describing. (2) A few names have been changed to protect privacy.

I have chosen a considerable level of courage to open up my private and sometimes intimate life so publicly to you. I invite you to participate with me in that courage with your generous and curious listening.

Please join me on my adventure now . . . .

Visiting Japan

5:30 p.m., Wednesday, April 28, 1999

Taken aback—delightfully. Through Angelina (the Chinese founder and owner of *East West Social,* an Asian dating agency here in the Los Angeles area), I had perused 50+ profiles and pictures and found 16 of interest. Sabrina (33, a Chinese lady who had lived in the U.S. for five years) accepted my request to call. I called her, but didn't expect to catch her in. I'd just planned to leave the message that I'd call her again when I return from Japan.

"Hello," she said.

"I'm leaving for a visit to Japan tomorrow. So I called to tell you I'll call again when I get back."

"May I come with you?" she asked.

"No!" I laughed, amused at my feeling flustered in the face of this audacious stranger.

We talked some. Her lighthearted, open, and friendly manner intrigued, perplexed, and amazed me. This woman seemed fearless!

"Suppose we set a date for when I return from Japan?" I proposed.

"I don't want to wait thaaat long," she stretched it out. "Can't I see you tonight?"

"I'd love to, but I have too much packing to do," I laughed.

"Let me meet you at the airport and see you off," she suggested.

"Splendid idea," I agreed.

2:35 p.m., Thursday, April 29, 1999

Liking at first sight. I just settled into my seat on this wide-body jet.

Flashback: Sabrina found me (in my blue-and-white-striped shirt) within ten minutes of my stepping into the sluggish serpentine check-in line. We extended our knowledge of each other as we progressed, and after check-in, moved to the food lounge for more conversation. It was not "love at first sight," but it was "liking at first sight." We both took risks with uncommon candor. It was fun!

"I look forward to our first date Sunday, May 16th," I said, grinning.

"Yes," she said simply, with a full body hop for emphasis.

Wow, and she lives in Manhattan Beach, just a mile from my apartment!

Let me off in Tokyo, okay? Just a step inside the passenger door, I've been assigned a window seat on this 400-plus-seat Thai Airways jet, final destination Bangkok. A steward told me they are 100 passengers short—so I can move around after takeoff.

Does your king love you? Announcements are in English, Japanese, and Thai. A Thai woman of 60+ sat to my right (she has three children ages 32, 30, and 28).

"What do you like most about Thailand?" I asked.

"I love my king very much and he loves his people very much," she replied.

I found this response most curious.

Thai women as compared to Japanese women. I've met enough native Thai women to get a feeling for their distinctive physical and cultural motif. But I'm at a loss as to how to describe it clearly. Japanese women have an allure, both physically and in the expression of a unique innocence (like a young child in a good way), that is not so evident in Thai women. Because of this captivating allure, my affinity for Japanese women is extraordinary.

"You are attracted to innocence because you exude a certain innocence yourself," Hitomi, my last Japanese girlfriend, once commented.

But when I try to further distinguish my own "innocence" or the "innocence" of Japanese women, I feel at a loss.

10:02 p.m., Thursday, April 29, 1999

My four any's. I've challenged myself to choose the courage and develop the skills to be able to talk with anybody, anywhere, anytime, about anything: My four any's. So I walked around the economy section of this jet and looked for an easy conversation to start. There were no "easy" openings. This last time around I "forced" myself to speak with a woman who had no headphones on. She was Thai. After a few words, she provided no feedback that invited further conversation. I gave myself credit for the attempt and felt content. Next time around the plane I will choose another person to speak with.

Better than average dancer? Just a week ago Joanna (my good friend visiting from Phoenix) and I went dancing at Alpine Village in Torrance. What spontaneous fun that was! The previous Saturday night I danced with Ella (my best friend in California, a veterinarian who practices alternative medicine for animals) at our Wisdom Course get-together (having fun is a mandatory part of the Wisdom Course, part of the Landmark Education curriculum). I used the two experiences to initiate a breakthrough in dance as a form of self-expression for me. In the past I've let fear of judgment that I'm inept and/or show-offish squelch really letting myself go. Those fears were still with me both Saturday and Wednesday nights, but I embraced them. Being with women I felt quite comfortable around made it a lot easier.

"You're a much better than average dancer," Joanna said. True or not, this simple comment solidified my intent to create more opportunities to dance.

My any's again. 10:40 p.m. An American man, probably in his late 50s, caught my interest this time around the plane. He's on his way to Thailand with the Christian Missionary Alliance. His "relationship with Christ" emerged at ten years old. We had a very enjoyable conversation until I was embarrassed to realize I'd been blocking some other passengers' view of the movie screen showing *Stepmom* with Julia Roberts and Susan Sarandon.

10:55 p.m. I just completed a seven-minute conversation with an Indian businessman who buys and sells property in India. He's returning from a visit to the U.S.

Go to Japan for only double the cost of calling! The one-way fare for this trip was $230. At 6000 miles, that's less than four cents per mile! At ten miles per minute, that's forty cents per minute and approximately twice what I pay per minute to telephone Japan from California. If I could drive my 1972 Oldsmobile to Japan, at $1.50 per gallon at fifteen mpg, the gas would cost me ten cents a mile, over twice as much per mile. And, at 60 mph, ten hours driving per day, it would take me ten days. I think I'll fly!

Climbing to the second floor. Upstairs in business class I visited a woman to whom I'd given the Servas telephone number while we waited in the boarding line. I found her absorbed in her book about Thailand, where she will vacation for the next two weeks. We talked about the Landmark Forum and I suggested that she check it out when she gets back to LA. (See the description of both Servas and the Forum in the Recommendations section at the front of this book.)

6:56 p.m., Friday, April 30, 1999 (Tokyo)

Zip! Zip! Zip! At Narita airport I breezed through baggage, customs, getting directions, and changing $200 into yen. The express train took me to Shinagawa Station, where I switched to the local line to Omori Station and then walked ten minutes to Iwai-san's home ("san" is an honorific that is almost always suffixed to a person's name when addressing or referring to them). The stay here will cost 1450 yen per night (about $12).

5:25 a.m., Saturday, May 01, 1999

A futon for my weary bones. As of last night at 11:00 I had been awake for over 24 hours, with only a few short naps. I felt my body sagging. I took some melatonin, and that, combined with my need for sleep, knocked me out quickly.

The sun was in full splendor when I awoke around 5:00 a.m. Four young Japanese men lay asleep on their futons in this large upstairs room. I've come and gone several times (ate a Promax bar, brushed my hair, found and put my socks on) without awakening them. I cannot say the same for them, as they arrived at several ungodly hours of the morning (I think from Osaka). I awoke to lights and chatter several times. I think they are in the IFLP (Introduction to the Forum Leader's Program) for Landmark. Breakfast will be served at 7:30. Last night, Iwai-san (I don't know her first name yet) invited me to attend her Seventh Day Adventist church services at 9 a.m. this morning. I accepted. What kind of adventure will that be?!

I paid Iwai-san 12,000 yen (about $100) for the six nights. The money she charges probably just meets her daily expenses. In addition to breakfast, she provides clean sheets and bedding, clean towels, etc. This is definitely a labor of love for her. She did the Forum eight years ago.

The Tokyo people are glad I am here. A few Japanese friends in America warned me that I would not experience the open friendliness from the Japanese people in Tokyo that I relished on my previous trips to other cities (namely, Sapporo, Kutchan, Yokohama, Yamato, Fujisawa, Chofu, Hakusan, Yokkaichi, Obama, Kyoto, Osaka, Kusatsu, Hiroshima, Kure, Yanai, Kitakyushu, Oita, Taketa, Nagasaki, Sasebo, and Tadotsu). So far their assertions have proved false. During my one-and-a-half-hour trip on two trains, I initiated conversations with at least ten Japanese people (both men and women).

"Hi, do you live in Tokyo?" I'd usually ask. "I live in Los Angeles and I'm vacationing in Tokyo for the first time." The "worst" response I received was a friendly, shy "I don't speak English."

Gum ambassador. I bought about 60 five-stick packs of Big Red Cinnamon gum at Costco in Los Angeles as small gifts for Japanese people that I might meet (cinnamon is an uncommon flavor in Japan). Already I've given out three. Across the aisle from me on the train into Tokyo, a father, a mother, and their children delighted me. The girl (about nine) was teasing and giving her younger brother (perhaps six) a lot of attention. The girl also played a bit with her *tamoguchi* (electronic toy pet). I "talked" mostly with the father.

"Your daughter is *totemo kile* (very pretty) and your son is *kawai* (cute)," I said. His daughter's reaction to me was so shy that I asked, "What do you call the way she is behaving?"

"*Uchikina* is the word for shy," he said. A new word for me.

I gave the father some Big Red gum.

"Say 'thank you' to the man," he said, pointing at me after he gave his son the gum.

Japan seems even cleaner to me this time than I remember from before. Everything is immaculate. The mother's action epitomized this commitment. Carefully she removed the piece of gum from her son's mouth, wrapped it with a piece of paper, and slipped it into her purse. He could then chew the new stick of gum that I had given him.

Déjà vu. When I returned to the U.S. after spending three months in Hiroshima last year, I'd planned to move to Japan. Later I talked myself out of it. However, just a few hours here interacting with the Japanese people got me back in touch with why I wanted to move to Japan before.

Keep the restaurant open for me? After I arrived and got settled in last night at Iwai-san's, I persuaded Toshio, a 22-year-old man who was already here for the IFLP, to go out for a bite to eat. After a five-minute walk we found a place that appealed to me. I ordered a Jen-Tendon (I think!?) which was tempura shrimp and vegetables over rice. About half way through our meal a youthful waiter came to our table. He fidgeted on one leg then the other, scratched his head, opened his mouth, but no words came out. I guessed (accurately, as it turned out) he was striving to figure out how to ask me something, but lacked the English. Toshio's command of English was equally undistinguished. Another server and then the cook came out of the kitchen, their aprons splashed and smeared with the food from a full day's work. Both looked at the floor. They shot bursts of speech at each other, but they, too, were at a loss for English words. I handed them my Japanese-to-English dictionary, and they searched through it to no avail. A Japanese man from down the counter volunteered, "Perhaps I can help."

"Is there anything else you want to order before we close the kitchen?" he translated with a broad smile.

So that's what was so important for them to ask me. The restaurant closed at 10:00 p.m.—and it was already about 9:50! This sort of politeness and consideration is so typical here (at least for gaijin, their word for Westerners)!

11:59 p.m., Saturday, May 01, 1999

Breakfast with seven Japanese women! This morning I savored Japanese fare and the pleasant company of seven women ranging in age from cute nine-year-old Saho-chan ("chan" is the honorific given to children) to 61-year-old Iwai-san (who looks 42). Afterwards, Iwai-san, Saho, and I took a taxi to church.

Sleeping with the Adventists. Because of Iwai-san's limited English, another lady at the church explained to me that Iwai-san would not return to the house directly, and that someone would open her house for me at 3:30 p.m. They had two services: Japanese and English. I was tempted to attend the Japanese service because there would be more Japanese people there, and, in hindsight, it would have given me justification for what I ended up doing. However, I chose the English service, attended mostly by Filipinos. Before the service was underway, I fell asleep!

Near the beginning of the service, I was startled awake when Iwai-san brought Saho to sit with me. Even though Saho was uncharacteristically reserved with me, I think she "feels" me and my connection with her. I was surprised and pleased when, in the course of changing chairs, she took my hand to lead me to our new seats.

The presumption of sin. At 12:30 p.m., after the church service, I was led to Sunday school. "How can the perfect God create a Lucifer who created sin?" was the issue under discussion. A vegetarian potluck smorgasbord followed (Seventh Day Adventists are vegetarians).

Romping in my playground. After lunch, I was ready to start my trek back to Iwai-san's house. The spring sunshine felt delicious on my skin. I approached a woman who was finishing her lunch on the church steps.

"Would you direct me to the nearest JR (Japan Railway) station and then to Omori Station?" I asked.

"I don't . . . ! Wait!" she said, pointing to the place where I stood. She fled and returned almost immediately with a friend (who was evidently eating on the street nearby). Together they gave me excellent directions.

Out on the sidewalk of a major street, torrents of people flowed by each minute. I stopped two high school girls in uniform.

"Where is the nearest bank?" I asked. I wanted to exchange

more money, since the banks would be closed on Monday, Tuesday, and Wednesday as part of the Golden Week holiday. They quickly commandeered three more classmates to help me in my search (the Japanese seem to want to collaborate whether it's really necessary or not). The five of them spent 20 minutes finding me two banks (both were closed, except for the ATM machines). I wasn't too worried. Iwai-san had said she could change some money for me.

Well before 3:30 p.m. I arrived at the house.

"*Konnichiwa* (How are you?)," I said to those who seemed interesting, as I stood on a much-frequented part of the street near the house. Some picked their way past me in non-response.

"Hello," said Satsuki (22). "Do you speak Spanish? I have just returned from a year in Spain."

We had the greatest 45-minute conversation. By the end, we both felt and expressed our sense of soul-to-soul connection.

"I dream of studying to become a graphic designer in Spain and to fully enjoy right now," she said wistfully.

"Would you say you are 'in resignation' about your life and your dream?" I asked. "And would you care to 'take the risk' and go for it?"

My first date in Japan. At 7:20 p.m., I met Yumiko Yoshida at Tokyo Station for a date. She is a member of the Friends Network, the first Asian dating service I joined in California.

I arrived almost 30 minutes early to meet Yumiko at the Tokyo JR Station, and was engaged in a delightful conversation with a young couple when she arrived. We enjoyed dinner (*Yakisoba* for me and cold buckwheat noodles and tempura for her) and later shifted to a small coffee shop to continue our conversation. I ordered hot milk at 350 yen (about $3.00) and she had a coffee at 450 yen. We were content to pay mostly for a place to sit. Even though I offered, she paid for her own coffee.

Yumiko is 39, lives with her mother, and has visited the U.S. about ten times since she was in her early 20s. I like her. She was shy and, I think, a little defensive. But by the end of the evening we had good rapport and had talked openly about a lot of things (like the differences between men and women). She will come as my guest on Friday evening for the Landmark Forum graduate event.

How about black teeth as a fashion statement? Japanese women occasionally have some blackness to their teeth that American women don't. It appears to be from decay. Yumiko's teeth are like that. Perhaps it is more acceptable in Japan because a few hundred years ago women dyed their teeth black as an expression of beauty. For myself, I notice that I've fairly easily accepted crooked teeth in Japanese women (my former girlfriend Hitomi had rather crooked teeth). I noticed, however, that I'm dismissive of a woman as a "romantic partner" if her teeth have much blackness to them.

Pictures show the way. "I'm shy and have difficulty 'asserting myself' with people," Yumiko said. I opened my picture album of family and friends to show her how I would not have a friendship with Stephanie (back in LA) if I had not "asserted myself" by sitting down next to her in a seminar and then asking her to work for me. Then, as I looked at the other pictures of friends in my album, I realized that I had chosen courage in some significant way to create a friendship with every one of them.

I get an apology (gomen nasai). I'd left a note for Iwai-san, telling her I'd be back about 11 p.m. When I returned home I showered, prepared for bed, and joined her, four other women, and three men in the den area for conversation. Most of the conversation revolved around me (they were all surprised and delighted I was bringing a guest on Friday evening) and the questions I asked ("What do you like/dislike about yourself?" and "What do you least understand about men/women?") One of the things I like so much about Japan is how easy it is to be the center of attention and for me to give the attention back to others in a way that they accept. The women and the men were from Osaka and are participants in the IFLP. I asked one woman what difference the Forum made for her. She said that before the Forum her life was tired and boring. Now she experiences herself as very powerful.

The three young Japanese men from Osaka apologized for being so loud when they arrived last night.

"We didn't see you asleep on the other side of that table," their spokesman explained, as all of them looked at the floor.

"I appreciate your apology," I said. And I do acknowledge to myself that it was quite probable they didn't know I was there.

11:05 p.m., Sunday, May 02, 1999

Bringing intimacy to Japan. After breakfast with the women this morning, I took a 1.5-hour nap, then strolled off to Hibiya Park. At the park I talked with three young women for about 45 minutes, and exchanged e-mail addresses with one of them. Then I called Keiko Inaki (who I had been unable to reach earlier). She is another contact I made through the Friends Network. She gave me directions and I arrived at her subway stop a little after 2 p.m. We spent until almost 9:30 p.m. together. Near the end of our visit I suggested that we do the Spiritual Intimacy Process. After much soul searching and many questions, she agreed. I much admire and appreciate her for her choice of courage to do it with me. She experienced a lot of embarrassment and was constantly afraid she was "doing it wrong." I very much enjoyed my time with her.

Very briefly, the Spiritual Intimacy Process™ (which I invented) has these five components: (1) the participants look into each other's eyes, without looking away, with an intention to create a soul-to-soul connection; (2) each participant continuously looks to see if there are any RAFTS to share (see page 336 for description of RAFTS); (3) each participant notices anything and everything s/he appreciates about the other and expresses that to h/im; (4) if neither has anything to say, then the process continues in silence; (5) the process continues indefinitely until either participant says, "stop."

6:05 a.m., Monday, May 03, 1999

Discovering the pockets in my yukata. This morning my roommates slept on their futons on the other side of this table and I had my Brother DP-530CJ word processor powered up. I quietly prepared and consumed a morning drink of psyllium husks and my 40-30-30 Balance drink. Finally, I discovered where the "pockets" are in this *yukata*: in the sleeves! I've stored my vitamin packet there so I won't forget to take it to breakfast. (A *yukata* is an informal man's kimono worn around the house.)

12:40 a.m., Tuesday, May 04, 1999

Tigers of two kinds. After the first day of the Forum (called the Breakthrough Technology Course here in Japan), I'm present to an intent that is both exciting and unsettling: I feel compelled to live in Japan. Being here and present to how people here are with me (and how that empowers me to be with them) has awakened me to how much I feel at home here and how much I miss it when I'm in America. Japanese women support and encourage my full self-expression in ways that feel so easy and right for me. In the U.S., it's as if I'm swimming upstream, whereas in Japan, I get what I want just by flowing and steering with the stream.

Yet, a move to Japan evokes for me a parade of tigers, both paper and real. Two seemingly real tigers are how to satisfy the Japanese immigration authorities and how to maintain my life coaching practice from Japan. And I will have to make the commitment, without any final answers, on how those issues can be addressed!

5:40 a.m., Wednesday, May 05, 1999

A major fork in my road. Even though I was VERY tired last night, I slept for only four hours. Was it due to jet lag, excitement about being in Japan, and/or the effects of being in the Forum? Whatever! I'll live in Japan by year's end. To think about it more would just postpone the fears associated with this decision. To empower myself by publicly declaring my intention, I stood up in the Forum yesterday. After being provided with a microphone, I announced to the Forum leader and to the 99 Japanese participants, "I am moving to Japan." (The Forum translator interpreted this into Japanese.)

"By when?" the Forum leader asked.

"By the end of the year," I responded. It felt great!

When I returned from three months in Hiroshima last year, I said I'd move to Japan. Then I equivocated and thought I could find a "Japanese intimacy companion" and be around Japanese and other Asians by moving to California. And I wouldn't incur the associated drawbacks and challenges of moving to and living in Japan. Being back here, I'm fully awakened to how truly SPECIAL my relationship with Japanese women is. Several factors work together to birth and support these "phenomena of relationship":

(1) I am in their country.

(2) I am a Caucasian American male.

(3) The Japanese see me as a "tourist" and not someone who tries to be Japanese.

(4) I am intensely attracted to and fascinated by how they look, their intensity with and interest in me, and their innocence.

(5) I have the ability to combine gentleness with realness.

(6) I have the interest in and commitment to continuous choices of courage to ask them questions that they have never been asked before.

(7) In Japan I love taking advantage of the "cross-cultural freedom effect" (see page 365 for a full explanation of this extraordinary phenomenon that I have identified and documented). This effect is a special feeling of safety and freedom to express oneself that often occurs when two people of different cultures relate to each other. Since each person is outside of h/is own culture, the background cultural rules of what can be expressed or not expressed are greatly relaxed (as compared with talking with someone from the same culture). As a result, the two can enjoy the type of freedom that young children (before they are fully culturalized) often experience when first meeting each other.

Not a single American I've met has shared with me a close facsimile to what I experience with the Japanese people. The primary reason, I think, is that they have not consistently chosen the courage to "intrude" themselves into the Japanese culture the way I have.

Yukata x 2. 6:30 a.m. I must complete my Forum homework before breakfast at 7:00. Last night Iwai-san granted my request to stay another six nights. After my shower, I came into the living room to say goodnight to the other people, while wearing my *yukata.*

"Would you like another *yukata?*" Takako (Iwai-san's sister) offered.

"That would be great!" I said.

"I will bring one from home today," she promised.

1:10 a.m., Thursday, May 06, 1999

Yukata x 3. Takako gave me two *yukatas*! They both look great!

7:30 a.m., Thursday, May 06, 1999

Tokyo: the city of crows. The Forum is over, except for tomorrow night. All Iwai-san's guests except for me have departed and the house is quiet. Out this second-story window golden rays pierce, then break through, a light overcast. Housetops, large apartment complexes, and office buildings define the skyline. Somewhere close by an unseen train's hypnotic sound announces its passing. Distinct from that, the cacophonous caws of crows give notice of their ubiquitous presence. This could be called the city of crows.

"I wash?" Takako asked and pointed at the *yukata* I had worn for several days.

"Thank you," I nodded.

The advantages of poor communication. 11:10 a.m. Takako and I navigated a tricky communication about my day and how it will interface with hers (Takako's English is quite limited). Both of us seemed to be amused by and to enjoy this challenge. It continues to amaze me that the slow and sometimes circuitous process of communication with the Japanese who speak limited English seldom frustrates me. In fact, the process gives me keen enjoyment and an excuse for us to get to know each other in ways that would not occur if we were fluent in each other's language.

The scooter woman. 8:00 p.m. When I returned to the house, it was locked. I called Takako from the local convenience store, and she roared up on her scooter five minutes later to let me in, along with two of the four cats who share this house.

Even though I'm a feminist, I like . . . . 10:25 p.m. Upon entry to my room, in front of me hung my *yukata*, washed and meticulously ironed! I attribute Takako's actions to four interweaving factors: an attitude of service that the Japanese people, and especially the women, have; the attitude Japanese women have of being in domestic service to "their men"; a desire to look good to and to be of service to Caucasians (especially to visitors); and her particular affinity for me.

Takako has her own apartment a 5-minute scooter ride from here. Through some arrangement with Akira Iwai-san (her sister), Takako "manages" this house, at least when her sister is out of town. She's 59 (but looks 45), and has three grown children by a husband who is gone. Although her sister is a Seventh Day Adventist, Takako is an atheist. Early in her life she dreamed of marrying an American man.

Frolicking in my playground. If I was amazed at my ability to start on-the-street conversations with Japanese last year when I vacationed in Hiroshima for three months, I'm now astounded. Yuriko, Tomoko, Arisa, Chie, Hideko—the list goes on and on. I have found surprisingly little defensiveness.

Earlier this evening at a Japanese fast-food restaurant, I sat one bar seat away from a young attractive woman (Arisa). She was about finished with her meal.

"Hi," I said. "I'm vacationing in Tokyo for two weeks from LA. I'm thinking of moving to Tokyo. Might you know the prices of apartments in this area?" I asked. She moved herself over to the stool next to me.

"I'll wait for you to finish your meal and then we'll find an agency that can provide you this information," she offered.

Later, coming out of the Ebisu JR Station, I approached another young woman.

"Might you know the way to this conversation lounge called the COM INN, at this address?" I asked as I held forth the address, handwritten (in Japanese) on a piece of paper.

"Yes," she said with a demeanor I interpreted as eager, shy, and innocent all at once (a powerful elixir for me). She walked with me, asking directions of other pedestrians along the way until she found the location for me. These examples are typical!

6:40 a.m., Friday, May 07, 1999
Location, location, location. This house is five stories high and has an elevator, in addition to the stairs! The horizontal

dimensions are roughly 50 feet by 55 feet. The top floor is only half size and is largely a rooftop patio. Half of the bottom floor is a double-car garage. If this house were located in Phoenix, Arizona on a half acre of land, I'd guess its market value at less than $350,000.

"How much do you think this house would bring if it were sold?" I asked Takako.

"340,000,000 yen," She replied.

"That's roughly $3,000,000 US dollars!" I exclaimed.

Nine "problems" of moving to Japan. I've been pondering the issues to address in my move to Japan:

(1) The weather gets cold in the winter and hot and muggy in the summer.

(2) I would have to face many obstacles in order to become legal, or deal with the uncertainties of being illegal.

(3) Living space is expensive—the money I pay now for an apartment in California will afford me only one-third the physical living space in Tokyo.

(4) Other costs will also be higher, especially supplements which I may want to have shipped from the States. Some costs will be lower. I won't need a car. The price of restaurant food of the quality and kind I want is significantly lower here. Cut flowers are cheaper here than in California. And a very short local telephone call costs 10 yen (8 cents)!

(5) Finding my way to new places and acquiring the local information I'll need to function here will challenge me and consume much more time than in the States. However, I will enjoy the process immensely, because it's an excuse to interact with the Japanese and for them to be helpful to me, which they, as well as I, love. What to do if I have a medical problem feels more confronting than some of the other issues.

(6) The potential for dangerous earthquakes may be greater here than in California! But, perhaps because I love earthquakes, that's not a significant worry.

(7) If there should be significant Y2K social unrest, it might be dangerous for me to be in a foreign country at that

moment in history (now less than eight months away). Actually, I feel that I would be safer in Japan on that count. The Japanese people are much more gentle and slower to violence than are Americans. And Americans have such prestige with the Japanese people.

(8) Doing my business from Japan could be problematic. We're getting into "legally gray" areas because technology makes obsolete the contexts in which the alien work laws were made in the first place. If I understand them accurately, my work in Japan, the way I plan to do it, will not violate Japanese alien work laws. Actually, I will not technically "work in their country." Japanese citizens will not pay me for services or products provided to them. My American clients will be coached via phone as they have been, and the money they pay me will be deposited into an American bank! A "work schedule" from 7 a.m. to 3 p.m. Japan time will translate to 3 p.m. to 11 p.m. the previous day in California and 6 p.m. to 2 a.m. in New York; that seems workable. I'm confident I can arrange to talk with my clients with these as my U.S. work hours. International telephone rates are plummeting. The rates to talk with me in Japan will not be very much different from the rates to talk with me in California. E-mail and Internet service here can be set up so that communication will be as easy and quick as it is in the States.

(9) I will miss my friends in the States. However, I have maintained my Arizona friends quite well with letters and phone calls from California. That will be no different in Japan.

My own matchmaker, no charge! 7:50 a.m. Breakfast will be ready in ten minutes. A new woman came in late last night and I want to meet her. So I'll continue with this later.

9:25 a.m. I think Takako has "set me up!" Akie Tanaka (31 on Sunday and pronounced: Ahh-Key-A with a long last "a") is big boned, tall by Japanese standards (about 5 feet 8 inches), has a rather attractive full face, generous lips (which I like very much), and long straight black hair that falls just below her shoulders.

"Akie will 'show you the town' today," Takako said with a beyond-typical smile.

"If it's up to me, we'll just talk and/or find other Japanese people to talk with," I thought to myself.

"Akie is single and very pretty," Takako said. Then she turned to me in front of Akie and very explicitly asked, "Dwight, you are open to marriage, right?"

I nodded, took the hint and asked, "Akie, what plans do you have for today?"

"She is freeee," Takako cooed in a tone I interpreted as triumph.

Akie's English is very limited, but I doubt there would be any possibility for a lasting romance even if her English were excellent. She's physically attractive enough, but there's a protectiveness that projects a "jadedness" that I doubt I will get past or heal. She's friendly, but it feels "surface" and ultimately that would leave me very unsatisfied. Regardless, I will have fun and adventure with her today and I will push her to the limit in her willingness to open up.

A translator for a romantic conversation! 12:05 p.m. I just participated in a very interesting and most unusual conversation. Isao Yamamori (68) makes this room (where I sleep and keep my things) his office once a week. His English proficiency (the product of four years of study) is a vast improvement over Takako's or Akie's. Isao arrived at 10:00 a.m., and Akie showed up smartly appointed soon after. Two attributes made this dialogue unique:

(1) Isao translated a singularly intimate conversation between Akie and me.
(2) It was obvious that Akie and I explicitly explored the possibility of a romantic relationship together.

"What do you want in a woman?" she asked me.

She was also unabashed about her loneliness and desire for a man in her life.

I found it quite interesting that Akie and I had to be very direct and blunt with each other—because exchanging subtleties through a translator proved impossible.

Isao didn't seem uneasy in his role as translator between the two of us. From this experience, I assume that the Japanese are much more open about issues of romantic interest than are Americans. I also assume that third-party matchmakers are valued, respected, and appreciated.

Takako fixed Akie and me a picnic lunch.

In California I worked very intentionally for over two months and joined three dating agencies to get only a few initially interesting dates going. After being here in Japan less than a week, I'm being set up with a certainly beautiful (and definitely interested-in-me) woman, without my even trying or making any specific request. That's incredible!

7:10 a.m., Saturday, May 08, 1999

Necking in the park. Notwithstanding my first impressions of Akie, we've had a great time together. I have never spent such intense time with someone I could barely speak to. We constantly refer to either the English-Japanese or Japanese-English dictionary. We sat on the one bench in a small wooded park, which overlooked a pond of ducks and Japanese *koi*, and ate our picnic lunch of *nigiri*. We taught each other words for simple things like sky, road, car. Soon we abandoned words for a more universal language that our bodies knew, which included gentle horseplay, teasing, and eventually quite a bit of kissing and necking. It was also a game for me to fully enjoy the necking while remaining on the lookout for passersby to avoid a full case of embarrassment. What, again, was so amazing to me was how unabashed we were in our expression with each other. Whenever I felt something or wanted something I, to the best of my dictionary-assisted ability, expressed that to Akie. Our very limited command of each other's language required me to express myself very directly.

Akie has to "power down." That evening Akie (a five-year graduate of the Forum) and I went to the Forum Evening Session. It was great to see all my new friends and to introduce Akie to many of them. Yumiko and Keiko showed up to learn about the Forum. I think both of them will register for the course.

Akie teased me about being an "old man" and I responded in a way that created fun for both of us.

"I'm 'power down'," she said, on the way home, not knowing the word for sleepy.

"You're an 'old woman' and I'm a 'young man'," I teased.

We bade each other goodnight.

Is my testosterone speaking? For breakfast we had curry and rice, grain tea, fresh lettuce, and tomato. About 8:25 Takako left to visit someone. Akie lay on a massage bed in the living room area, luxuriating in a "machine massage." I added a surprise foot massage to her treatment, which led to deep kissing and to slightly more than necking.

Even without language and cultural differences, relationships are often problematic because of assumptions and misinterpretations. A translator for some important and even more frank communication is becoming essential for Akie and me. My projections and/or concerns about a "continuing relationship" with Akie may or may not be founded.

"Are you interested in getting married?" Takako had asked me before. And, with much qualification (e.g., not living together, having separate money, etc.), I would say the answer to that is "yes." However, at this point, with Akie, it doesn't seem likely. And I'm definitely open to discovering things about her that would change my mind! The way my relationships are, with Akie or any woman, no matter what the "relationship status" is, I always want to be able to say, "If this romantic relationship should end tomorrow, I would be totally happy that I had what I had with her up to this point." If Akie is to explore a romantic relationship with me, I want (if possible) to know if she is willing and committed to have a relationship on this basis. So that's what I/we need a proficient translator for.

I could just go with, "Well, Akie can take care of herself. She's 31 tomorrow, after all. She's a mature, sophisticated woman." And if my testosterone were allowed to operate by itself, that's probably what I would go with. (That testosterone is powerful stuff! If it weren't built into our bodies, I'm sure the FDA would put it on the same prohibited-substances list as heroin.)

Sleeping with a cat. 10:05 a.m. Akie is still making up her face. I must have misunderstood her regarding when we were leaving.

2:20 p.m. Takako just handed me the key to the house. I came back by myself to take a nap and she'll be going out soon. I feel very trusted.

4:20 p.m. One of the four cats very agreeably cuddled up and slept with me. It's been too long since I slept with a cat.

11:35 p.m., Saturday, May 08, 1999

Still a teenager at 54. When I'm the flotsam in the "flow" of life, the ride never ceases to amaze. As I approached Omori JR Station (a 10-minute walk from the house), I was surprised and happy to meet Akie coming the other way. I thought she would not be back until late. We walked back to the house, snacked, engaged in a little horseplay, and then I told her I wanted to gift us a movie for her birthday. We "saw" the movie *Shakespeare in Love* in English with Japanese subtitles. I put "saw" in quotes because Akie and I were rather busy, stretching the limits (at least for me) of what I'm willing to do sexually in a public theater with people all around. I was pleasantly surprised by Akie's aggressiveness.

When she and I are out in public, if I'm aware of a communication impasse, I approach the nearest young Japanese woman and ask her if she speaks a little English (the answer is "yes" 80% of the time). Then I request some translation help. I've done this three times already to facilitate discourse with Akie. Akie hasn't initiated this kind of contact, but once I do, she gets right in there.

I'm beginning to have second thoughts about the need for "the big conversation." (Is this my testosterone speaking?) Akie's way of being with me has not been congruent (to the best of my interpretation) with a woman who considers me marriage material (at least at this stage in our relationship). From all indications, she's definitely less romantic than I am and more matter of fact about sex.

Will I get a visitor in the night? 12:10 a.m. I'm going to bed. I invited Akie to come to my bed in the middle of the night. Did she understand my invitation? I didn't put that one through a translator! Whether or not she will want to take me up on the offer is another question. It would be very nice and I'm not attached to it (I masturbated to help with my non-attachment).

6:50 a.m., Sunday, May 09, 1999

I get reverse culture shock. I seem to need less sleep than in California. At least so far. No visitor during the night.

Last night about 10:40 Takako was full, but she asked Akie and me if we'd like something to eat. By the time I'd showered and donned one of the *yukatas* that Takako had given me, the two of them had a light meal prepared. The fare included boiled squid, *wakame* (seaweed), licorice-flavored (at least to me) shiitake mushrooms, one patty of a meat-enriched potato pancake, a small piece of fried chicken, some other slightly nutty and delicate vegetable, and rice.

How I experience Japan is synonymous with how I experience the Japanese people. During each of my three previous visits to Japan, I have felt excitement, peace, and affinity, and absolutely no culture shock. I felt culture shock only upon returning to America!

The way the Japanese people are with me continuously fulfills my particular "unanswerable question" (no matter how many times it gets answered in the affirmative, the question reoccurs, as if I need constant reassurance): "Will you see me as uniquely special?"

I ???? Akie! 9:30 a.m. Akie was still lying under the covers on her futon when I went downstairs this morning. I sat on the floor at the foot of her futon and massaged her feet. Takako smiled at me when she saw what I was doing.

"What do you like about Akie?" I asked Takako during breakfast.

"What do you like about Akie?" Takako countered.

"I like her lips, her playfulness with me, and the feeling of soul-to-soul connection I feel in looking into her eyes," I replied.

"You said 'like' rather than 'love'?" Takako seemed to search my face for meaning.

"Yes, 'like'," I confirmed. Our eyes met for a moment, and then

I lowered mine. That response will perhaps communicate partially what I wanted to say to Akie with the "big conversation." Even if a sexual relationship with Akie doesn't go any further than it already has, I consider that I've had a delightful, adventurous affair with a very attractive and special woman.

6:15 a.m., Monday, May 10, 1999

She teases the most when it's the safest. I can't tell if Akie has her own business or acts as a rep; probably the latter. Her company is based in Hokkaido. She reps lingerie (we did some window shopping in a lingerie department in the Ginza yesterday). About half the time she is home in Fukashima City; the rest of the time she travels all over Japan. Right now she's "on vacation" and doing a little business (her mobile phone rings a lot). Everyone knows her in this neighborhood. She stops to talk with many people.

Akie loves to tease me. When we are outside and more in public, she gets even more sexual. Probably because she knows she can tease me (she's very good at it!) and it's "safer" for her. I fully engage in and enjoy the game; I even pretend that the frustration of it bothers me more than it does (she loves my being "bothered"). She has also found that she can embarrass me in public (by how and where she touches me). Prior to being with her, I thought that I was not easily embarrassed in public. But she has found my limit and exceeds it on purpose! When she touched me in a way that embarrassed me in a department store, I started a play-fight with her so she couldn't use her hands to embarrass me! I quickly looked up the word for "shameless" (*haji-shirazu no*) and called her that. She looked at me, mirth brimming her eyes and nodded.

I'm shameless, too. In a different way I could be called "shameless" in Japan. Because I easily say "Hello, how are you?" to anyone I pass on the sidewalk. Often I get a smile or "Fine, thank you" back. But if I get back no visible response or change in behavior from the person I spoke to, it doesn't bother me. My saying "hello" to strangers doesn't bother Akie. She finds it amusing.

Akie with the poker face. This experience with Akie is unique in at least three aspects:

(1) She's the first woman I've had a romantic relationship with where we essentially can't speak to each other.

(2) She's the first woman I've been with who has aggressively teased me sexually.

(3) She's the first woman I've been with who has that "aloof, model demeanor." Akie, I think, falls into the "gorgeous" category here. And she's a woman who knows she's gorgeous. It's obvious I find her attractive, but my personal taste would have me pick many other Japanese women over her. Her often expressionless face discomfits me. It's the face models put on as they strut their fashions on the ramp.

"You don't let your face tell me what you're thinking," I accused. She answered in a lyrical stream of Japanese. Assuming I understood her response, she denies that she keeps her feelings from showing.

So it's a puzzle for me that I have this romantic proclivity with a woman such as Akie. In the U.S., her way of being and behavior would have bothered me to the point of unacceptability. Here, for now, it's satisfying, nurturing, exciting, and a glorious adventure. And I like her.

How can I live (legally) in Japan? Yesterday I called my new friend Ruth Shields, an American I met at the Landmark Center. She teaches English here and she assists a lot at Landmark. I offered to treat her to lunch so we could brainstorm the best approach for achieving legal residence in Japan. Ruth, Akie, and I enjoyed a leisurely lunch, and Ruth (who is semi-fluent in Japanese) helped Akie and me learn more about each other. Then Ruth and I brainstormed. We came up with a number of avenues to explore. The fresh conclusion of most immediate use was that I could come to Japan on the automatic tourist visa for 90 days. At the end of the 90 days, I could go out of the country (e.g., to Korea or to the U.S.) for a day or more and then return to Japan for another 90 days. If I attempt to stay here for more than 180 days in this manner, there may be some questioning from the immigration authorities.

However, 180 days is a rubber stamp. In half a year I can make the contacts and develop the relationships that are needed to get a more permanent visa and/or sponsorship. The risk that I couldn't do that in six months feels negligible.

Taking care of a stranger's kid. 8:10 a.m. No one stirs downstairs. I'm glad. I don't want to miss anything. And I have so much to catch you up on in this journal.

Last night Akie and I walked to the video store to rent a video. A two-year-old boy was crying. As we approached him, Akie swooped him into her arms to comfort him. The boy's mother was next to him with an infant in her arms. This seemed completely natural (Akie did not know this woman or her children) and the mother just expressed gratitude for Akie's help. This attitude of assumptive assistance is just part of the Japanese culture.

Iwai-san's back from her trip. It was a surprise to learn that she went to Boston and back! She was animated and not tired at all. Her vitality at 61 amazes me.

10 p.m. Takako entered bearing little cakes to celebrate Akie's birthday.

I told Iwai-san (who is a vegetarian Seventh Day Adventist) and Takako (who is an atheist) that I was very impressed with their love and affinity for each other given their "differences." Takako is two years younger than Iwai-san.

My feelings about this journal. As I have been writing this journal with the intention of sharing it with you, I've had some background thoughts that I think are important to include: sharing these in-process thoughts, attitudes, and responses, not only regarding Akie, but also in other areas, is often very confronting for me. There it is, right in front of me, hard evidence of my attitudes toward myself such as that I "should get it right," "should not have changing perceptions and perhaps even changing standards," and "should know what I want 'from the beginning'." And I project this meta-attitude onto you, when I imagine that you'll be critical of me. Also, I am aware that what I report as "facts" out there in the world, even though others may readily corroborate them as "facts," are, more to the point, just a mirror of my soul, evidenced by my choice to report some "facts" and not others. The idea of "objective reporting" feels like a very slippery concept.

Akie chickens out. 10:10 p.m. Akie and I went our separate ways today until we arrived "home" about 3:00 p.m. We then sat on the sofa and, even though Takako was somewhere in the house, Akie teased me (with my permission) to the point that I was uncomfortably hard.

I decided to turn the tables on her in this teasing game. I looked down and said, "Look what you've done!" She chuckled happily.

"I'm going upstairs to masturbate," I said (I find it very interesting that she understood the word "masturbate"—which was good since I couldn't find it in my English-to-Japanese dictionary). I was one surprised lad when Akie followed me upstairs and into the toilet room! I locked the door and closed the blinds, which overlooked the patio. When I began to ready myself, she chickened out. She unlocked and exited the toilet room and returned downstairs. I came down to the kitchen several minutes later with a grin on my face. Akie asked me if "it" was good. I replied that it was very good and that I thought of her the whole time.

The gifts of life. 11:10 p.m. I've showered and bade Akie and Iwai-san "good night."

Over the few days we've known each other, I've developed a growing awareness that Akie has a lot of self-confidence, is quite outgoing for a Japanese woman, and carries herself with a certain aplomb. Yet, when I think of how Akie and I act with each other, it reminds me of a delightful teenage game.

One dilemma for me is how to dance with/between "what I say I want" and "what shows up" in my life that adds such zest to my life right now. I had previously put to paper in explicit and specific detail what I want in a woman. And then Akie showed up, someone who does not fit my idea of the woman I want. Heaven help me! I could just dismiss her and say, "No, this woman doesn't fit my plan on several counts." Or I could argue that, while I'm preoccupied with her, I reduce the likelihood of "the" woman showing up in my life because I have already filled the vacuum. Or I could take the attitude that Akie showed up for a reason and that to disdain my pleasure in her presence would be a slap in the face of "providence" and a sabotage of the fun, affection, and self-expression possible for both of us. This last approach appeals to me more than the first two. I can still remain fully aware of what I want in a woman and why I want it. AND I'm open to discovering, through Akie, new things about myself and the dynamic possibilities in relationships.

6:35 a.m., Tuesday, May 11, 1999

Keeping the hunger alive. This is my last full day here in Japan.

Yesterday, soon after our teasing episode, Akie and I took Choco (a small beagle) for a walk. It seemed that all the residents of the village were being walked by their dogs. These back-alley-ways have a cozy, country-village feel to them. At least 30 dogs walked their masters to meet us. In addition to the poop bag, Akie brought doggie snacks, which she fed to the other dogs, as Choco and the other dogs smelled each other up with tails wagging. I exchanged e-mail addresses with a young Chinese lady who was born in Taiwan, spent eight years in San Jose, and then 2.5 years here in Japan. Then Akie and I met Yumie, a 21-year-old, university student majoring in English. I started the conversation and then Akie joined in. We enlisted Yumie to translate for us. Akie invited her to Iwai-san's house for "tea time." Yumie accepted and visited/translated for over an hour, while Akie fixed *hiyashi* rice for the three of us. Akie, through Yumie, satisfied her curiosity about my 1996 divorce from Yuko. And through Yumie I was able to share with Akie that I do not believe a man and woman should ever live together if they expect to be able to maintain romance with each other. I told her that if I were with her much longer than the several days we've been together, I would need to be away from her to get hungry for her again. I also said that part of the reason we weren't tired of each other yet is that we are so new to each other. Whereupon Akie and Iwai-san became preoccupied with their own separate conversation—so Yumie and I had an avid conversation of our own about passion, sex, romance, and how to keep it alive. Yumie has had boyfriends since she was 18 and she's had her current boyfriend for three months. She was very interested in my ideas about how to keep the passion alive and deepen the intimacy. Yumie doesn't have an e-mail address so we exchanged regular addresses. I like her.

You don't have a fax machine at home? Fax machines are ubiquitous in Japan, not only in businesses, but in homes as well. Having a fax machine is seen as vitally important.

"The system for assigning addresses for houses and businesses is the cause of this urgency," Ruth Shields explained. Typically the first building built on a street becomes the #1, the second building #2, etc. Consequently, the number on a building has no correlation to its physical position on the street. Hence it's impossible to predict location of a building from its address. People are compelled to fax each other maps that depict their home or business position relative to local landmarks. The upshot is that a fax machine is essential for business and a social life!

Whenever I hand my business card to someone, they look on the back for a map, which, in my case, is not there.

Shouting and no tipping. Whenever you enter a store in Japan (except for really big stores, like department stores), one or more of the clerks shouts out to welcome you into the store.

There's no tipping here—which I absolutely love.

Me "Dwighto-san"? Except in family relationships, people typically refer to each other only by last name (I think I am going against tradition by using people's first names, although I always put the honorific "-san" at the end.) For example, nametags for participants in Landmark programs in the States always show the first name in big letters and the last name in small letters. Here in Japan it's reversed. They put the last name in big letters and the first name in small letters. Bill Palmer, the Forum leader, always addressed the participants by their last name (with "-san" as in "Tanaka-san"), although he asked the participants to address him as "Bill." I noticed that, during the Forum, one of the participants addressed Bill as "*sensei*," which means "teacher." In Japan, if a person has a position of respect, as a teacher does, they are not addressed by their name; they are addressed by their position. Even though Bill doesn't speak Japanese, he caught the reference to himself with the honorific "teacher," and, through the translator, asked the participant to refer to him as "Bill" and not "teacher."

Yumiko Yoshida, who was my date on my first day in Tokyo (and who came to my Forum Evening Session), called two days ago. She expressed a desire to see me again before I fly back to the States. We'll meet for dinner tonight. I have no romantic interest in Yumiko. And I like her.

Tokyo or or or or or . . . . 8:00 a.m. I've asked myself the question: why move to Tokyo instead of some other Japanese city? Here are my reasons for Tokyo:

(1)   Tokyo and Osaka are the only cities that have direct flights to the U.S., so it makes it more convenient to live in one of these two cities. My experience of Osaka is limited, but I found the pollution there intolerable when I hitchhiked through the city two years ago. Tokyo is surprisingly pollution free.

(2)   I want to be near the Landmark Center for classes and meeting Japanese people who have been stimulated by the Forum technology.

(3)   Tokyo has an abundance of opportunities to discover and use, which is important to me.

(4)   I've found that Tokyo people are just as friendly as people in other Japanese cities.

(5)   Prices do seem higher in Tokyo (than Hiroshima, for instance), but only marginally so for food and there is not really any major difference in rent prices. Besides, I plan to find and make a special deal in renting a portion of a house (perhaps with some trade for English conversation). This way I will bypass the requirements of having a non-tourist visa and sponsor in order to rent an apartment.

I REALLY like the neighborhood I'm in now (admittedly, I haven't checked out the thousands of other neighborhoods in Tokyo) and it's only 30 minutes (walking and train included) to the Landmark Center from here.

Two major factors apply in my developing a timetable for a move to Tokyo:

(1)   How and whether to finish the Landmark Wisdom Course, which ends in January. I really don't want to wait until January to move to Tokyo.

(2)   My need to get myself financially and logistically ready to live well and to effect a seamless transition for my clients and my business.

The lease for my apartment in Hermosa Beach is up at September's end. Although I would have to be very focused and intentional, I think I could have everything ready to move by the end of September. I might see if Iwai-san is open to my staying at her place for a maximum of two weeks while I get set up to live here. If I spent most of my time meeting people in the neighborhood and asking if they knew of someone who might have some house space for rent, I'm sure I could have a place to stay within that two-week time frame. Then, allowing for moving in and getting set up (computer, phone system, e-mail, appliances, etc.), my break with my clients in the States could be kept to about three weeks. In addition, I would make many friends with my neighbors even before they officially became my neighbors.

10:50 p.m., Tuesday, May 11, 1999

When did you last cry? I'm all ready for futon (bed). I'll write until the melatonin kicks in and I begin to get sleepy.

Today, Akie took me to a restaurant owned by a Forum friend of hers. The restaurant specializes in myriad entrees based on daikon. The outing required a long train ride (past Yokohama). I like daikon, but this was a bit much for me. While at the restaurant, however, I stumbled upon a way to learn Japanese that keeps me in the present, is fun, and is easy for me. For example, at the restaurant, Akie, Eda (Akie's friend), and a woman customer chatted among themselves. I did my best to repeat what each of them said (even though I didn't understand it). I repeated it loudly enough so I could hear myself, but quietly enough so that they couldn't hear me.

Tomorrow I'll return to LA, and I think Akie and I are ready for a break from each other. If she were more expressive, I think I could enjoy her more; but her face is often inscrutable to me.

"When was the last time you cried?" I asked her.

"In 1991 I was a cry baby," she said dismissively.

She was 23! I think eight years is too long for anyone to go without having a good cry, especially if that person is a woman. (Is that a double standard?)

6:05 a.m., Wednesday, May 12, 1999

A life of regret. Yesterday, after our day trip, Akie left me for an overnight stay with a friend or on business, I'm not sure which. She'll return just in time to see me off today. I continued on the train to Gotanda Station, and arrived over an hour early for my dinner appointment with Yumiko. I strolled around a bit and bought a few gifts for friends back in California.

Yumiko and I found a small restaurant and monopolized a table for two hours. I imagined that the servers were impatient with us for doing so (Japanese servers do not receive tips to possibly compensate for extra time spent). I justified our behavior to myself by noticing that there were always empty tables in the restaurant.

Our discussion covered a wide range of topics. We even did the Spiritual Intimacy Process for a bit. The theme of our discussion, however, was her incompletion and regret that she had not moved to the U.S. fourteen years ago when she was 25. And since then she has continued to be "on the fence" about moving to America. So she has "kept the wound open." She "radiates" a timidity and pain that is an expression of her incompletion and not being true to herself. I encouraged her to take the Forum, either here or in the U.S.—where she plans to vacation in July. I think she will. And we'll stay in touch.

Serendipity strikes again. At Shinagawa Station I picked my way down the steps to the train platform and bid my eyes to select a lady to approach. Four had promise. I picked the one who looked the most interesting. As I approached a position on her right, I faced half toward her and half toward the tracks.

"How are you?" I said. Our conversation continued as we boarded the train. I asked if she had an e-mail address. And Tokiko Nanba exchanged e-mail addresses with me.

Serendipitously her home is in Iwai-san's neighborhood, so we exited the train together and continued to talk as we walked. When we reached Iwai-san's (Tokiko had an additional five-minute walk), Tokiko asked for my assurance that I would e-mail her. She is in her 20s, works as a buyer for Denny's Japan, and wants to be a lawyer. I write about these "spontaneous" meetings, not because they're unique, but because they happen 2 to 3 times per day with miniscule effort.

I returned home to an empty house. Iwai-san assisted at Landmark last night, so she's not likely to stir until after 8 a.m. It's 7:50 now. I think I'll get dressed (I'm in one of the *yukatas* that Takako gave me) and take a walk around the neighborhood. I will leave the house at 1:00 p.m. today, allowing two hours to get to the airport. My flight leaves at 4:55 p.m.

To pay for the extra meals they've graciously served me, I'm going to offer/give Iwai-san an extra 5,000 yen (about $40); the 2000 yen per night included only breakfast.

Choco walks me. 8:05 a.m. It took a while to find the leash for the dog who lives on the outside patio of the top floor of this house. He doesn't care, he'll walk anybody who takes him. At first I was concerned about losing myself in the maze of back-alley-way roads of this neighborhood. Then I realized that, worst case, I could ask someone how to get to the Omori Station and from there I could get back to the house. The flow of people walking through the system of merging alleyways led me out of the maze to Omori Station without asking a single direction. What a satisfying mini-adventure.

I noticed some automatic fear associated with making this request, but I asked Iwai-san if I could stay at her place for 7 to 14 days when I first arrive in Tokyo around October 1st. She said yes!

The Japanese bank remembers me. 11:30 a.m. Just finished a late breakfast. Iwai-san slept in this morning.

Iwai-san said that Akie called to say she'd be "home" here at 12:30 p.m. She wanted to make sure I didn't leave before she returned. That pleases me.

Whenever you exchange money here, the banks require that you write down the contact address and telephone number for where you're staying in Japan. This morning I forgot to bring Iwai-san's information to exchange another $100. The bank lady remembered me from before and found the required information in the bank records. I gave her a packet of gum, which she blushingly and effusively accepted.

Akie's lucky money is all wet. Japanese people love their fresh-cut flowers and florists do a brisk business on nearly every major block. On the way back to the house, I stopped to buy a sunflower for Akie. They wrapped it, put a bow on it, and gave me a gift card, all for 210 yen, about $1.80! Flowers are one of the few items that are less expensive in Japan than in the U.S.

After Akie and I ate at the daikon restaurant yesterday, we went to a shrine. People took out coins and bills to wash them in the "special water." It is believed that this will bring good luck to "multiply your money." Akie washed her money. I declined to wash mine. Later, at the train station, the machine to buy a train ticket would not accept her 1000-yen bill because it was still wet. I traded her for one of my dry ones.

Just when I start to drown in her eyes . . . . 12:40 p.m. Akie arrived "home" and received the flower I bought her with a moment's searching eye contact and a happy hug. She brought me some candies "to eat on the plane"—which I will not eat on the plane. Akie and Iwai-san surprised and charmed me when they insisted they walk me to the Omori Station. Each one carried a bag. Akie then went on the train with me to the Nippoli Station to make sure that I got on the through train to Narita Airport.

I kept asking Akie to look into my eyes. She'd look for a little bit, usually in a mocking way. But then she'd say "end" and look away.

I was glad she came with me, and I was glad I was "by myself" when she put me on the final train. I introduced myself to Keiko Shoda, an 18-year-old university student studying economics in Tokyo, and spent almost the entire 50-minute trip in avid discussion with her. We will e-mail each other.

After I checked my bags, I found a table next to three Japanese women and chatted with them while I ate a light Japanese lunch. Then I bought a few final Japanese gifts and proceeded to gate for boarding.

Twelve days that changed my life 4:28 p.m. My window seat is on the left side of the plane just behind the wing. An elderly Laotian man with a cane sits to my right. An American woman in her early 50s has the aisle seat; she's just returning from a month in Nepal.

5:08 p.m. Moving. Faster! Faster! Faster! Liftoff! Retracting landing gears. 700 feet. 1000 feet. I see rice paddies everywhere with islands of trees and houses in between.

8:40 p.m. Passed over the International Date Line. 3166 miles to go. 669 mph; 96 mph tail wind; 37,000 feet; minus 65 degrees.

10:40 p.m. (Still Japan time) The just-discernable dawn twilight quickened as we raced into the sun. Flying east, as we are, we had less than five hours of darkness.

Are we living in the same world? 10:55 p.m. May, the woman returning from Nepal, and I had a lengthy discussion. She's spent considerable time in Japan and her experience of the Japanese is exactly the opposite of mine. Whereas she experienced them as almost always not helpful and not especially friendly, for me they were very helpful, generous, and friendly. Perhaps the Japanese pick up on my preconceived attitudes about them and respond accordingly.

Starting the next millennium in Japan. 12:30 a.m. Just finished my *okonomiaki* (a "pancake" containing various meats and vegetables, covered with a special sauce) for the last meal on this flight.

10:05 a.m., LA Time. Touchdown in LA. Fifty minutes early!

ഇ

Plans for Japan

8:07 a.m., Friday, May 21, 1999

I am now irresistible. Even though I don't have "the woman for the rest of my life" in my life, my coach, Charles Sung, and I have declared the "finding a woman" project complete, because I've made the transition from "needing a woman" to being "irresistible to women"!

Gourmet conversations? Yesterday I enrolled a new client who owns the restaurant/bar immortalized by the hit play *Rent,* called "The Life Café," on the lower east side of Manhattan. We will explore the possibility of reinventing her eatery as a "Gourmet Conversations" restaurant.

I know it could be very successful. I've already asked people if they would go out of their way to try such a restaurant at least once if they heard about one. Nine out of ten of them have said, "yes!"

Although delectable food and friendly atmosphere would be vital, what would set this restaurant apart would be "Gourmet Conversations." People would come with the expectation of being seated with a person they did not previously know. Getting to know another person would be the meal's destination. Whether you ever saw that person again would be up to you and the other person.

To spark conversation, placemats, or special menus would prompt questions grouped by category. Some examples:

(1)   Casual (What kind of work do you do? Who do you think will win the NBA this year? What movie did you like recently?)

(2)   Vulnerable (What do you like best about yourself? What do you dislike most about yourself? When did you last cry and what was it over?)

(3)   Casually curious (You have such an interesting last name! What are its origins? I can't quite place your accent?)

(4)   Stretching the limits (What do you least understand about men/women? What was the most passionate experience of your life? What do you dislike about your mother?)

(5)   Looking for wisdom (What is the most important thing you've learned about living life fully and joyously? If you could give advice to your 10-year-old self, what would it be?)

You could even ask the server to bring you a list of questions not available from the "main menu" (specialized categories like "questions about music" or "questions about travel" or "questions on philosophy").

I can imagine that people might often have the most fun just discussing the questions that were given as suggestions to start the conversation!

I love getting paid for sharing questions and ideas with people! It's absolutely the perfect "job" for me.

12:40 p.m., Saturday, May 22, 1999

The importance of honesty. I cherish Sabrina's innocence and funny spirit. I really like her, but I don't see us having a forever relationship. On our second date (after Tokyo), I told her it was unlikely we would marry. She was (pleasantly?) surprised by my honesty. She wants to get married and have four kids. I will support her in doing that—after our time together!

Inspired to cry. Three days ago Sabrina's 74-year-old father participated in his U.S. citizenship ceremony. He wept unashamedly.

5:20 p.m., Sunday, May 23, 1999

129 days until "Goodbye, America." The tasks I've set for myself to accomplish between now and October 1st are daunting. And very exciting! As I create my outline of things that I need or want to do before I move to Japan, the magnitude of this endeavor intimidates me. Yet it's my experience that when my clients or I have a "deadline" date, it's amazing what can happen. And my commitment is to do it with leisure. At this point getting many of the tasks/projects done appears quite problematic. That's one reason I'm taking on Charles Sung as my coach for this project. Our first session is tomorrow.

9:24 p.m., Wednesday, June 02, 1999

We're not going to Las Vegas. Sabrina is so funny.

"Why don't we drive to Las Vegas and get married?" she said with some heart.

In the past I'd be defensive and withdraw, but I looked in her eyes, and stayed in touch with my appreciation for her.

"Thank you for loving me so much, and we're not going to Las Vegas," I said.

I am SO blessed to be a life coach. The intensity I have with each of my clients fuels my love for my coaching practice. If my interaction were just with an employer or one or two clients, the intensity level I'd achieve (both ways) would be a mere shadow of what I experience now with about 40 clients at a time. This intensity enlivens me, challenges me, and puts a zesty spring in my step.

5:00 p.m., Thursday, June 03, 1999
An Ayn Rand stamp!!! In 1964, three books by Ayn Rand changed my life. She was considered a pariah by much of society, the media, and the intelligentsia. Today, I bought Ayn Rand stamps at the post office! Ayn Rand vehemently opposed a government monopoly post office both on principle and practicality. If she were alive today, I doubt that she would allow her name to be associated with that government monopoly.

8:25 p.m., Thursday, June 03, 1999
Sabrina's resistance to fishing. I've told Sabrina that I'll teach her to fish, but I won't give her fish, yet I feel pressured to rescue her. My challenge is to stay centered in my affection for her while maintaining my boundaries. I've coached her in job seeking and, to a point, she's coachable, but then she impresses me with her ability to change the subject!

"You widen my horizontal," she says, meaning, you widen my horizons.

10:23 a.m., Friday, June 04, 1999
God bless those endorphins. Exercise slipped from my routine for a few months. Today I deliberately reinstated this truant activity and a few others. It intrigues me what stimulated this new resolve. In the past, whenever I've had scarce time to do a multitude of tasks, my approach was to eliminate as many activities as I could, so that I could be certain I'd get the most important or essential tasks done. This time, however, I'll take a stand to "do it all" and

"have it all," even though, at this point, it doesn't seem possible. I realize that "having it all" means that I will exercise regularly over the next 118 days. (Please note the essay on page 406 for my views on "having it all" as they have evolved since June, 1999.) I will also experiment with regular self-administered rebirthing sessions until I leave for Japan!

10:50 a.m., Monday, July 05, 1999

A world apart, yet so close. In August 1995, I spoke to Yui Hasegawa's high school English class in Sopporo on the northern island of Hokkaido in Japan. We exchanged e-mail addresses and kept in occasional touch. In December 1996 she contacted me from a small college she was attending in Pennsylvania. She and a college friend (another Japanese woman) visited me in Arizona for four days over the Christmas holidays.

About two months ago, the e-mail exchange quickened and deepened. My Chinese friend Sabrina was challenging me with interesting times, and Yui's ex-boyfriend in Hokkaido was confronting her with problematic issues. E-mails zip-zipped over the Pacific Ocean in seconds, at least once per day! We plumbed each other's character and cherished our mutual transparency.

Her dream of writing for a 1700-employee newspaper in Japan is now a heady new reality. Seven hundred and seventy-two applied and Yui was one of the eleven hired!

Yui invited me to wake her at 12:30 a.m. their time this morning, which was 8:30 a.m. here. It was great to celebrate with a ten-minute chat.

1:45 p.m., Monday, July 05, 1999

A problem created by every culture. It's simple, it's a bargain, and it's easy to implement. It would eliminate billions of heartaches and save trillions in currency. Children would be wanted. Starvation would fade away. Why wouldn't everyone support this idea? On an individual-choice basis, it's primarily the attitudes of men (and some religious anachronisms) that prevent this idea's implementation.

Imagine a culture where men, as a "rite of passage" into puberty, underwent a vasectomy before intercourse. The man's ejaculate would be stored for optional use when a baby was wanted. To refuse would make a man a pariah.

The downside could be the likelihood of increased incidence of sexually transmitted diseases, because without the motivation of pregnancy prevention fewer condoms might be used.

Overusing the post office. I've created a new service policy for my clients. Every time I have a telephone session with a client, I mail them a handout (essay), which is usually relevant to what we addressed that day. As a result, I'm mailing 60+ letters a week. This new feature adds a very nice panache to my service and I really enjoy the process. For a bonus it spurs me to write all those essays I still have in my head. Every day I jot notes about new essays I'm eager to write so I can send them out to clients as needed.

Calling Hiroshima. At half past midnight, Sunday, May 23rd, my time, I called Hitomi in Hiroshima where it was 4:30 p.m. the same day. It was so good to hear the smile in her voice. I find it interesting that I cannot say that I am "in love" with either of my two former wives or any of the girlfriends that I had prior to my marriages. However, in some real sense, I am still "in love" with both Hitomi and the girlfriend I had before her (my last two girlfriends) and I suspect I always will be. All it takes is to hear either of their voices and my heart melts as my spirit takes wing.

2:19 a.m. Friday, July 09, 1999

Eating too good feels "bad." Forty-five minutes ago, I awoke and finally took some melatonin. There's an fidgety feeling over the surface of my body, especially on my arms and legs. This feels familiar from past juice fasts when my body was cleansing. I assume that the same physiological response is occurring now. I've been eating better and better. Yesterday, especially, I ate in a very healthy way, with no hunger, while restricting my calories to only 1400. This crawly/fidgety sensation disturbs me. If I returned to a less healthy eating program, the unpleasantness would vanish almost immediately. However, I'm at a new level of inspiration about the life I want to live and where I want to go. As a result, I choose curiosity about this adventure, notice the sensations, allow them to be, and maintain an ongoing inquiry into the costs and benefits of various eating strategies.

I needed to whine. Last weekend I got into a funk. I often recommend "The Whine List" to my clients, so I called Maren and she was willing to participate in the process with me. I bitched, moaned, and complained, holding nothing back. Maren listened and encouraged me to whine more. Within ten minutes I was all whined out. Afterwards, I was able to see that if I give up trying to make myself feel better and am present with my body and my needs, allowing myself to whine fully and completely, then the funk disappears and my exuberance is renewed.

7:48 a.m., Saturday, July 17, 1999

"Why are you moving to Japan?" Ruth Alice (my mother's cousin) asked via e-mail. Thanks, Ruth Alice, here it is:

(1)   My life inspirations are connection, adventure, playfulness, innocence, and romance.

(2)   I relish the presence of and conversation with women.

(3)   My bliss is the rapt attention of attractive women.
Japan's attractions in ascending order:

1%   -> Safety; Japan is physically safer than the U.S.

2%   -> Japanese cuisine ranks a ten in terms of taste, presentation, and healthfulness.

3%   -> Psychological/cultural adventure has high value for me. Being "outside" their culture, yet inside their country, I experiment with behavior in ways that, submerged in my own culture, wouldn't occur to me. Outside my culture I'm freer to express my authentic self.

94%   -> I **love** the "dance" that occurs between me and Japanese women.

How Japanese women show up for me:

(1)   Three quarters of them are physically alluring.

(2)   They express a child-like innocence that enchants me.

(3)   At least with me, they seem non-defensive. In a train station, I can say, "How are you?" to an attractive lady,

and twenty minutes later, we've exchanged telephone numbers and e-mail addresses and she's made it clear she'd welcome friendship.

(4) I experience them as great listeners. They make special sounds to indicate their active interest.

(5) They embody a gentleness that evokes serene safety and willing vulnerability.

How we interact together:

(1) They're exotic for me and I'm a "movie star" to them. The mutual intensity is immediate and I totally love it!

(2) I love our eye-to-eye, soul-to-soul contact. The Japanese caution against eye contact. However, when I meet Japanese women, prolonged eye contact is often spontaneous.

(3) We enjoy the freedom to be ourselves. Because we're both "outside our respective cultures" we experience a freedom to connect and communicate with a candor improbable within our own cultures. I call this the cross-cultural freedom effect. This phenomenon absolutely amazes me.

How I show up for Japanese women:

(1) I am like a celebrity for them.

(2) Simply because I'm a native English speaker, I'm valued.

(3) Gentleness is a highly valued trait in Japan and, even though my approach is often forward, they are very appreciative of my gentle and considerate manner.

(4) As an American with gentlemanly bearing and manner, they accord me keen attention, respect, and admiration.

The upshot? I feel powerful and accepted. To me, why I'm moving to Japan is a no-brainer. It just makes sense.

On the slow boat to Japan. The twelve-pound test package went out today to my friend Keiko Inaki in Tokyo. I included items that would represent most categories that I would ship in the future:

books, paper, soy protein powder, a can opener, Post-it notepaper, a sweater. The package was marked as a gift and cost $27.93 to ship. ETA is within eight weeks. I'm testing three things: how long it takes for the package to get there; what custom duties, if any, are charged; and if the package is delivered to her door or she has to pick it up at the post office.

Today I quizzed my "air consolidator," from whom I intend to buy my roundtrip ticket, about fees for extra luggage on my flight to Tokyo. With a payment of $77 for each extra piece of luggage, the number of pieces I can take is limited only by my pocketbook and desire. The usual luggage size and weight limits apply to each piece.

4:19 a.m., Tuesday, July 20, 1999

How to express unpopular ideas powerfully? Until my mid-teens, I argued and debated with relish, but enjoyed few friends. In *How to Win Friends and Influence People* by Dale Carnegie, I discovered why I had few friends and stopped arguing. However, I also stopped disclosing my opinions and sharing myself openly.

The Landmark Wisdom Course encourages us to move private thoughts into dialogue. Last week (in my weekly Wisdom community group) we discussed a couple whose son was born with severe congenital disabilities. The mother split. The father started a foundation to address his son's type of condition, and created something great in himself. We honor his type of action (as we should). However, we don't honor the courage to quit, especially to quit powerfully and with dignity. I don't know if the woman exercised courage, but we didn't ask. I kept my thoughts private. Then someone in the group asked, "Are you withholding something?"

"Our culture doesn't celebrate the courage to choose endings," I risked alienation to say. "Divorcing my last wife was the biggest act of courage of my entire life. Marriages are celebrated, but not divorces. Yet, it's endings that make new beginnings possible."

And alienate it did! One lady apologized afterwards for her strong reaction to me.

I thought, how could I share my ideas, which are often radical, without shattering rapport? I requested coaching and received helpful feedback. My new approach:

"What you said about that woman's lack of commitment to her family suggests an idea I'd like your feedback on. Okay? . . . I know from personal experience that it is possible for divorce to be a choice of considerable courage, clear vision, and follow-through. I'm in an ongoing inquiry about this. I'd love to receive your candid feedback on pros and cons in celebrating divorces and other endings and honoring the courage to make life's tough choices and walk a difficult and perhaps lonely path with dignity. What do you think?"

Mutual inquiry, instead of statements of opinion, encourage what I desire: self-expression and inquiry for others and myself, and enhancement of our mutual connection.

6:05 p.m., Friday, July 23, 1999

I'll never cook for them again. Yasuhiko and Kumiko Ito will come from Japan to visit in September. I laugh when I recall (in the spring of 1997 when I stayed in their home for two days) how I cooked a meal for them "my style." Poor Kumiko watched in horror as I, with no inkling, desecrated her culinary rules. Judging by their one dainty helping, my "treat" was outside their gustatory boundaries.

They were amazed at how famously I got along with timid Mio (their three-year-old daughter). It'll be a special joy to see Mio (now five) again.

૭૦

_____

_____

_____

_____

_____

_____

_____

_____

_____

_____

Questing and Questioning the World

6:51 p.m., Sunday, July 25, 1999

The power of the "lazy" man. Since reading Stephen Covey's *The Seven Habits of Highly Effective People*, I've incorporated ample free time into my schedule. I now take time to "sharpen the saw," explore opportunities and ideas that I wouldn't have the leisure or energy for if I designed my life with scant buffers and packed it with must-do's.

Someone said that if a person is to make a major difference in the world, they must be a little underemployed. Whether or not I end up making a major difference in the world remains to be seen, but I've got the underemployed part handled!

I'd read about great people who engaged in lengthy correspondence with colleagues, discussing issues and problems that intrigued them.

"I'd never have patience for that," was my attitude prior to a few years ago.

Yet, today, that's what I do. I send e-mail around the world in a split second and receive a reply within hours. Computers, e-mail, built-in spelling and grammar checkers. Wow! Do I love the opportunities and thoughts they bring to me with such ease!

The dialogue generated by my journals and *Courage Now* (an e-mail newsletter that stimulated the writing of this book) educates and excites me, and this is ample reward to stimulate me to put ideas on paper. It's fun. I "steal" time from other areas of my life. It takes no patience at all.

2:01 p.m., Friday, July 30, 1999

Me become a minister? My friend Ceci, who's getting married on September 5th, invited me to be the minister who presides at her wedding to her fiancé, Reid. I feel so honored and touched that she asked me. (Just twenty-five dollars would make me a minister with the Universal Life Church of California!)

However, I'm just as amazed at how confronted I am by this

idea: "What!? Me a minister who marries people?!" Exploration of this automatic reaction provided Ceci and me with some fun. (My brother-in-law became a minister through the Universal Life Church just so he could preside at my first wedding.)

"I'm leaving the invitation open," Ceci said with an irresistible smile while she searched my face for reaction.

I think someone else will preside at her wedding.

The power of paper. A graphic artist and I are designing my new stock stationery paper. This is so exciting. Michael Schnell, a graphic arts college student, works as an intern for an architectural firm in Santa Monica. Is he good! At least for what I want. We have one or two more drafts to go and then the stationery will go to press. It look's so good! I'm eager for you to see it.

I'll order 10,000 sheets; that will last me for over three years.

8:00 a.m., Saturday, July 31, 1999

A secret partially unveiled. I haven't mentioned it before. It was too fresh—perhaps too fragile. Three and a half weeks ago I received this e-mail from a former client/friend in Cleveland whom I have never met.

"I will regret it for the rest of my life if I do not meet you face to face before you leave for Japan," she wrote.

Ever since then we have exchanged e-mails at least once per day and many phone calls. Never before have I felt as romantically close to someone whom I have never met nor even seen a picture of yet!

We are both excited and scared about her impending arrival on the sixteenth for a three-day visit. We know there's little likelihood of our relationship continuing in a way where we can be physically together. Given our other desires and commitments, we'll take what we can get. Our "relationship purpose" and our "relationship's direction" have been teased out in our discussions.

"Historically, I'd have asked myself, 'Would I marry this man?' 'Would I want this man to father my children?'" she said. "The purpose was elsewhere. My motives were elsewhere, not of the present," she added.

"I've operated in similar fashion, looking to the future to justify the present," I replied. "But now, in this moment, I suggest we consider asking ourselves this: Is there anything about this projected intimacy that would damage either of us or be costly into the future?" We contemplated it.

"No!" we concluded and leapt at the opportunity to embrace the present with each other.

"Is our 'purposeless' relationship sufficient unto itself (via e-mail and phone)?" My move and her plans precipitated the need for this discussion. We've resolved to have the present be enough, and don't know how this tryst will evolve. No guarantees. Actually, this way of being with relationships (especially romantic relationships) keeps romance zesty.

In *Getting the Love You Want*, Dr. Harville Hendrix says the power struggle commences when couples commit. Before that, it's all honeymoon. I say it's possible to keep the honeymoon going indefinitely. However, lovers must share willingness to remain at risk. The feeling of love and romance is so strong, we demand its guarantee. Yet, the guarantee itself most often kills what it was intended to protect.

6:25 p.m., Tuesday, August 03, 1999

The first shower of my life. At Ceci and Reid's couples' shower, I was enlightened by discussions with Lena and Corina, with whom I spoke separately. I projected that my unusual questions ("What do you find most confusing about men?") made Lena uncomfortable, because her eyes flitted about the room. Corina seemed uncomfortable also. I asked Corina for feedback, emphasizing the value of her candid disclosures.

"Coach me on how I might act differently so you'd enjoy our conversation and feel more rapport," I requested.

"Jumping right in with deep sharing is uncomfortable for me. Try a slower approach," she advised.

I then quizzed Lena.

"I loved your questions. They weren't the boring party type. I felt 100% rapport. I've no suggestions to offer." Then added, "You might arrange these discussions in settings with fewer distractions. Focus is difficult when a party is swirling around me."

Two women. Similar behavior. Two entirely different realities.

It's amazing what I discover when I don't assume I know what is happening!

8:00 a.m., Friday, August 06, 1999

My friend in Japan does the Forum. Keiko Inaki called me from Tokyo this morning at 7:15 my time. It was 11:15 p.m. tomorrow her time. She'd just finished her first day of the Landmark Forum. When I completed a review of the Forum in Tokyo in May of this year, she was one of two people who came as my guests to learn about the course. She signed up for it. Just now she called to ask a few things about her homework. I'm eager to hear how it goes for her. She will complete the three full days of the Forum at about 7 a.m. my time tomorrow.

❧

From Sunset Days in the USA to the Sunrise Days in Japan

8:20 a.m., Wednesday, August 11, 1999

Fear at Magic Mountain. Yuko (my ex-wife) and Lucas, her son (age 11), arrived from Phoenix for a visit. Lucas wanted to experience Magic Mountain (a first for both of us) and Yuko had some business to attend to. I let Lucas lead and didn't know if I'd take any rides. Under the theory that fewer inches represents less scary, I decided to try a 42-inch height requirement roller coaster (a minimum height requirement is set for each ride). I did okay, and took more rides. The final ride, however, was the 54-inch Riddler's Revenge! I balked. Twenty-seven minutes in line and I still planned to step aside when it was time for Lucas to board the roller coaster, but I began to argue with myself.

"There's no point in taking this ride. It's just scary." Then another voice countered, "But there's no point in not doing this, either. It's only fear. There is no danger. It's a perfect opportunity to practice courage." I took the ride and felt disappointment. It wasn't as scary as I'd anticipated!

8:50 p.m., Thursday, August 12, 1999

Mea culpa! A breakthrough with Lucas. I took Yuko and Lucas to LAX (LA International Airport). Shortly after returning home I received a call from Lucas, from Phoenix, thanking me for the fun. However, I could hear his Dad in the background pressuring him to share something, and Lucas's voice sounded strained with resisted tears. I created a safe space for him.

"I admire that you've considered sharing with me. I understand your fear, and I'm safe to share with," I said.

"I left $25 and some change on a side table at your apartment. Did you pick up my money?" Lucas asked, trying to act casual.

"No," I said. But later I remembered picking up the $25 (thinking at the time it must have been mine). I mailed the $25 to him immediately. I called back and apologized with the same casualness he'd used, laughing it off as a funny mistake.

Lucas was more distressed than I thought and, with his father's encouragement, called me again to share his upset. I apologized profusely.

"Lucas, you are very important to me. I always want to know if I've upset you, or if I've treated you unfairly. Is there anything I could do or say to make things whole for you again?" I asked.

"Everything is okay now," he said.

8:41 p.m., Sunday, August 29, 1999

We are the people around us. One of the ideas that is promulgated again and again within Landmark is that who we are is a function of the people in our lives. How we "show up" in the world for ourselves and for others is strongly influenced by the "environment" of the people around us. When I went from the 9th grade into the 10th grade in high school I changed communities, from Flatrock, South Carolina (a small provincial, lower middle-class community) to Shelby, North Carolina (a somewhat larger, middle-class community). When I was "inside" the Flatrock community, in addition to my parents and siblings, the people of that community were my world. Yet I had no sense that who I was "being" was, in large measure, a function of those people. After moving to the new community, and later gaining perspective on that move, I began to see that who I had "become" in moving to Shelby was a significantly "different" person (whom I liked better) than the person I had been in Flatrock.

Landmark's "action approach" on this idea is to encourage people to transform their "people environment" by enrolling those people into the Landmark work. Makes a lot of sense.

I notice for myself, however, that I am able to pick people to be my "environment" (i.e., my friends and clients and family) who constantly inspire me with their lives (regardless of whether or not they've done Landmark work).

A very interesting action expression of this principle is coming up for me. Fundamentally, the number-one reason I am moving to Japan is because "who I am" and "how I show up for myself" in the "environment" of most Japanese women is someone that I totally love to be. I can be "more myself" with ease and grace and adventure in a way that does not usually occur for me in the United States. And, I am sure, as I find and choose my friends in Japan, that effect will be even more enhanced!

The bottom line is this: I am moving to Japan because I so much like who I "become" in the presence of the Japanese women in Japan.

9:42 a.m., Saturday, September 04, 1999

My "Boing Kangaroo Boots" arrived. Walking or running with these is similar to a workout on a tightly stretched mini-trampoline. I strode (seven inches taller) to the bank and the teller, rather nonplussed, said,

"Have you grown or something?!"

What fun! I played with how fast I could boing, and passed runners, overtook skateboarders, passed bicyclists and received several cheers! After a few minutes, however, I needed to walk. When I passed the weekend bands, I boinged to the music. Kids grinned and I boing-skipped.

An hour of boinging was the best workout I've ever had without using will power!

In Japan, I will already stand out as a tall American; boinging might be too much! I'm not sure even I can stand that much attention.

The five fears of Dwight. My friend David Saxby has been an effective guide for me through multiple breakthroughs. Today I presented him with a chronic stressor. At issue is a conflict between five parts of me that bicker and fight over "limited territory."

The "Impeccable Dwight" wants to do all tasks to his total and complete satisfaction.

The "Responsible Dwight" wants to keep agreements and promises that he needs/wants/should keep. He appreciates the benefits of consistency in kept agreements.

The "New Idea Dwight" wants to put Michelangelo Buonarroti to shame. (I looked up the full name to satisfy "Impeccable Dwight"!) Not that I feel competitive with Michelangelo, but I want to do so many things!

The "Comfort/Pleasure Dwight" wants to do whatever he wants, whenever he wants, without regard for plans, ideas, promises, obligations, reasonability, health, etc.

The "Spontaneous Dwight" thirsts after the freedom to always be able to act on the excitement and intuition of the moment.

All five Dwights are strong components of who I am. Often they collide in competition for my time and focus. Clients and friends are seldom aware of this conflict. My own selective awareness of it is rare; the conflict just clutters up my mental-emotional background.

David suggested logic: make a choice, choose what's important and decide what costs and benefits I am willing to trade off. I felt the answer wasn't in that direction.

A fundamental principle that I've discovered in life coaching is this: if you have a continuing issue or problem/complaint in your life, the source is most probably your resistance to fear.

So I looked for the resisted fear, asking these questions:

What does Impeccable Dwight fear will happen if he doesn't get his way enough?

I'm frightened I'll bypass the juice of life by not following every item to the end of the road. I'll miss the full sense of completion and celebration earned through doing a masterful job.

What does Responsible Dwight fear will happen if he doesn't get his way enough?

If I don't keep agreements with myself and others, I won't do what it takes to create the essential accoutrements of life (like good health and enough money). Or I will miss out on exciting experiences (like the state of mind that results from practicing my Deep Awakening Renewal process).

What does New Idea Dwight fear will happen if he doesn't get his way enough?

What if I don't have the time to develop this/that/those ideas? To consider that I won't do these things, or at least some of them, distresses me. It frightens me to accept the disappointment that I don't have time to do, or even start, everything I think of.

What does Comfort/Pleasure Dwight fear will happen if he doesn't get his way enough?

Sometimes I just want to feel good. I don't want to persevere, be fearless, or choose courage. I want some down time to veg out. If I can't have that time, especially when I really want it, I'm frightened life will seem a treadmill, that I'll feel like I'm constantly going nowhere.

What does Spontaneous Dwight fear will happen if he doesn't get his way enough?

I'm afraid I'll miss that "in-the-moment" opportunity, or that a special feeling of excitement will escape. I'm frightened I'll miss out on what God is trying to hand me, because I'm not paying attention.

My breakthrough is the acceptance that, with this dilemma, there's no way to allay the legitimate fears of the five Dwights. There is, however, a way through: recognition and acceptance of each Dwight's fears as they arise through using the "Making Friends with Your Fear" process, honoring the five-year-old Dwight for the courage he chooses to stay engaged with life while he experiences these fears.

Here's my plan: The Responsible Dwight will put together an overview process, which details the passions, fears, and reminder items for each of the five "kingdoms of Dwight." Periodically, I'll review these five kingdoms and give proactive recognition to each kingdom's fears.

In the past, much of my successful function depended on disregard of each kingdom's sacrifices. And, with dissonance among my five kingdoms, I paid a price in my performance and fundamental peace.

I'm excited about this new project! I am so thankful to David for helping me create this breakthrough.

10:24 a.m., Wednesday, September 08, 1999

I was there in history. Yesterday, at my local Blockbuster Video store, *The Passion of Ayn Rand* was a featured new release. I gawked. My friend Maren noticed my astonishment and said she wanted to watch the movie with me.

The film spotlights Ayn Rand, her husband Frank O'Connor, Nathaniel Branden, and Barbara Branden. In 1967-68, when I was single in New York City, I met all of them, took classes from Nathaniel and Barbara, and Ayn Rand autographed my copy of *Atlas Shrugged*. Of the four, my closest contact was with Nathaniel Branden. After his break with Ayn Rand, I attended "weekend intensives" and did some one-on-one work with him.

The movie spanned the period from 1951, when Nathaniel and Barbara first met Ayn Rand and Frank O'Connor, to the 1968 breakup between Ayn and Nathaniel.

As I watched the movie, I found myself feeling uncomfortable. The movie portrayed unsettling aspects of Ayn Rand's personality— things I'd noticed in person, but had written off as aberrations. I found these things disturbing, although they did nothing to negate her philosophy. Back when I knew her, I had tried to justify her frequent condemnation of peoples' motives, should they appear to be tainted by altruism. At the end of Dr. Branden's seminars on Objectivist philosophy, Ayn Rand was sometimes present to entertain questions from the audience. If she were asked a question that implied an altruistic presumption, she would publicly excoriate the questioner—something that always troubled me. After a few years of attending Objectivist lectures and mixing with Objectivists, I drifted away. The harshness and lack of gentleness and compassion among most of Ayn Rand's students repelled me. I found myself attracted to people that I often disagreed with intellectually, but felt a deeper affinity with emotionally.

What impressed me in watching the movie was how actress Helen Mirren portrayed the personality and features of Ayn Rand. From my experience, Helen was right on!

What my ex-wife taught me. My primary strategy for survival in life had been accommodation. I might have appeared assertive sometimes, but it was inside of being an accommodator. My second wife Yuko's primary strategy for survival was assertion. She appeared accommodating sometimes, but it was inside of being an asserter. Given our life-survival strategies, our selection of each other made perfect sense. People often choose partners who embody an aspect of themselves that they've disowned.

Yuko's most precious gift to me was an unintentional one. She compelled me to step outside my "safe" box of accommodation. To leave her (she wouldn't leave me) was the biggest choice of courage of my entire life. It required that I dismantle my self-image as the good-guy accommodator.

What is interesting is my life-long pattern of attraction to assertive women. Ayn Rand was the archetype of assertion, a woman who had scarcely developed any capacity for accommodation at all. Loretta, my first real girlfriend, was highly assertive. All my significant girlfriends and the woman I was married to before Yuko were also in the assertive camp, at least in comparison to me.

This pattern disintegrated after my breakup with Yuko. The women I've fallen in love with since then haven't been more assertive than I and, perhaps in some cases, have been a little less assertive.

$473 roundtrip to Japan! Korean Airlines Flight #2 will leave

LAX at 10:00 a.m. on November 4th. Total cost with taxes, delivery charge, etc. is $473! Absolutely amazing. For a roundtrip, one-year, open-ended ticket!

I could have waited longer before I purchased the ticket. However, I knew that to purchase the ticket early would feed my excitement, and that my heightened anticipation will release a bonanza of energy that I can use as I focus on preparations for the move.

6:09 p.m., Wednesday, September 15, 1999

I can't wait for computers to be smarter than me! *The Age of Spiritual Machines: When Computers Exceed Human Intelligence* is the most exciting (and in some ways terrifying) book I've read about the future of the human race.

Moore's Law (Gordon Moore, inventor of integrated circuits, and former chairman of Intel) states that the speed of computers available at a given price doubles roughly every eighteen months. Ray Kurzweil, in The Age of Spiritual Machines, cogently demonstrates that Moore's Law has been in operation since 1908, when the Hollerith Tabulator (the first calculating machine) was invented. From 1908 until 1950, roughly every three years the number of calculations per second per $1000 of machine cost doubled. From 1950 to 1966, the doubling accelerated to every eighteen months. And since 1966, the doubling has been occurring roughly every twelve months!

In 1997 the computer (Deep Blue) beat Gary Kasparov, the Russian world chess champion. That means that it was possible to program a computer to be smarter than the smartest man in the world in the domain of chess.

Ray Kurzweil conservatively predicts that by the year 2010 a computer will exist that will be judged by the Turing Test (a test in which humans are asked to decide whether or not the "intelligence" on the other end of an "Internet chat" is a human or a computer) as being as intelligent as a human being! By the year 2020, a desktop computer costing $4000 or less will be equal to your intelligence. By the year 2060 one computer will equal the intelligence of all 12 billion humans on this earth combined.

What are the implications? Read the book!

6:10 a.m., Thursday, September 16, 1999

How to recognize myself? All my life, when looking at that man in the mirror, I'd feel surprise that the face associated with me looked as it did. As if "that's not what I look like!" If anyone were to ask what I "really look like," I would not be able to easily tell them. I just wouldn't be like "that man in the mirror." It's not that I'm displeased with what I look like. If I had complete and easy free rein, I might play around with my body some, but basically I'm happy with my looks. My looks just don't reflect me as I "feel and conceptualize" myself. It would be fascinating to sit down with a computer program that allows one to modify faces. I'd like to see what face I'd create to express my essence.

Perhaps I'm disassociated from my body, and this represents an opportunity to "fully own" my body. Or perhaps it's an expression of my spirituality such that I'm experiencing self as distinct from my body. That's something I could rejoice in. Ha!

1:43 p.m., Thursday, September 16, 1999

Too much boinging! This is a totally new experience for me. With an extra long break looming deliciously, I boinged down to the boardwalk. On the boardwalk I stretched my boinging out to a glorious full stride. What fun! But not for long. The front muscles in my upper legs began to hurt. Wow, so much intense exercise so fast! Knowing that if I continued, even though I wanted to, I would pay for it, I decided to turn back. Bounce by bounce I returned home. Always before, I stopped my exercise because I didn't feel like it anymore or because I'd put in my allotted time, not because it was prudent to pace myself. I love it!

6:00 p.m., Friday, September 17, 1999

The Internet strikes again. One project I'm choosing to complete in the next 47 days is the "Find a Place to Live" project. The way I've structured it, I will be fine if I don't find the place to live before I get to Tokyo, because I've allotted two weeks in the plan to find a place once I'm there. Yet it's a rewarding challenge to explore how much I can move in that direction from here in Hermosa Beach, California, using the Internet.

Two English websites published in Tokyo allowed me to place free ads. Here is what I wrote: "English speaking (U.S.) male, 55 years old, professional consultant, seeks 20+ *tsubo* living area, no more than one-hour train ride from Shinagawa Station. Able to pay up to 150,000 yen per month for indefinite residency. References available. Need to rent from November 15th. E-mail: Dwight@GoldWinde.com or fax 206-312-0071 (USA)." (A "*tsubo*" equals about 3.3 square meters.)

Although not essential, I plan to participate in some Landmark Education events, and the Landmark center is near Shinagawa station. If I can't find any affordable living unit within a one-hour radius, I will content myself to make my home where I find the best deal.

Already I've received three responses (one each from an American, a Japanese, and a Korean) about apartments, after subscribing to the "Living in Yokohama" mailing list and sending out a broadcast e-mail requesting information on a place to live! I now have their private e-mail addresses and can correspond with them directly. It feels great to be in action!

8:36 p.m., Wednesday, September 22, 1999

So many great women in my life! In two days my mother will arrive from Tennessee!

6:15 p.m., Wednesday, October 06, 1999

Mama helps me leave our country. Mama and I packed and shipped eleven boxes and one mailing tube (over 400 pounds total), to two friends in Japan, one in Tokyo and one in Yokohama. I'm hoping to keep the total number of bags I have to check when I fly to five (I'll have to pay the $77 extra-bag charge on three).

My mother and I were a joy for each other for all ten days. We are always the best of company for each other, and this time seemed better than ever.

3:18 a.m., Saturday, October 16, 1999

A wish come true: an earthquake.

"LOS ANGELES (AP)—An earthquake struck Southern California, a long rumbler that shook buildings from Los Angeles to Las Vegas. No reports of damage or injuries yet. That was a bad one, but we're fine. Lucy Jones of the California Institute of

Technology said the quake measured 7.0. It struck about 3 a.m." — The Associated Press.

I awoke to a sway, slight enough that I wasn't sure what was causing it. As the swaying increased, however, my window blinds began to swing in arcs and rattle against each other, and I said to myself, "Yes! This is an earthquake!" Next I heard a splash outside my open window and thought, "Someone must be very excited about this earthquake to jump into the pool!" I opened my door and saw waves of water actually splash out of the pool, up onto the pool deck, and gush down the steps and corridors toward the street below. My next-door neighbor, Lori, was outside her door in pajamas talking on a cordless phone. Others congregated outside.

Out in front of my complex I met the Hermosa Beach Fire Department. They had come to check out a report of a broken water main, but it turned out to be just our pool splashing onto the street!

I'd looked forward to experiencing some California earthquakes, but had given up hope. Well, I got my wish.

Natural disasters excite me. My mother describes an experience from when I was about one year old and our family lived in Guam. She says she remembers sitting on the bed with my father and me during a raging typhoon: the water was one foot deep on the floor. She says she loved the experience. I suspect that I learned my love of storms from her.

5:23 p.m., Saturday, October 16, 1999

From California to Arizona to Tokyo (at the speed of light).
Using three-way calling, I put a call through to my friend Yoko Facundus in Scottsdale, Arizona and then Iwai-san in Tokyo. For the first two weeks, while I look for a place to live, I plan to stay with Iwai-san. However, Iwai-san is 61 and like most of the older generation in Japan, doesn't speak much English. I wanted to confirm that everything was still okay per my previous arrangements with her, and to let her know when I will arrive. That's why I needed Yoko as interpreter.

Although my flight will arrive at 2:40 p.m. on Friday, November 5th, through Yoko, I told Iwai-san that I will arrive at her house between 5:30 and 8:00 p.m. I will be going through customs, but the main reason I'm allowing such a wide margin for my arrival time is that I will have between four and six pieces of checked luggage (in addition to my carry-ons)! I plan to just take my time moving the pieces in multiple trips as I get on and off the trains. Other Japanese travelers are likely to help, but I don't want to count on that. The final train stop brings me within a twelve-minute walk of Iwai-san's home. From that point I'll try to see if I can get all my bags into a taxi (maybe more than one trip)! That it will be a magnificent and uncertain adventure, I'm sure.

Yoko mentioned my search for my new home to Iwai-san. She said Iwai-san volunteered to help me in my quest.

8:30 a.m., Tuesday, October 19, 1999

Fifteen days until Japan. I'm going to be embarking on the biggest change of my entire life! What an adventure!

Always time for romance. My tight schedule just got tighter. My Cleveland girlfriend arrives on the 31st and departs at midnight on the 2nd. I'm so excited to see her again! I'll shut down the office and the "rest of my life" for three days. I'll then have one day, Wednesday the 3rd, to let everybody pick up their "yard sale" purchases, have Noe (my computer expert) pack my computer, ship final boxes, throw away or put out for Goodwill items that weren't sold, and clean the apartment spotlessly in order to get my security deposit back in full! Except for these few things, I have to have everything complete by the 31st.

5:10 a.m., Friday, October 22, 1999
A visit from yesteryear.

Frank Jorgensen is flying in for a three-day visit. It's been twelve plus years, at least, since I saw him! In Shelby, North Carolina his mother, Solveig, from Norway, and my mother were best friends. The past two-plus years I've had the pleasure and honor of brainstorming ideas with him for the resort and railroad he runs in West Virginia.

9:42 a.m., Sunday, October 31, 1999
Skipping my Wisdom class. To get things complete before my girlfriend from Cleveland arrives at 9 p.m., I called in to take the

day off from my Landmark Wisdom Course. Wow, what a full day I have ahead!

I made the confirmation call for my flight on Korean Airlines leaving at 10:00 a.m. on Thursday. They gave me seat 34G.

From this point on (until further notice), everything I share will have been transcribed from long hand, since my word processor requires a wall plug, and I won't be around one of those for a day or two.

8:36 a.m., Wednesday, November 03, 1999

A lifetime in three days. I'm thrilled she came back! And now she's left and I may never see her again. It was special beyond description for both of us. So much opened up; it seems long ago that she arrived.

9:50 a.m., Thursday, November 04, 1999

10, 9, 8, 7, 6 . . . blast off! The flight is only a little over one-third full, so I have two seats to myself.

Of the thousands of things that could have gone wrong in an undertaking of this complexity, so far the only mishap I've noticed is the loss of one cufflink on the shirt that I'm wearing. (I'm using a paper clip to keep my cuff together!)

I just asked the stewardess for some water. I will drink at least one cup each hour. I also took my first homeopathic "No-Jet-Lag" tablet, with others to follow every two hours.

10:02 a.m. Backing out of the gate. Flight time is estimated at 11 hours and 15 minutes.

I stretched the limit on baggage: seven checked pieces (with a 70-lb limit each). One box exceeded the 70-lb limit by several pounds. (I had already packed the bathroom scales in that box!) Each piece of luggage exceeding the two I get with my ticket cost me an extra $77. Officially they were supposed to charge me triple for the one box that exceeded the limit. However, with my explanation about having already packed the bathroom scales inside the box in question, and a gentle request to talk with someone about the issue, the penalty was waived and I paid $385 extra for the five boxes, as if they were all within the weight limit.

As I boarded the plane with my four bags, the gate agent suggested that I was exceeding the carry-on limit of two bags. I asked him if it would help if I could stuff one bag inside another. He passed me on through. Perhaps if the flight had been more fully booked, he would have insisted I check something as regular luggage.

10:40 a.m. A menu is handed out. For lunch we have the option of *pibimbap* or fillet of salmon. For dinner a choice of *pulgogi* or chicken curry. Of course, I'll take the *pipimbap* and *pulgogi*.

10:50 a.m. Hot, wet hand towels are being served.

10:10 a.m. (Japan time). We just passed over the International Date Line. Four hours and 40 minutes to go.

In just a few days Japan will essentially (right after New Zealand and Australia) be the first country to welcome the new millennium.

8:40 p.m., Friday, November 05, 1999 Tokyo, Japan

Watch out, Japan! Here I am! Our jet arrived only a few minutes late at Narita airport; it was a long walk to passport control and then to baggage claim. The airport luggage carts are free at Narita, seemingly supported by advertisements on the carts. Three carts were necessary to carry my seven checked bags and four carry-ons. I was the last in line for customs control and I got a little more than the customary brush through. But after several questions as to the purpose of my visit (long vacation) and who I would stay with, the customs officer passed me through without examining anything. I really didn't want to open even one of those boxes. I imagine the customs official felt that way, too.

Take the subway with seven bags totaling 210 kg (about 460 lbs)? In relays I managed to walk my three carts to where I could exchange $500 for yen. The QLine Baggage Delivery Service relieved me of the difficult time, not to mention the probable upset of many Japanese commuters who I would have inconvenienced, if I had used the public train system to move my bags. I don't know how I would have made it. The QLine Baggage Delivery Service promised delivery of my seven bags between noon and 8 p.m. the next day. The cost was 1600 yen each (the best way to guesstimate the dollar equivalent is to knock off two zeros, i.e., $16 in this case). There was a 30-kg limit on each bag, so the one 38-kg bag cost 2100 yen. I didn't object to that charge, since the additional fee was roughly proportional to the extra weight involved. The total cost was 11,620 yen—a bargain!

3:40 a.m. in California. My Brother word processor works! It's 8:40 p.m. here and 3:40 a.m. in California. I'm wearing my *yukata* (a traditional informal man's kimono worn around the house) that Takako gave me when I stayed here last May. I'm tired! Good night.

1:30 a.m., Saturday, November 6, 1999

I'm in your tomorrow. It is 8:30 a.m. yesterday in California and my body is savvy to that. Ten minutes ago I awoke and, oddly, I feel rested. On the second story of this five-story house I'm alone and I'm thinking of you, my friends, back there in the States.

Serendipity on the train. At my request, on my trip from the airport, two young Japanese women assisted me in purchasing my train ticket from a vending machine and rode with me the ninety minutes to Shinagawa Station. They'd just returned from sightseeing in China.

"As a woman, what is most confusing for you about men's behavior?" I asked Keiko (age 22).

"I'm a traditional Japanese woman. We don't like to talk about the really important feelings between a man and woman. But I like to assume that my boyfriend and I understand each other," said Keiko.

Then she surprised me with the ease with which she shared with me in depth about her 30-year-old American boyfriend, who will return to the States in March. About her mother (53) who doesn't live with Keiko's father. And how Keiko, her mother, and her mother's father (88) live together in a rather strained environment, with a quiet resentment between her mother and her mother's father. Keiko gave me her e-mail address. I will invite her to check out Landmark Education, and maybe get her mother to check it out as well.

12:05 p.m., Saturday, November 6, 1999

Takako feeds me twice. Dawn barely showed itself over the skyline of Tokyo. About 3 a.m. sleep overcame excitement and I slept until 4:45 a.m. As my new world awakened, I jotted down first impressions and organized a "things-to-do" list with the zest of an adventurer.

Three out-of-towners (two women and a man) came in last night, one from far off Hokkaido. They all slept downstairs, giving me privacy. My friend Iwai-san opens up her home for out-of-towners who are participating with Landmark Education.

At breakfast we (four) savored grilled salmon, rice, seaweed salad, a mushroom stir-fry, miso soup, fresh sliced cucumber and daikon, a tofu dish, various condiments, and bancha tea. Takako conjured this gustatory bonanza for us, and then ate afterwards.

Takako (57) may have a crush on me. The circumstantial evidence: (1) she gave me two *yukatas* when I was here in May, (2) she wore a rather elegant dress just to wait for me when I arrived last night, (3) she's awkward around me, spilled a glass of water, and (4) her apology was excessive (even by Japanese standards).

12:33 a.m., Sunday, November 7, 1999

A Japanese faux pas. Seated on the sofa, I donned my Boing Boots to take Chaco (the dog) for a walk. Entering the foyer, I spied all the shoes lined up, and realized I'd made a major faux pas (Japanese *never* wear their shoes in the house). I apologized to Iwai-san instantly both then and when I got back. ("*Gomen-nasai*!")

The Japanese response to my boinging was interesting, yet predictable. Such a sight is surely more unusual in Japan than in California, yet response was subdued. The Japanese are both less expressive and less intrusive than Americans. If I stop to talk with them, however, I predict that I'll get a more engaged response. And it's possible the boots are too far out.

8:50 p.m., Monday, November 08, 1999

I am now a resident of Tokyo! I signed a letter of agreement and paid a deposit for my place to stay. It's a 10-tatami-mat room (which I later learned comes to about 180 square feet), with abundant storage and use of a common living room, kitchen, and bathroom. Currently only one tenant shares the house. The permanent tenants will max out at three. It's graveyard quiet, because my second-floor room overlooks a peaceful Buddhist graveyard. Yet all this is in the heart of Tokyo and convenient by train to everything.

I get all this for 100,000 yen per month (about $800). I've investigated, and that's a steal. The landlord, Kenichi Anazawa (27), will be my guest tomorrow night at a Landmark graduation. This old house is his fixer upper and is a new business for Kenichi (he was a timber importer). I think he's eager to get his expenses covered. Kenichi and I found each other through an ad I placed in the Tokyo Classifieds (a website), and we've swapped e-mails for a month.

Wednesday, I move in with a truck Kenichi has arranged for. We'll pick up my boxes from Keiko's and Iwan-san's (who live in Tokyo) and from Shigeto's (who lives in Yokohama). Kenichi and I (with help from Ichiro, the other tenant) will move my things. (Ichiro is pronounced Itch-y-lo.)

4:02 p.m., Tuesday, November 9, 1999

Am I making the right choice? Even though I'm solid in my decision, I notice that I am taunted by a stream of automatic fears: What about this? What about that? To acknowledge them I shall list the advantages and disadvantages as I see them now:

Advantages:

(1) The price is very good, even exceptional. A 100,000-yen-per-month apartment is almost unheard of in Tokyo.

(2) The terms are exceptional. If I rented through an agency, the move-in costs would be five times the monthly fee! I'll only pay one month's deposit and the first month's rent. Also, I can move out with three month's notice and Kenichi can only raise the rent at two-year intervals. Also, most landlords/rental agencies require a Japanese guarantor for foreigners. Kenichi has enough confidence in me to not require this, even though I do not have a residency status visa!

(3) Utilities, a house computer with around-the-clock

Internet access, a refrigerator, a microwave, and a clothes washer are included. Two toilets are available: both Western and Japanese style (nothing to sit on, just a "hole" in the floor that requires good squatting skills). Decorating and furnishing the common room to our taste is encouraged.

(4) Kenichi is a searcher and I feel that we will get along great. He understands and appreciates the Western mind and I think we'll be able to maintain a win/win attitude.

(5) The location is fantastic. In terms of accessibility, I could not have chosen a better location. Twenty minutes from Shinagawa station, so I can easily attend Landmark courses if I choose. Looking at my Tokyo map I see that I will be within easy walking/bicycling distance of the National Museum, Ueno Zoological Garden, the Aquatic Zoo, Ueno Park, and Tokyo University. Within a 90-second walk from my front door is a major thoroughfare, with restaurants, banks, stores, etc.

(6) The immediate environment is superb. I am amazed at how quiet it is inside the house. A beautiful Buddhist cemetery is below my balcony windows.

(7) Kenichi has a section of the house set aside for transient international guests. And I have a passion for meeting and making new friends. So this flow of new people to visit with as they come and go, most probably from different parts of Asia, is perfect!

Disadvantages:

(1) I don't have as much private living space as I would like.

(2) There may be some spatial boundary problems in sharing the kitchen, etc.

(3) There may be noise boundary problems. Ichiro Gunji-san, the rather shy, retiring man who lives upstairs in the alcove room, expressed concern over my having guests too often.

(4) There is no heating or cooling provided. I am concerned that the wiring will not provide sufficient power for these things.

All in all, the advantages far outweigh the possible disadvantages. And, worst case, or if I find a much better place, I can give notice and probably be able to exit gracefully, perhaps in less than the three months stipulated in our agreement.

3:45 p.m., Tuesday, November 9, 1999

From California to Tokyo, from dollars to yen, in ten minutes. Even though I had no reason to fear it wouldn't work because it worked fine in Hiroshima last year, I held my breath a bit when I handed my Visa debit card and passport to the Sumimoto Bank money exchange clerk and asked for 300,000 yen. The ten minutes stretched long in my anxious mind, but I got it! The power of electronic communications, free markets, and international agreements amazes me.

Cross-cultural freedom effect with a beautiful woman

This morning I met Hiroko over breakfast. She's up from Nagoya. She's trained to introduce people to Landmark's Breakthrough Technology Course (the course known in the U.S. as the Forum) here in Japan. We hit it off, and I was delighted when she suggested we talk some more before the session tonight. I'll meet her at 5:30 at the Landmark Center and we'll find a place to eat dinner together. The cross-cultural freedom effect operated big-time with us. If she weren't married, and if I didn't live in another city, she'd be a romantic interest.

8:36 p.m., Friday, November 12, 1999

I must avoid "absurd action." Kenichi and I drew up a two-page agreement (in English!) and I paid him the deposit and the money for the remainder of this month. I'll make deposits directly to his account at Citibank. I laughed when I read the section that gives landlords cause for eviction ("if the tenant engages in absurd action"). In the U.S., this clause would be unenforceable. In Japan, however, such a clause is acceptable, since every Japanese knows what "absurd action" is. I can guess what absurd action might be and I may engage in some, like boinging around the neighborhood. I didn't argue.

My environment at "Liberty House." That is Kenichi's name for this home. My 10-tatami-mat room feels smaller than I had imagined it would. The way I've had to arrange the desk I bought puts my computer up pretty high. In fact, I have to stand up to type. The Internet hook-up is not yet accomplished and I must buy a high stool to sit on when I use my computer, but my computer is powered up and it works!

To my immediate right I hear the hum of my electric/kerosene heater. It's set to 20 degrees centigrade and it tells me that the current area temperature in here is 18 degrees. Wearing a long-sleeved turtleneck, I am comfortable.

Must the neighbors approve? Japanese society is very consensus oriented, something I have known for a long time. Still, it surprised me when Kenichi told me he'd invited all eleven immediate neighbors for a meeting tomorrow, to share with them about the foreigner (namely me) who is living in their midst. He requested that I join them.

"I'd be delighted," I said. "But I have that 2 p.m. appointment with Shigeto Omori in Yokohama."

"Go ahead. Keep your appointment. I'll handle everything okay," he said. He then added, "Smile and say hello to each neighbor you pass in the alleyways."

"I've been doing that," I replied.

Getting a haircut, Japanese style. Yesterday I saw a barber shop that offered haircuts for 1000 yen (usual range is 1800 yen or more). First, I had to feed a vending machine 1000 yen to get a ticket. Then I gave my ticket to the lady who seated me in the barber chair. She prepped me (gown, etc.). Once I was properly cosseted and packaged, the barber swept in with the air of a master. Moments later my shag was shorn and he moved on; the lady, with an eye for detail, clipped a little extra and sucked all the loose hair off me with a vacuum cleaner. The sides are a little shorter than I wanted, but it will grow.

1:07 p.m., Tuesday, November 16, 1999
Japan as a check-less society. Japanese typically pay their

bills through ATM machines, through the post office, and through other means I've not yet discovered. Today I needed to pay ASIST corporation 21,000 yen for the setup of my two phone numbers (using a single ISDN line). Through Kenichi's fax, they sent me their bank name and account number and suggested I use an ATM machine to make the payment to their account. Asahi Bank is a two-minute walk from my house. I went to the teller instead of the machine. She smiled graciously.

"No problem. Just fill out this form in *kanji*," she said, as though it was the simplest thing to do. (*Kanji* is the Japanese system of writing based on borrowed or modified Chinese characters.)

"No way!" I declared, feeling consternation. She excused herself and returned, still smiling, with a lady who seemed to be in charge of general customer assistance at the bank. I was escorted to the ATM machine and taken through the process step by step. The machine accepted my 25,000 yen and gave me change, along with a receipt.

Valere, the Frenchman I've worked with to get my phones set up, was able to tell immediately that I'd made the payment, and sent me, via express mail, a device I will need to get everything going on my end. NTT (the rough equivalent of AT&T in its heyday, before it faced competition) is scheduled to install my telephone tomorrow afternoon.

I can now "play" with money. I'm as prudent with money in Japan as I was in the U.S. However, it's less painful to spend in Japan. I seem to have a painful early-childhood association with "giving up" money (specifically dollars). It's as if my survival is in question, unless I associate pain with spending dollars. However, I spend yen like monopoly money, without the pain response. I like the freedom to spend without pain!

Adventures in food shopping. Every time I go grocery shopping I buy at least one mystery item. When I get home, I ask Ichiro or Kenichi what I bought. So far I like everything. I am very thankful that the Japanese use the same numerals as we do, so I know how much items cost before I buy them.

Some neighbors are in an uproar. Kenichi, in general, and I, in particular, appear to have created a crisis in the neighborhood. When Kenichi welcomed Ichiro, a month ago, they visited all the neighbors bearing gifts and everything seemed okay. In the meeting he had with the eleven neighbors on Saturday, three were very favorable to the idea of foreigners as well as Japanese living here, some—like myself and Ichiro—on a semi-permanent basis, with others to be more transient. Three neighbors, however, were adamant that Kenichi's plans for this house are unacceptable. One threatened legal action. Tomorrow Kenichi will consult a lawyer to be certain he's on solid legal ground. But we'd prefer to have our neighbors feel good about us.

Kenichi views the hostile neighbors as prejudiced against foreigners. This neighborhood is old, and most of the people have resided here for over 40 years. More than 98% of the residents of Japan are Japanese. Until recently, the rest (primarily Koreans) were required to carry identity cards to testify to their "Korean-ness," regardless of whether or not they were born here.

The disparity in attitude between people over 45 and those under 45 is much more prominent in Japan than in the U.S. Japanese youth are pro-foreigner, especially with regard to Americans. Their attitude could almost be characterized as infatuation, whereas members of the older generation are often xenophobic.

Ichiro, Kenichi, and I have adopted the following strategies: (1) I will continue to say "Hello" (in Japanese, "*Konnichiwa*") to all the people I pass in the neighborhood. (2) I will not throw a housewarming party or entertain foreign guests until Kenichi returns from Asia in mid-January. (3) I will not buy kerosene for my heater (Ichiro will buy it for me), since a neighbor expressed fear that I, as a foreigner, would not understand the buttons on my electric kerosene heater and might start a fire. (4) Kenichi won't rent to anyone else while he's away. (5) We'll let the neighbors get used to me. (6) We will encourage any police, fire, or health inspectors to come to the house as desired or requested by the neighbors. (7) Kenichi suggested we say that he and I have known each other for a year via e-mail so that the fearful neighbors might find comfort in the assumption that he knows me well. We already know and trust each other better than many people who have known each other a long time.

On Kenichi's request, I coached him on how to talk/listen to the neighbors so that they will feel confident he has really listened to them. This impressed him. And I lent him the book, *Instant Rapport*.

I bought flowers for Kaiko Miharu, the lady next door who is on our side. She was gracious in her appreciation.

I notice that, although I'd like the neighbors to feel good about me living here, it doesn't concern me in the same way that it would if I were living in America under similar circumstances. Even though I'm surrounded by Japanese culture, it doesn't have me in the same way that the American culture has me. For Kenichi, however, the Japanese culture does have him, even though he thinks it doesn't. His actions are more in rebellion than in transcendence. Hey, he's only 27! I'm 55 and I'm still working on it!

9:38 a.m., Wednesday, November 17, 1999

Walk right in: don't bother to ask. The door was unlocked and the deliveryman opened the door and walked right into the foyer without any permission. This is not considered rude or unusual in Japan. In fact, it would probably be considered unusual if he knocked and waited for me to answer. He delivered the special telephone equipment (which I signed for) that is needed to get my ISDN line operational once the NTT people come to install the equipment this afternoon. Until then, I will organize and put away my things.

Nurses in the night. Last night on my 25-minute walk to Asasuka I talked with two nurses (both 21). The 15-minute conversation was a thrill for me. For a man to start up a conversation on the sidewalk in a big city at night with two 21-year-old women (where there's no defensiveness, just delight) is something that would be rather atypical in the U.S. After today, I'll focus on exploring the city and socializing, since my infrastructure is in place for living and doing business in Japan—all accomplished in under two weeks! Amazing!

Translation by phone to get my phone. About 11 a.m. I got a call on my mobile phone (which my friend Keiko had helped me get when I first arrived in Japan). I could tell it was from the NTT man. But, aside from that, we weren't able to communicate much. After he hung up, another NTT man, this time one who could speak English, called me. He told me that the NTT man who had called me before was downstairs waiting for me! I don't know why he didn't try the buzzer or knock loudly (strange, given my experience before).

Once I let him in, using his mobile phone, we communicated with the translator the few things we couldn't do with sign language. I now have my two numbers installed and tested.

8:45 a.m., Thursday, November 18, 1999

We won't accept your trash. When I went out this morning to put out more empty boxes (actually filled with Styrofoam popcorn), I found a box still there that I'd left on Tuesday. On the box, I noticed a sticker in Japanese. I brought all the boxes back into the house.

"What does this sticker say?" I asked Ichiro.

"It says this is unburnable trash and it was put out on a burnables-only day," Ichiro explained, as he picked up a hand full of the Styrofoam popcorn and let it slip through his fingers.

6:32 a.m., Friday, November 19, 1999

Brrrrrrrr!!! I still have thin blood from living in Arizona. It's 7.2 degrees centigrade outside and 13 degrees inside. Three insulating layers encumber my torso, but do not give me the comfort I'm accustomed to (after living 18 years in sunny Arizona and one year in southern California). I traded in my kerosene heater for an electric one. It doesn't have quite the power, but it doesn't stink, and I don't have to pay for the kerosene (electricity is included in the rent).

Dinner with Ichiro. In his hesitant, shy way, Ichiro suggested we go out for dinner. I accepted. I think it helped solidify our friendship.

"What gives you the most pleasure in life?" I asked him.

"Drinking beer and singing (karaoke)," he said.

My strategy to meet women. How do I meet the women I want to meet? How can I maintain contact so it can develop into friendship and/or romance? These are the questions that interest me.

So far, an enjoyable conversation develops with one in four/ five women that I approach on the train. I have five basic requirements for a friendship/romance prospect: (1) I find her physically attractive, (2) she is unmarried, (3) her manner of conversation is charming or alluring, (4) she speaks English, and (5) she has e-mail. Of course, I don't even approach a woman unless she meets the first and second criteria (absence of a wedding ring is what I go by for the second criterion). In talking with her, I quickly find out if she meets the third and fourth criteria. And, if she meets the first four criteria, I ask her if we might exchange e-mail addresses and discover if she meets the fifth.

Here is my plan, which will require the choice of courage (again and again): I'll buy the cheapest train ticket at 130 yen and board the Yamanote line at Uguisudani Station. The train completes a circle, with twenty-seven stops, in roughly an hour. I'll board the first car and find a woman who passes criteria one and two, and approach her with a request for directions. Then if she meets the first four criteria, I'll talk with her for up to five more minutes for the potential exchange of e-mail addresses. Once I've exhausted the possibilities in one car, I'll exit the train at the next stop, and enter the next car on the same train, so as to appear to have just entered the train. Then repeat.

I may complete the circuit several times. My estimate indicates I can make a new potential friend every thirty minutes or less. In half a day I'd have ten potential friendships I'm eager to pursue!

Looking over the above I'm embarrassed to notice how calculating it appears. Interesting, because from inside me it feels very different. Selfish, absolutely, because I love the adventure of pursuit along with the pleasures of friendship and romance. But also magnanimous, because I know that when I befriend a woman my motive is to create such a mutually beneficial relationship that, at its conclusion, she will feel that the day she met me was her luckiest. Given my life coaching experience and recent romantic relationships I know the objective is within reach; several women have, in fact, volunteered this sentiment.

8:54 a.m., Saturday, November 20, 1999

Fear of cults in Japan. Last night I asked Ichiro to explain various pieces of mail I found in my mailbox. Two were for him.

(Since I put up the only mailbox here, I'm getting everybody's mail!) One flyer, he explained, was from a cult. He adjusted his nose a tad higher and swept the imaginary letter behind him and dropped it, a graphic indication that I should throw it away. This dramatic gesture conveyed the impression that Ichiro thought the letter might infect me. Landmark will have to be very careful here in Japan that it not be branded as a cult. In the U.S. this is usually not as much of an issue.

Accommodating the neighbors. I received this e-mail from Ichiro:

"Dear Dwight.

Today, I'll go back home around 6 p.m. and go to a supermarket for buying food or so. If you want some food, I will buy instead of you. Please let me know list. As you know, our neighbors are against your cooking by using Gas. I really think that you feel inconvenience. I am sorry about that thing.

I guess that this kind of intolerable matter cannot seen in U.S.A, these days. But, long time ago, U.S.A used to has similar problem against women and black pepole. However, they could get rid of their constant effort. In near future, Japan may bacome liberal country like U.S.A. or Canada. I beleive so.

Thank you for your patience.

Regards, Ichiro Gunji"

Kenichi's in a crucible. His plan is to accommodate the fearful neighbors where possible. He presumes that they'll soon get used to seeing me around the neighborhood, and calm down. Then I can go about my business without restrictions.

"Let Ichiro buy groceries for you. Ichiro likes you and is happy to do this," Kenichi said.

"No!" I objected. "This is too much. If we need to, we can tell the neighbors that I only cook with the microwave (which is 85% true)."

Ichiro got home, and we came up with the following plan. I'll not shop at the local market (where the neighbors are likely to see me). I'll walk to a market five minutes farther down the street. I'll put my groceries in containers the neighbors won't recognize as grocery bags. What a gas!

Kenichi's already on his trip to Asia. Before he left, the lawyer declared that his legal position is solid.

No waiting for your order: a merry-go-round of sushi. I met Kyoko and her friend Hajime at the Hachiko exit of the Shibuya JR Station. I first met them last May, when I visited Tokyo for two weeks and made my decision to move to Japan. This time they introduced me to a restaurant where the chefs stand in the middle and make small sushi and sashimi dishes, then put their creations onto a big revolving platform that passes the seated customers. The edible art on the yellow dishes cost 120 yen, pink—180 yen, and blue—240 yen. When you want a dish, you take it and eat. I stuck to seven yellow dishes and enjoyed a satisfying, healthy meal. When you've finished, the assistant counts the dishes of the different colors and tallies up your bill.

Afterward our meal I invited Kyoko and Hajime (both 23) to see my new place, mess and all. They're my first official visitors, and they'll be friends.

9:01 a.m., Sunday, November 21, 1999

Is this really my home? All my actions are directed toward becoming a permanent resident here, but it feels like I'm just visiting. Interesting.

Kindness, kindness, kindness. I have mentioned this before about the Japanese, and it still amazes me. Every time I ask someone why s/he likes someone else, the number one reason is, "They are so kind."

Surreptitious buying. I did my first surreptitious grocery shopping today. I hid my groceries in a box.

Each time I shop I want to learn something new about what I buy (or don't buy). Today I asked a woman in the store what was in a package (whose contents I didn't recognize).

"Pig intestine," she said.

No wonder it was so cheap!

Strategy exercise #1 to meet the women I wasn't in the mood.

I avoided it. Yet, once I got into it, it was fun. I rode the Yamanote Line one full loop, followed my plan, and approached 15 to 20 women. Four spoke English well enough for a rewarding conversation. Two had e-mail addresses. I'm interested in one as a friend, and the other has romantic potential. She manages an architectural office. I am pleased with this first foray into my new adventure.

To continue reading about my adventures
    in Japan and my enchantment with Shanghai,
    see www.GoldWinde.com/Cbook/More/Journal.

ॐ

Courage around the world

Although my intention is that this book eventually be translated into many different languages, for now I have satisfied myself by including the translation of my courage definition into a few of the world's major languages. If you can read one or more of these languages (Chinese, Russian, Spanish, French, or German), I hope you will enjoy the translation!

Acknowledgmentsand List of Contributors

Without my literary and artistic collaborators, this book would be a shadow of its final form. In addition, working with each of them has continually inspired me, making the process all that more enjoyable.

Recommendations

Movies, books, workshops, and travel—I've got some stimulating suggestions for you in all these areas.

Table of Contents—Unabridged Version

This unabridged version of the table of contents doubles as a non-alphabetized index. As such, I have placed it at the end of this book.

Books on the Back Burner

The provisional title of my next book is *Romance AND Family: How to Have It All*. Other books that I am excited about, but I may or may not get to, are listed on the last page of this book.

๛

My Courage Definition in CHINESE

什么是勇气？

勇气是意志和意愿
　是正视内心的恐惧
　是为了实现最崇高的承诺和最深切的渴望
　而去积极行动，勇于冒险

勇气被创造，被抉择
　瞬间的抉择
　它始终垂手可得
　它随时随地对你敞开大门
　跨过门槛只在一念之间
勇气无法储存也不能累积
与其认为"拥有勇气"或"没有勇气"
不如认为"选择勇气"或"选择暂时的安逸"

只有当如履薄冰时，
人们才选择勇气
人人都善于压抑、否认、掩饰、对抗、排斥内心
的恐惧
（或驳斥它的存在）

以期待缓解甚至麻醉恐惧
真正的勇气是对恐惧认识体会阐释后
而采取正确的行动
更要为勇敢的行径而自诩和骄傲
无论结局是好是坏
勇气傲然独立

是否选择勇气并无是非对错之分
不过是一个抉择
一个关于付出和回报的抉择
总是选择勇气的生命
将拥有一个自己热爱的生活
总是选择安逸的生命
生活将只是退缩和苟延
安逸人皆向之
但若成为生活的目标（往往是潜意识的）
生命将则畏头畏尾
而非灵感激扬。

Lily Pan (Chinese translation of the Courage Definition—with the help of her classmates)

Lily was born in Shanghai, China in 1979, and is now "a training doctor majored in endocrinology in Shanghai Sixth People's Hospital." (lilypii@yahoo.com.cn)

For my courage definition in Russian, Spanish, French, and German, see www.GoldWinde.com/Cbook/More/Languages.

Acknowledgment and List of Contributors

How can I ever know the profound influence that my mother, father, sister and brother, and my maternal grandfather and grandmother have had (through the long reach of time) on the creation of this book!?

How can I ever know the often untraceable but definitive effect that all my friends and colleagues over many decades have had upon this book?!

Many books and workshops have played a major role in my life development—far too many to count or even completely remember. A few, however, stand out. For these, I am deeply grateful to:

— Ayn Rand (novelist, essayist, and founder of the philosophy of Objectivism)
— Nathaniel Branden (psychologist and self-esteem expert)
— John Grinder et al. (creators of Neuro-Linguistic Programming or NLP)
— Werner Erhard (progenitor of Landmark Education and its technologies for life)
— Fernando Flores (discoverer of the four fundamental ways of speaking: assertions, requests, promises, and declarations)
— Anthony Robbins (NLP evangelist, personal development consultant, author, and public speaker)

Since April 2000 and the inception of the *Courage Now* service, I have been blessed by countless acts of encouragement and suggestions from thousands of subscribers. My decision to write this book was shaped by contributions from more people than I can name in this space, but I do want to mention several who were particularly persistent and persuasive in encouraging me to share my insights with a broader audience: Beth and Jim Gehring, Chi Newman, Mary Silva, and Susan South. And Trish Coffey and Michael Arri have been by my side all the way to the final submission to the publisher.

A special corner of my heart is set aside for John Bowling, my trusted business assistant in Arizona who has made it possible to me to live both in Tokyo and Shanghai while continuing to do business in America.

The following contributors to the book have been my treasured partners in its creation:

Michael Arri (book format design and implementation)

Michael decided to move to Shanghai after graduating from Hamburg University in Chinese Studies in 2001. After translating Dwight's definition of "Courage" into German, he helped to format and edit the book in return for some most valuable coaching sessions. Now he lives in Beijing, but he dreams of retiring at a fishing village in Cornwall, England, one day. (urban-china@gmx.net)

Christina Chen (graphic artist for all but one of the illustrations in this book)

Christina is a 23-year-old Shanghainese girl, who is "still on her way to exploring the unknown world, due to her curiosity." She says that when she was a little kid, she seemed to be interested in unusual things and that her life now seems a little bit different from others. She finished her high school and university courses all by herself, as she says "with a strong will," and is now "an undergraduate of English language." As a language student of Shanghai Foreign Studies, she explains, "art isn't anything familiar with me," but I chose the courage to "take a try on this unfamiliar field." The illustrations in this book are her first artistic works. She says, "Although with much efforts, I was interested and enjoyed making these illustrations. I believed that courage, interest, and patience compile a desired life. Sometimes, courage is dangerous, but it does make a change in your life. At least that is true to me." (northeurose@yahoo.com)

Joel Hanson (initial editing of the Poetic Essays)

Joel dreams of finishing his first marathon, putting the final punctuation mark on his first novel, and mastering the cello. He is a musician and former band member, a dream chaser, and potential moviemaker. A Minnesotan by chance, a Seattleite by choice, Joel spent the past year in Shanghai, teaching spoken English classes and assiduously editing the poetic-essay and "Toxic Word" sections of this book.

A University of Minnesota graduate in philosophy and cultural studies, Joel has combined his educational experience and creative interests to follow a path of his own design. He has written collaborative music for television documentaries and live theater, published political essays and music reviews, and is currently working on a book about his experiences in China. Despite his many projects, thinking is his favorite hobby, especially while staring at the ceiling at night and trying to solve the problems of our beautiful, chaotic world. (petitfrere30@hotmail.com)

Calvin Shine (graphic artist for essay "Are you a giver or a trader?")

Born in Shanghai, China in 1978, Calvin is a cartoonist and is currently employed as the chief designer of Shanghai Dahong Advertising Co., Ltd. (rainworks@etang.com)

Anne Stanford (final editing of all parts of this book)

Born and raised in Connecticut, graduate of Smith College, veteran of the publishing industry, Anne has for the past 15 years brought up her two children (and several horses) on her farm outside Charlottesville, Virginia. A person for whom physical activity has always been central, she worked on this book at a time when she was recovering from an injury that had kept her sedentary for three years. Living with limited physical mobility has given her a deepened appreciation for the privilege of health and movement on many levels and a renewed commitment to her dream of building her farm into a vibrant center for discovery and partnership.

She says that editing the courage essays was a particularly powerful experience for which she will always be grateful, that by reading the essays slowly and carefully on a daily basis she experienced a profound shift in who she was being and the choices that she saw in her life as well as her ability to contribute to those around her. (stanford49@earthlink.net)

May Wang (assisted Michael Arri in essay formatting)

May describes herself as "a Chinese girl, who is admiring Dwight and having a dream to be a coach like him one day, living in Shanghai now." She works for a training company, likes reading and "outward sports" and making friends. (yuanmay5@sina.com)

Vanessa Xu (layout design and wardrobe consultant for book cover picture)

Vanessa was born in Shanghai and now lives in Toronto, Canada. She has a special interest in both fashion and art. (shxuwen@yahoo.ca)

I want to make special mention of others who have contributed to this book in various ways: Keith Varnum, John Rice, Rachael Bao, Amy Chou, Isabella Qi, Susan South, and Chi Newman; language translators for my courage definition (see www.GoldWinde.com/Cbook/More/Languages) Vladimir Legkostup, Dmitri Samoilov, Martha Young, Mary Silva, Jimmy Molea, Danny Chane, Olivier Henry, Michael Arri, and Pia Christina Heisele. During the final review of the book (before submission to the publisher), I received much appreciated and detailed feedback from "eagle eyes" Pete Maclean and Gregg Roberts. Other final reviewers whose feedback was much appreciated include Lee Shinefield, Doug White, Peter Gradjansky, Lily Zhu, Karen Doughty, Julie Zhou, John Stob, Debbie Blackmon, and Mayumi Hara.

❧

_____
_____
_____
_____
_____
_____
_____
_____
_____
_____
_____
_____
_____
_____
_____
_____
_____
_____
_____
_____
_____
_____
_____
_____
_____
_____
_____
_____
_____
_____
_____
_____
_____
_____
_____
_____
_____

Recommendations

In making these recommendations, I am struck by several thoughts:

(1)   If I didn't stop it somewhere, the whole content of this book could be consumed just by this recommendation list.

(2)   I have undoubtedly forgotten many important recommendations.

(3)   I can often take specific exceptions with many of my own recommendations, even though I think they are, in general, very good recommendations.

(4)   I am restricting my recommendations (most of the time) to movies, books, and services, which relate in some significant way to the focus and theme of this book.

Movies have been a deep source of enjoyment and inspiration in my life. This lists only a few that I found exceptionally interesting and inspirational.

Pleasantville—directed by Gary Ross, with actors William Macy, Joan Allen, Jeff Daniels, Tobey McGuire, Reese Witherspoon

Chocolat—directed by Lasse Hallstrom, with actors Juliette Binoche, Johnny Depp, Lena Olin, Judi Dench, Alfred Molina

Dangerous Beauty—directed by Marshall Herskovitz, with actors Catherine McCormack and Rufus Sewell

My Big Fat Greek Wedding—directed by Joel Zwick, with actors Nia Vardalos and John Corbett

The Truman Show—directed by Peter Weir, with actors Jim Carrey, Don Taylor, Laura Linney, Noah Emmerich, Natascha McElhone

American Beauty—directed by Sam Mendes, with actors Kevin Spacey, Annette Bening, Thora Birch, Wes Bentley, Mena Suvari

My Dinner with Andre—directed by Louis Malle, with actors Wallace Shawn and Andre Gregory

The Bridges of Madison County—directed by Clint Eastwood, with actors Clint Eastwood, Meryl Streep

Scent of a Woman—directed by Martin Brest, with actors Al Pacino and Chris O'Donnell

After my parents and perhaps the Landmark Education courses, **books** have influenced my life more than any other stimulation.

Non-Fiction

Real Moments by Barbara De Angelis

Radical Honesty: How To Transform Your Life By Telling The Truth by Brad Blanton, PhD

When I Say No, I Feel Guilty by Manuel J. Smith

Virtue of Selfishness: A New Concept of Egoism by Ayn Rand

Passionate Marriage: Love, Sex, and Intimacy in Emotionally Committed Relationships by David Schnarch

Mama Gena's Owner's and Operator's Guide to Men by Regena Thomashauer

You Just Don't Understand by Deborah Tannen

Flow: The Psychology of Optimal Experience by Mihaly Csikszentmihalyi

Awaken the Giant Within: How to Take Immediate Control of Your Mental, Emotional, Physical & Financial Destiny! by Anthony Robbins

First Things First: To Live, to Love, to Learn, to Leave a Legacy by Stephen R. Covey, A. Roger Merrill, Rebecca R. Merrill

The Fifth Discipline: The Art and Practice of the Learning Organization by Peter M. Senge

Getting to Yes: Negotiating Agreement Without Giving in by Roger Fisher

Anti-Aging Zone by Barry Sears

Truth Cannot Be Rehearsed: Talks, Sessions and Essays About the Art of Being Fully Human by Robert Augustus Masters (out of print)

The Black Butterfly: An Invitation to Radical Aliveness by Richard Moss

The Power of Now: A Guide to Spiritual Enlightenment by Eckhart Tolle

The Seven Spiritual Laws of Success: A Practical Guide to the Fulfillment of Your Dreams by Deepak Chopra

Fiction

Atlas Shrugged by Ayn Rand
The Fountainhead by Ayn Rand

Coaching, counseling, workshops, and trainings, have played a major role in my life development. I mention here only a few that are still generally accessible and I consider to be of the highest value and quality.

The Forum and other related programs by Landmark Education have made more difference in my life than any other single factor. Landmark Education provides their programs in six different languages around the world and has offices in every major city in the United States. You can check out www.landmark-education.com.

Neuro-Linguistic Programming or NLP. I originally studied this discipline (the science of subjective experience) under its founders John Grinder, Richard Bandler, Leslie Cameron-Bandler, and Robert Dilts back in 1979-1981. Although I have taken numerous trainings from various sources (including Anthony Robbins, who got his start in NLP), I have no particular workshop or book recommendation at this time. There are plenty out there to choose from. NLP has made a huge difference in my life. Its approach is a nice compliment to the Landmark Education approach (NLP is more content focused; Landmark Education is more context focused). Just search on "NLP" on the web and you'll find plenty of options to check out.

Servas, founded in 1948 in Denmark, is an international home stay organization. Currently they have about 14,000 families around the world in over 135 countries who are waiting for you to come stay and visit with them in their homes. No money exchanges hands. The standard stay is two nights, unless otherwise arranged. The Servas mission is international peace and understanding. In the U.S. you can join as a host or a traveler or both. The yearly fees are very reasonable (less than $100).

In the spring of 1997 I took the vacation and adventure of

a lifetime, staying with 18 separate Japanese families in 18 different cities—from Yokohama to Nagasaki—over forty days. Including all my travel by air from Arizona to Japan (I flew into Osaka), all my train travel within Japan, all the gifts I brought for my host families, I spent less than $3000 for the 40 days. I made many great friends and ended up understanding the culture much better than expatriates who had lived in Japan for years.

You can contact Servas for more information at www.usservas.org (the USA branch) or www.servas.org (the international web site). Or call them in New York City at 212-267-0252.

Rebound exercise is the easiest, most efficient, safest, and (perhaps for you) the most enjoyable form of exercise currently available to mankind. In only seven minutes per day with this indoors exercise (no need to worry about the weather), I keep myself in good physical shape with my rebounder. A type of mini-trampoline, the rebounder exercises **every** muscle in your body **at the same time**. Don't buy a cheap one. The bounce will be tight and the springs will break. You can buy a good one for under $200. It will last you a lifetime and will be the best buy you'll ever make. There are a number of good competitors out there. I bought mine through www.reboundair.com. Their web site will also provide you with a wealth of information on the miracles of rebound exercise.

Holosync® audio technology provides an effortless way to release and dissolve resisted fear and pain. Find out more at *www.centerpointe.com.*

જી

_____

_____

_____

_____

_____

_____

_____

_____

Table of Contents

—Unabridged Version—

Special Note: In the following Table of Contents, the letter "c" is used to denote the word "courage." An asterisk* is used to indicate that a web site link is provided for further non-essential reading.

Table of Contents -Unabridged Version-

Courage: The Key to a Thousand Doors
(Choosing the Third Cornerstone of Courage)

My journal is continued at
www.GoldWinde.com/Cbook/More/Journal to include

Appendices

෨

Books on the Back Burner

My next book, already in the works, is provisionally titled, *Romance AND Family: How to Have It All.*

Working titles for some of the other books that I think would be fascinating to research and write are listed below. I may or may not get around to writing these books—and I invite others to consider writing them before I do.

- How to Say "No" Gracefully in Any Situation or Occasion
- If You Are Human, Then You Are a Victim: The Insidious Addiction of Victimhood
- How to Create a Divorce You Can Celebrate
- How to Create Great Endings (for schooling, friendships, romances, marriages, jobs, projects, and life)
- Fatebeliefs to Build Your Life On: A Foundation for Joy, Accomplishment, and Self-Expression
- Toxic Words: The Hidden Pollutants of Our Mind
- How Remnant Behaviors Will Kill Us: Our Rational Mind Is a Small Boat on the Tempest of Our Genetic Programs
- Structures That Will Make Your Life a Breeze
- Dancing on the Edge with God: Playing with Time and Causation
- Redesigning the House of Culture: The New Challenge of the Twenty-First Century
- City, Sweet Home: The City You Always Wished Existed So That You Could Move There: Designing Our Environment from the Bottom Up
- A Vasectomy for Every Man: A Simple Cultural Solution for the Oldest Problem
- A Dictionary of Positive/Negative Connotations: How Words are Rarely Innocent
- What 150 Years Has Wrought: Why the King of Yesteryear Would Envy the Slum Dweller of Today
- Sloppy, Tasty, Healthy and Quick: A Guide to Preparing Great Meals in Twenty Minutes or Less